NEPHROLOGY AND GERIATRICS INTEGRATED

Nephrology and Geriatrics Integrated

Proceedings of the Conference on Integrating Geriatrics into Nephrology, held in Jasper, Alberta, Canada, July 31–August 5, 1998

Edited by

Dimitrios G. Oreopoulos
The Toronto Hospital, Toronto, Ontario, Canada

William R. Hazzard
J. Paul Sticht Center on Aging, Wake Forest University School of Medicine, Winston-Salem, NC, U.S.A.

and

Robert Luke
University of Cincinnati Medical Center, Cincinnati, OH, U.S.A.

Publication of this book was supported in part by the John A. Hartford Foundation through a grant to the American Geriatrics Society entitled "Integrating Geriatrics into the Subspecialties of Internal Medicine".

KLUWER ACADEMIC PUBLISHERS
DORDRECHT / BOSTON / LONDON

Library of Congress Cataloging-in-Publication Data

ISBN 0-7923-6181-4

Published by Kluwer Academic Publishers,
P.O. Box 17, 3300 AA Dordrecht, The Netherlands.

Sold and distributed in North, Central and South America
by Kluwer Academic Publishers,
101 Philip Drive, Norwell, MA 02061, U.S.A.

In all other countries, sold and distributed
by Kluwer Academic Publishers,
P.O. Box 322, 3300 AH Dordrecht, The Netherlands.

Printed on acid-free paper

Printed in the Netherlands.

Contents

DISCUSSION / RECOMMENDATIONS / EPILOGUE

List of Participants

Darrell R. Abernethy, MD, PhD
Clinical Director
Chief, Laboratory of Clinical Investigation
National Institute of Aging
Gerontology Research Center
5600 Nathon Shock Drive
Baltimore, Maryland 21224-6825
U.S.A.
Tel.: (410) 558-8611
Fax: (410) 558-8318
E-mail: abernethyd@grc.nia.nih.gov

Laurence H. Beck, MD
Department of Internal Medicine
Cleveland Clinic Florida
3000 W. Cypress Creek R.D.
Ft. Lauderdale, FL 33309
U.S.A.

William M. Bennett, MD, FACP
Division of Nephrology
Hypertension and Clinical Pharmacology
Mailcode PP262
Oregon Health Sciences University
3314SW U.S. Veterans Hospital Road
Portland, OR 97201-2940, U.S.A.
Tel.: (503) 494-8490
Fax: (503) 494-5330
E-mail: bennettw@ohsu.edu

Margaret J. Bia, MD
Professor of Medicine
Director of Transplant, Nephrology
Yale University School of Medicine
Section of Nephrology
2073 LMP
P.O. Box 208029
New Haven, CT 06520-8029
U.S.A.
Tel.: 203-785-4184
Fax: 203-785-7068
E-mail: margaret.bia@yale.edu

Wendy Weinstock Brown, MD, MPH, FACP.
Professor of Internal Medicine
St. Louis University School of Medicine
Director, Clinical Nephrology
St. Louis VA Medical Center
915 N. Grand Blvd.
St. Louis, Missouri 63106
U.S.A.
Tel.: 314-289-6485
Fax: 314-289-6303
E-mail: wendy.brown@med.va.gov

Richard J. Glassock, MD, MACP
Professor of Medicine
Department of Internal Medicine
University of Kentucky
Lexington, KY 40536
U.S.A.
Tel.: 606-257-5499
Fax: 606-323-1197
E-mail: cwtown1@pop.uky.edu

William R. Hazzard, MD
Professor of Internal Medicine
Senior Advisor, J. Paul Sticht Center on Aging
Wake Forest University School of Medicine
Medical Center Boulevard
Winston-Salem, NC 27157-1207, U.S.A.
Tel.: 336-713-8585
Fax: 336-713-8588
E-mail: whazzard@wfubmc.edu

William L. Henrich, MD
Professor and Chairman
Department of Medicine
University of Maryland Hospital
22 So. Greene Street (N3W42)
Baltimore, MD 21201, U.S.A.
Tel.: 410-328-2488; Fax: 410-328-8688
E-mail: Whenrich@medicine.ab.umd.edu

Heidi Hoeben, MD
Resident Renal Division
Department of Medicine
University Hospital
De Pintelaan 185
9000 Gent, Belgium
Tel.: 32 9 240 4524
Fax: 32 9 240 4599

Keith A. Hruska, MD
Ira M. Lang Professor of Medicine
Barnes-Jewish Hospital at Washington University School of Medicine
216 S. Kingshighway
St. Louis, MO 63110, U.S.A.
Tel.: 314-454-7771; Fax: 314-454-5126
E-mail: khruska@imgate.wustl.edu

David Humes, MD
John G. Searle Professor and Chair
Department of Internal Medicine
University of Michigan Health System
3100A Taubman Center
Ann Arbor, MI 48109-0368, U.S.A.
Tel.: 734-936-4495; Fax: 734-615-2645
E-mail: dhumes@umich.edu

Sarbjit Vanita Jassal
Clinical Lecturer
Department of Geriatric Medicine
University of Liverpool
UCD, Daulby St.
Liverpool, L69 3GA
U.K.
Tel.: +44 151 706 4062
Fax: +44 151 706 4064
E-mail: vanitajassal@hotmail.com

Saulo Klahr, MD, FACP, FRCP
John and Adaline Simon Professor of Medicine
Washington University School of Medicine
Barnes-Jewish Hospital
216 S. Kingshighway Blvd.
Suite 4300
St. Louis, MO 63110-1092
U.S.A.
Tel.: 314-454-7107
Fax: 314-454-5110
E-mail: sklahr@imgate.wustl.edu

Norbert Lameire, MD, PhD
Chief Renal Division
Department of Medicine
University Hospital
De Pintelaan 185
9000 Gent
Belgium
Tel.: 32-9-240 4524
Fax: 32-9-240 4599
E-mail: Ingrid.Verslycken@rug.ac.be

Andrew S. Levey, MD
Professor of Medicine, Tufts University School of Medicine
Director, Division of Nephrology Clinical Research Center
New England Medical Center
750 Washington St., Box 784
Boston, MA 02111
U.S.A.
Tel.: 617-636-2372
Fax: 617-636-8329

Julia Lewis, MD
Associate Professor of Medicine
Division of Nephrology
Vanderbilt University Medical Center
S-3223 Medical Center North
Nashville, TN 37232-2372
U.S.A.
Tel.: 615-343-6105
Fax: 615-343-7156
E-mail: julia.lewis@mcmail.vanderbilt.edu

Robert Luke
University of Cincinnati Medical Center
Department of Internal Medicine
231 Bethesda Avenue
Cincinnati, OH 45267-0557
U.S.A.
Tel.: 513-558-4231
Fax: 513-558-3878

Anke Nelde, MD
Resident Geriatry
Department of Medicine
University Hospital
De Pintelaan 185
9000 Gent, Belgium
Tel.: 32 9 240 2345
Fax: 32 9 240 3895

Dimitrios G. Oreopoulos, MD, PhD, FRCPC, FACP, FRCPS(Glasgow)
Professor of Medicine, University of Toronto
Past President of the International Society for Peritoneal Dialysis
Director, Peritoneal Dialysis Program
The Toronto Hospital – Western Division
399 Bathurst Street, 6E-539
Toronto, Ontario M5T 2S8, Canada
Tel.: 416-603-7974; Fax: 416-603-8127
E-mail: dgoreopoulos.msn@attcanada.net

Thomas Rashid, MD
Urology Resident
William Beaumont Hospital
3535 West 13 Mile Road, Suite 501
Royal Oak, Michigan 48073, U.S.A.
Tel.: 248-551-2250
Fax: 248-551-2240

Larry T. Sirls, MD, FACS
Director
Urodynamics Laboratory
William Beaumont Hospital
3535 West 13 Mile Road, Suite 501
Royal Oak, Michigan 48073
U.S.A.
Tel.: 248-551-2250; Fax: 248-551-2240
E-mail: Lsirls@beaumont.edu

David R. Staskin, MD
Assistant Professor of Urology and Surgery
Harvard Medical School
Director, Continence Center
Beth Israel Deaconess Medical Center
330 Brookline Avenue, Libby 130
Boston, MA 02215
U.S.A.
Tel.: 617-667-5619
Fax: 619-975-5295
E-mail: dstaskin@bidmc.harvard.edu

Theodore I. Steinman, MD
Professor of Medicine, Harvard Medical School
Director, Dialysis Unit
Beth Israel Deaconess Medical Center
Renal Division
330 Brookline Avenue (FD220)
Boston, Massachusetts 02215
U.S.A.
Tel.: 617-667-5278
Fax: 617-667-5595
E-mail: tsteinma@caregroup.harvard.edu

Perry M. Sutaria, MD
Fellow in Reconstructive and Female Urology
Harvard Medical School
Beth Israel Deaconess Medical Center
330 Brookline Avenue, Libby 130
Boston, MA 02215
U.S.A.
Tel.: 617-667-5619
E-mail: psutaria@pol.net

Raymond Vanholder, MD, PhD
Assoc. Prof. Renal Division
Department of Medicine
University Hospital
De Pintelaan 185
9000 Gent
Belgium
Tel.: 32 9 240 4524
Fax: 32 9 240 4599

Martin G. White, MD
3525 Turtle Creek Blvd. #20De
Dallas, TX 75219-5514
U.S.A.
Tel.: 214-334-5613
Fax: 214-853-5034
E-mail: mgwhite@swbell.net

James F. Winchester, MD, FRCP(Glasgow), FACP
Professor of Medicine, Director of Dialysis Programs
Division of Nephrology and Hypertension
Department of Medicine
Georgetown University Medical Center
PHC 6003
3800 Reservoir Road
Washington, DC 20007
U.S.A.
Tel.: 202-784-3662
Fax: 202-687-2808
E-mail: jwinch@ix.netcom.com

Introduction

DIMITRIOS G. OREOPOULOS[1], WILLIAM R. HAZZARD[2] and ROBERT LUKE[3]
[1] *The Toronto Western Hospital, Toronto, Ontario, Canada;* [2] *J. Paul Sticht Center on Aging, Wake Forest University School of Medicine, Winston-Salem, NC, U.S.A.;* [3] *University of Cincinnati Medical Center, Cincinnati, OH, U.S.A.*

The 20th century was marked by breathtaking progress in almost all elements of civilization and humanity throughout the world. Nowhere was this more evident than in biomedical science and medicine, in which, especially in the post-World War II era, exponential growth in the sophistication of medical research and technology paved the way for its application in the diagnosis and management of mankind's most dreaded diseases with their untoward burdens of disability, disease, and premature mortality. Of these advances none was more dramatic than the advent of dialysis for the management of end-stage renal disease, a previously rapidly and uniformly fatal condition that has now been transformed into a challenge of chronic management with a focus on all aspects of quality of life.

However, just as dialysis has transformed the discipline of nephrology into the management of what was a previously hopeless condition into one of optimistic and positive attributes, the scientific and technological advances of medicine have contributed to the progressive survival of an increasing proportion of those born into middle and indeed old and, increasingly, old-old age. In the 20th century the average longevity in Western nations has increased from just over 45 years in 1900 to over 75 years by the end of the century, and the prospect of explosive growth in those over 75, 85, and even over 100 now dominates the thinking of health-care and social planners who look toward the burgeoning population of elderly citizens in the 21st century and the inescapable costs of their health care. Thus, paradoxically, scientific progress and improved general health have produced an unprecedented challenge to apply sophisticated medical technology to the benefit of the elderly citizens of the 21st century. Somewhat belatedly the medical establishment is coming to accept the challenge of caring for the elderly in a manner that is humane, efficient and of the highest medical and technical quality. Anticipating this challenge, the John A. Hartford Foundation has taken as its central mission improved geriatric care across all specialties. The project that formed the basis of this conference and the present volumes is a major element of the multifaceted Hartford strategy, in this instance part of the project entitled, 'Integrating Geriatrics into the Subspecialties of Internal Medicine'. In this

Oreopoulos et al. (eds.), Nephrology and Geriatrics Integrated, xvii–xix.

five-year initiative investigators at Wake Forest University, with the sponsorship of the American Geriatrics Society and the support of the Hartford Foundation, conducted a series of Geriatric Education Retreats (GERs), of which that for nephrology took place in Jasper, Alberta in August of 1998. As with the other GERs, this meeting followed certain common organizing principles:

(1) The central hypothesis is as follows:
   (a) Historically, internal medicine has been the largest specialty in medicine;
   (b) Internists (and family physicians) generally are the primary care physicians of choice for most elderly Americans;
   (c) However (until recently), most physicians who completed residencies in internal medicine pursued training and careers in the medical subspecialties (the largest and best compensated of which captured a disproportionate share of the 'best and brightest');
   (d) Therefore, to best serve the medical needs of elderly Americans now and in the future, we must enrich the training of medical subspecialists in gerontological and geriatric aspects of their disciplines;
   (e) Consequently the purpose of this initiative is to capture the interest and support of subspecialists through the development of research and teaching agendas and funding opportunities in the geriatric and gerontologic aspects of those disciplines.

(2) The strategy is as follows:
   (a) To incorporate geriatric content into the training of fellows in each subspecialty;
   (b) To 'gerontologize' faculty in each subspecialty to ensure training (as well as teaching) of medical students and residents;
   (c) To enrich the geriatric content of American Board of Internal Medicine (ABIM) subspecialty examinations;
   (d) To disseminate the concepts and experiences of these GERs at regional and national conclaves of subspecialists (as well in reverse fashion, of general internists and geriatricians from subspecialists to generalists).

(3) This educational experience, the GER, would combine one part geriatricians, one part subspecialists turned geriatricians (e.g., a nephrologist with a special interest in perhaps the aging kidney or urinary incontinence) and one part of subspecialist 'movers and shakers' as yet uneducated and uninvolved in the care of the elderly. At these GERs all three kinds of attendees would be brought together in a total immersion experience for one full week in pleasant surroundings for a mixture of didactic/Socratic, formal/informal, professional/social, intellectual/extracurricular interaction around a common focus on aging, geriatrics, and the care of the elderly in that subspecialty. In short, at the end of this experience,

'gerontologized' subspecialty leaders would emerge dedicated to the incorporation of geriatrics into their subspecialty and to the dissemination of their experience and enthusiasm widely throughout their discipline.

Five previous GERs preceded that for Nephrology: Endocrinology and Metabolism (August, 1995, Orcas Island, Washington), Cardiology (August, 1996, Banff, Alberta), Medical Oncology (February, 1997, Puerto Rico), Rheumatology, Infectious Diseases, and Immunology (August, 1997, Whistler, British Columbia), and Pulmonary/Critical Care Medicine (March, 1998, St. John Virgin Islands). Subsequently GERs in Gastroenterology (March, 1999, St. John Virgin Islands), and finally, in General Internal Medicine (Summer, 1999, Jasper, Alberta).

A common strategy has been employed for each medical subspecialty; individualized, however, to the challenges, nature, and tradition of the subspecialty. For nephrology, as elaborated in the succeeding chapters of this volume, this recognized areas of interest and philosophy common to both geriatrics and nephrology; areas divergent and dissimilar, and yet with a common commitment to the care of those progressively disabled by impaired function and concomitant morbidities in other organ systems that limit both the quality and quantity of life. As with previous GERs a remarkable convergence of spirit and goodwill marked the GER held at Jasper, Alberta for nephrology. All participants discovered a common interest, challenge, and commitment in providing the best medical care to a progressively aging population of patients under their charge. Geriatricians learned from nephrologists, nephrologists learned from geriatricians, and both recognized that they had much in common personally and professionally. The 'Spirit of Jasper', which was almost palpable, is sure to be sustained. This volume will add to the momentum generated in Jasper as not only the knowledge but also the spirit of this GER become disseminated broadly and through time to the many other physicians and health professionals, who will be challenged to provide the best in health care to a progressively aging population in the 21st century.

The Clinical Physiology of Aging

WILLIAM R. HAZZARD
J. Paul Sticht Center on Aging, Wake Forest University School of Medicine, Winston-Salem, NC 27157-1207, U.S.A.

Aging is a lifelong process, beginning at conception, ending at death, but largely genetically programmed and hence passed on to succeeding generations via gametocyte DNA. It is by definition a time-related process proceeding along a vector that is the resultant of genetic and behavioral/environmental forces, the former being defined as 'primary aging' and the latter as 'secondary aging'. Thus descriptions of the physiology of aging in the 'real world' reflect individual or population gene-and-environmental interactions. A corollary principle holds that the earlier in the lifecourse that a process passes the clinical horizon from 'normal' to 'abnormal' (in the clinical context, from health to disease), the more likely it is that genetic forces will predominate (e.g., the rare, almost purely genetic homozygous autosomal recessive diseases of infancy and childhood); conversely, the later the clinical horizon is crossed and – especially germane to geriatrics – the later dysfunction, disability, and death will ensue, and the greater the role of behavioral/environmental determinants. Or, put otherwise, at one extreme of the lifecourse, childhood disorders are more likely to be attributable to single, genetic and notably simply-inherited or homozygous recessive disorders. At the other end of life, diseases of old age rarely if ever are caused by single-gene abnormalities; in fact, all disorders of old age are multifactorial in origin. In between these extremes, diseases that express themselves throughout adulthood but before old age reflect varying proportions of genetic and behavioral/environmental influences. Although much has recently been written of so-called 'longevity genes', and whereas no doubt certain patterns of DNA confer particularly robust health and resistance to disease, such patterns are most likely to reflect the hybrid vigor of the 'wild type' (i.e., lack of mutant genes that increase vulnerability) and, in any event most probably are highly polygenic as well. Thus it appears to be more the absence of major disease-conferring genes than the presence of longevity genes *per se* that represents the genetic basis of long life. All this is by way of introducing the physiology of aging as a largely time-dependent, stochastic process, the efficiency of which generally increases rapidly during infancy and childhood (Fig. 1), reaches a maximum around age 30 (with much variance about that age among different systems

Oreopoulos et al. (eds.), Nephrology and Geriatrics Integrated, 1–16.

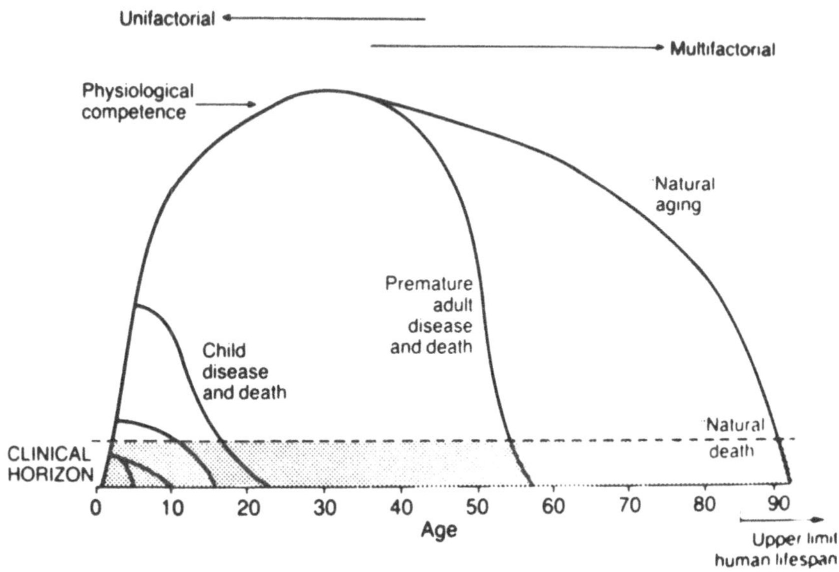

Figure 1. A cartoon depiction of the prototypical relationship between age and physiological efficiency. Note that peak efficiency is achieved at ca. 30 and that the control of all processes becomes progressively multifactorial with advancing age.

and especially among different individuals), declines slowly and almost imperceptibly throughout mid-life (defined by the author as 25–75 years, age 50 being a convenient midpoint of midlife that also coincides with the average age of menopause in women), and decreases in accelerating fashion in old age, often ending in a terminal cascade of vulnerability, frailty, dysfunction, dependency, and death.

Proceeding from these principles, and by analogy with elementary physics, the succeeding consideration of the summary of the general physiology of aging attempts to resolve the vector of the time course of aging, whether in the individual or in populations, into its primary/genetic/immutable and secondary/behavioral-environmental/potentially modifiable components. This exercise, also recently fashionable in lay and scientific publications, has led to concepts of 'Successful Aging' [1, 2] or 'preventive gerontology' [3, 4], both based upon principles articulated by Fries in a classic 1980 essay, 'Aging, Natural Death, and the Compression of Morbidity' [5], recently updated and defended in more contemporary terms [6]. All points of view emphasize, however, that barring a breakthrough in medical engineering on a population-wide basis (e.g., the harvest of stem cells during youth and their long-term preservation and reinfusion in late life) or chronic therapy that inhibits time-related pathological processes in a fundamental, multipotential fashion (e.g., long-term antioxidant ingestion), the human lifespan will continue to have a fixed absolute upper limit (defined for now by the death in 1997 of Jean Calmonde at 122). More cogent to the practice of geriatric medicine, for the population as a whole the 'barrier to immortality' will remain at a median upper limit at about 85 ± 7 years (skewed toward a lower average age at death) [6]. Hence, a fundamental principle of stochastic mathematics applies to interventions designed to maximize the duration of robust physiological efficiency: the later the intervention is introduced (e.g., exercise training in nonagenarians), the less its impact on added longevity. A corollary principle also holds across the entire continuum of adult life: given the progressive decline with advancing age in the difference between resting, steady-state homeostatic regulation and that which represents the maximal possible response to stress (e.g., maximal aerobic capacity during treadmill exercise), in order to minimize age-related declines in physiological function (e.g., exercise training), with advancing age a greater and greater effort will be required. When simply maintaining homeostasis in the resting, unstressed state requires maximal effort, frailty is defined, a condition common among the very old with their multiple diseases and disabilities, persons in whom an insult that would be trivial for a younger, fit person (e.g., influenza infection) can trigger an irreversible, terminal cascade.

Finally by way of introduction, physiology at the level of the whole organism reflects the net effects of integration of a complex array of control mechanisms, which regulate function and maximize efficiency and survival in a given environment. This regulation is exerted at multiple levels: the gene, the cell, the organ, and the organism. At each level, many processes operate in a manner that provides balance to the system in a way that is flexible, dynamic and highly adaptive, generally providing layers of redundancy and reserve, the state of the organism at any given moment reflecting the net of opposing ('Yin and Yang') forces. This may produce the appearance of a calm, 'steady state' of homeostasis, but it reflects a delicate balance of finely tuned, highly dynamic forces (sometimes called 'homeodynamics', a term perhaps in turn perverted by geriatricians who, faced by the inability of their patients to respond to even minor perturbations, have coined the term the 'homeostenosis' of old age). Progressive erosion of the aging person's ability to adapt to changes in their environment defines the 'physiology of aging'. This in turn challenges geriatric expertise to sustain life of acceptable quality through therapeutic interventions of a behavioral, dietary, environmental, pharmacological, surgical, prosthetic, social, or, most frequently multidimensional, multidisciplinary nature, a challenge that grows exponentially with the progressive frailty of the elderly patient.

The Physiology of Aging

Although general physiology is often detailed organ system by organ system, especially in the aging subject mechanisms of communication and transportation between such systems become of paramount interest and therefore will receive principal emphasis here. A detailed summary of this subject is beyond the scope of this treatise but has received in-depth review elsewhere [7, 8]. What follows is thus but a cursory summary, of necessity stressing those elements of the physiology of the elderly at such points of communication and transport as well as those physical changes characteristic of old age that render the elderly most vulnerable to environmental or iatrogenic perturbations.

These points and portals of vulnerability of the elderly to such perturbations are summarized in Table 1. These render the elderly individual more prone to the adverse effects of infections, autoimmune diseases, malignancy, and accumulations of toxic substances, most notoriously iatrogenic pharmacological misadventures.

Table 1. Physiologic defenses and their changes with age

Defense Mechanism	Age Change
Immune Function	
T lymphocytes	Impaired antigen or mitogen response
B lymphocytes	Decreased antigen-specific Ab production
Cytokines	Decreased IL-1, IL-2; increased TNF, interferon, IL-6
Antibody production	Autoantibody formation
Physical Barriers	
Skin	Thinning, loss of subcutaneous fat, decreased blood supply, fewer melanocytes to absorb UV light, decreased collagen and elasticity
Gastrointestinal tract	Hypochlorhydria and gastric atrophy
Respiratory tract	Decreased mucociliary transport and cough (?)
Removal of Toxic Chemicals	
Hepatic metabolism	Decreased first-pass and oxidative metabolism
Renal excretion	Decreased renal blood flow, GFR, and creatinine clearance
Avoidance Reactions	
Sensory awareness	Reduced high-frequency hearing, proprioceptive sensory receptors, visual accommodation, and lens transparency
Reflex motor responses	Increased reflex time and decreased nerve conduction velocity
Response to Environmental Perturbations	
Temperature changes	Decreased responsiveness to heat; decreased responsiveness to cold

GFR = glomerular filtration rate; IL = interleukin; TNF = tumor necrosis factor; UV = ultraviolet.

Immune Function

As knowledge of the complexity of the immune system and inflammatory response mechanisms expands exponentially, the vulnerability of the elderly to deficiencies in these systems at nearly every point becomes increasingly apparent. Perhaps first to be disclosed was the age-related progressive atrophy of the thymus, which decreases from its maximal size attained near puberty to but a fatty vestige by late middle age. The major thymic hormones decline *pari passu* and are no longer detectable after 60, while the proportion of immature, undifferentiated T-cells increase. Whereas the number of circulating T- and B-cells does not appear to decline with age, the T-cell response to a given antigenic or mitogenic stimulus is greatly diminished. Moreover, those that do respond and enter the cell cycle display reduced replicative capacity. Hence, the T-cell-mediated immune response to a given stimulus is substantially reduced in old age (and no doubt further impaired in the sick, malnourished, typical older patient).

The function of these T-cells may be diminished beyond that represented by their reduced number, especially in regard to secretion of cytokines (see, Table 1, also no doubt exaggerated and confounded by coexisting illness and malnutrition). Hence a vicious cycle of reduced thymic hormones, reduced mitogenic response to those hormones, impaired cytokine secretion, and altered response to those cytokines may be triggered by infections or other stimuli to this inflammatory cascade, a scenario especially common in the elderly patient.

B-cell production of antigen-specific antibodies may also be impaired in the elderly, with increased relative influence of suppressor T-cells. This dysfunction appears more a malregulation of intercellular communication and coordination between various elements of the immune system than dysfunction of the cells themselves. This dysfunction also more frequently leads to monoclonal immunoglobulin elevations in the elderly, which, while usually benign, can produce pathological accumulations and multiple myeloma, Waldenstrom's macroglobulinemia, primary amyloidosis, or heavy chain disease. It is also reflected in higher levels of autoantibodies, most of which appear as benign markers of the aging process but can also lead to diseases prominent in the elderly, notably pernicious anemia and autoimmune thyroid disease.

Nutrition and Energy Metabolism

A second system marked by decline in efficiency with aging and diminished intersystem coordination and communication is that devoted to energy metabolism. The universal cellular requirement for oxidative metabolism is met by systems of ATP generation, both locally and from more distant stores, or nutritional intake. The efficiency of ATP generation and utilization at the cellular level has been little examined with aging. More studied and hence reviewed here has been the efficiency of regulation of carbohydrate, fat, and protein metabolism, all of which gradually become eroded with advancing age. This generalization and the corollary principle that an abrupt or major decline prior to old age signals the advent of specific disease is perhaps best illustrated by glucose metabolism and diabetes, a critically important age-related disorder.

The maintenance of a blood glucose concentration sufficient to deliver this substrate to critical tissues, notably the central nervous system, yet not so excessive as to invite the untoward effects of severe hyperglycemia (notably hyperosmolar coma or, more chronically and subtly, advanced glycosylated end-product [AGE] protein accumulation) represents a prime physiological regulatory objective. This is accomplished via a continuously fine-tuned balance between carbohydrate intake, its digestion to simple sugars, absorption, and uptake by brain, liver, kidney, and peripheral tissues, and the breakdown of glycogen and release of glucose from stores in those tissues. These processes are modulated by the secretion of insulin and the counter-regulatory hormones – glucagon, catecholamines, cortisol, and growth hormone. A keystone of the fine regulation of this system is the sensitivity of the liver and peripheral tissues to insulin.

Careful studies of healthy young and elderly human volunteers have underscored the pivotal role of declining insulin sensitivity as a cardinal feature of aging (Fig. 2). Thus, at a given level of insulin, even when normalized for the reduced lean body mass characteristic of old age, less glucose is metabolized in older persons. Older subjects also characteristically mount a more sluggish insulin response to a glucose load, whether administered orally or intravenously. The combination of both leads to a decline in the efficiency of glucose metabolism with advancing age, reflected less in the overnight fasting glucose level (which on average rises about 1 mg/dl/decade) than in the two-hour post-oral glucose concentration (which rises ca. 5 mg/dl/decade).[1] Thus, the incidence of impaired glucose tolerance (defined by standards independent of age) rises with advancing age, and frank diabetes becomes increasingly prevalent in old age. Here also is illustrated the modulation of the age at which the clinical threshold is crossed as the resultant between environmental and genetic forces. In the case of Type I or insulin-dependent diabetes, which typically presents in childhood, this event reflects the person's genetic sensitivity to infection-triggered, islet-cell autoimmune destruction and a resulting absolute deficiency of insulin (without impaired insulin sensitivity). This response contrasts with the more complex, deliberate interaction between insulin, its receptor, and its intracellular effects in the case of the far more common Type II or non-insulin-dependent diabetes that occurs in adulthood but before old age – a disease that is heavily concentrated among obese, sedentary persons with diminished insulin sensitivity. However, among those who do not develop diabetes until old age, the defect that results in impaired glucose tolerance or the fasting hyperglycemia of frank diabetes proceeds from

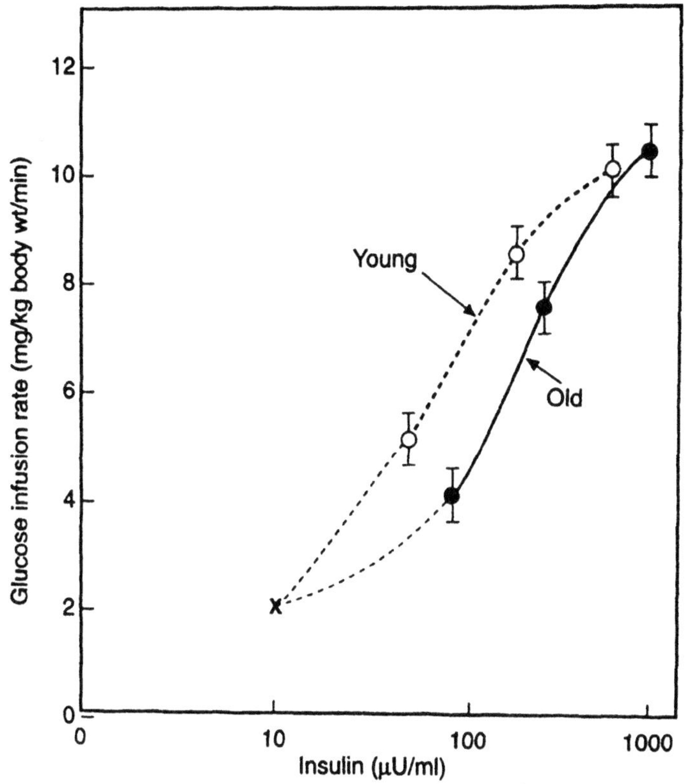

Figure 2. Dose-response curves for insulin-mediated whole body glucose infusion rates (expressed as mg/kg body weight) in young (dashed line) and old (solid line) subjects. Elderly individuals have reduced sensitivity to insulin but no change in maximal glucose disposal (Rowe JW, Minaker KL, Pallotta JA. Characterization of the insulin resistance of aging. Reproduced with permission from J Clin Invest 1983; 71: 1581)

a yet more complex interaction among genetic susceptibility, adiposity, physical activity (exercise enhances insulin sensitivity), and the diminished insulin sensitivity and delayed insulin secretion of old age per se.

Related to the efficiency of glucose metabolism are the progressive adiposity and decline in lean body mass that characterize the aging process across adulthood but can be traced back to about age 20 when, on average, peak lean body mass is achieved. As to total body mass, in a normative sense this increases progressively in 'the first half of middle age', 25–50 or so (Fig. 3), reflecting the greater continuous accretion of adipose tissue than the concurrent progressive decline in lean body mass. In the second one-half of middle age, when these two processes are in balance, a plateau in total weight is the norm, while weight loss is characteristic of the final phase of life as both fat and lean body mass decline. Plasma lipids characteristically parallel these trends in body weight (except for the 'post-menopausal over-

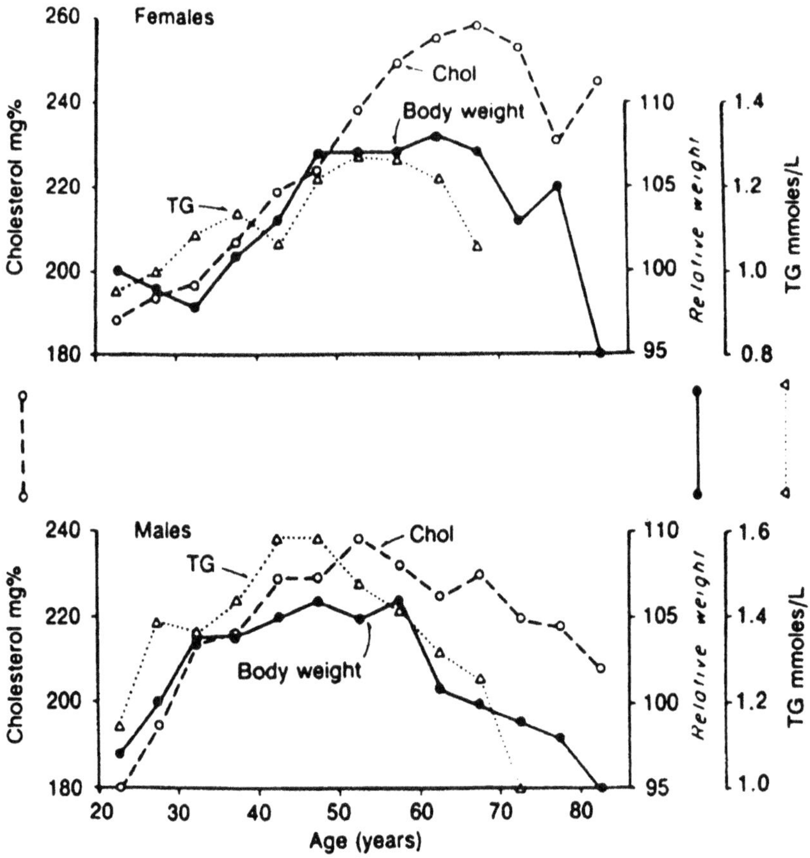

Figure 3. Superimposition of values throughout the adult age span for an index of relative body weight serum cholesterol from the Tecumseh study (Montoye) and triglycerides from the healthy subgroup studied in Stockholm (Carlson and Lindstedt). Reproduced with permission from Bierman EL, Glomset JA. Disorders of lipid metabolism. In William RH, ed., Textbook of endocrinology. Philadelphia: W.B. Saunders, 1974.

shoot' in women, reflecting the rise in cholesterol – specifically the low-density lipoprotein, LDL, cholesterol – that follows the decline in estrogen secretion at the menopause).

Much has been written on the physiological or patho-physiological implications of these changes [9]. Suffice it to say here that, characteristic of the blurred margin between 'normal' and 'abnormal' that defines much of the physiology of aging, the disease specificity of deviations from norms for middle age in both weight and serum lipids declines with advancing age, and variance increases; whereas maintenance of the lean body habitus and low serum lipid levels of young adulthood throughout midlife and beyond appears to confer robust health and vigor into advanced old age (often attributable in part to a high level of physical activity), a *loss* of *weight* and/or *decline* in blood lipids may herald impending disease, frailty, or death, notably when a catabolic downward spiral has been initiated by one or more processes activating the immune system, be it 'infection; infarction; or infraction' (the author's mnemonic for the triggers of the terminal cascade of geriatric complications that often follow: infractions to include falls, and other trauma, including surgery, perturbations in nutrition or fluid status, and iatrogenic misadventures). Thus, seasoned geriatricians (and all experienced clinicians) have learned to worry about older patients whenever weight declines, especially when the weight loss is involuntary, and when cholesterol decreases without hypolipidemic intervention.

In a related vein, nutrition in general appears to be well maintained with advancing age in the absence of active disease. However, just as the margin between 'steady-state' (resting) and perturbed or stressed homeostatic reserve declines with aging so, too, does the margin between adequate nutrition in the unstressed state and that required during periods of increased requirement, notably in the presence of active disease. This reduced margin of safety is based in part in the declining energy (and hence caloric) requirement with aging, which parallels the progressive decrease in lean, more metabolically active body mass that begins in the third decade. This decline is associated with a physiological and the counter-regulatory simultaneous reduction in caloric intake; while this coupling between caloric expenditure and intake is imperfect (accounting for the progressive rise in adipose mass until advanced old age), it does lead to a narrower margin of safety in micronutrient intake, given that the requirements for the vitamins and minerals ingested as part of a balanced, healthy diet are believed to remain undiminished with aging. Hence the population of marginally nourished persons grows as caloric intake declines among the elderly (however, the prevalence of vitamin and mineral supplementation among them, especially those of middle and upper class, is high and should be routinely ascertained as part of the clinical evaluation).

These micronutrient reserves become rapidly exhausted during periods of stress, especially with injury or illness. So, too, do body stores of glycogen, protein, and fat, and rampant malnutrition may ensue. What would appear perverse in terms of survival, such disease states, almost invariably accompanied by inflammation and immune activation, are associated not only with accelerated catabolism but also profound anorexia. Markers of the accelerated malnutrition that ensues include declines in albumin, prealbumin, transferrin, retinol-binding protein, and cholesterol – the last presumably reflecting impaired synthesis and secretion of the carrier apolipoproteins B (for LDL) and, ultimately, A (for HDL). Whether or not such apoprotein depletion results in functional deficiencies in such fat-soluble vitamins as A, D, E, and K at the tissue level remains to be elucidated in the elderly. What seems clear, however, is that such decreases carry an ominous prognosis, illustrated in a study of elderly hospitalized patients with acquired hypocholesterolemia, who, as compared with their normocholesterolemic comparison controls, suffered a twofold increase in complications, hospital stay (and cost), and mortality [10].

Maintenance of Structural Integrity

These issues of nutritional status and aging are closely related to the challenge of maintaining bodily structural integrity in old age, both of the musculature and the skeleton. Sarcopenia and osteopenia, terms describing inadequate muscle and bone, respectively, are extraordinarily prevalent in old age and threaten the health, mobility, and independence of the elderly.

The determinants of muscular integrity with aging have received much investigation but still represent research challenges. With aging there occurs progressive loss of muscle fibers, especially of the fast-twitch variety, and of the capillary vessels that supply their metabolic requirements. These losses can be overcome only in part by exercise training (although, even among nonagenarian nursing home residents, active training improves strength and general function [11]). Here, too, the disease-related, protein-calorie malnutrition that is associated with immune activation, catabolic hypermetabolism, and diminished caloric intake, almost invariably accompanied by reduced physical activity, rapidly produce muscular atrophy. All these changes contribute to the profound weakness and the delayed recovery from acute illnesses and surgery characteristic of the elderly. This underscores the critical role of early and active physical rehabilitation and aggressive nutritional therapy in the acute and subacute care of older patients.

The skeleton, too, suffers progressive loss in strength and integrity with advancing age. This loss begins shortly after peak bone mass is reached during adolescence. Indeed, given the long time course of age-related bone loss and relatively low absolute threshold of skeletal mineral content below which risk of osteoporosis-related fracture rapidly escalates, a sound long-term strategy is to prevent (or at least delay) such fractures by maximizing skeletal mass through nutrition and exercise during adolescence and throughout adult life.

Preservation of skeletal integrity to withstand the stresses of physical activity is an essential physiological task accomplished through a delicate interplay of multiple organ systems and cells, hormones and growth factors, cytokines, and related biochemical mechanisms that regulate bone mineral content and its organization into bone that is both strong and resistant. The hormones involved include parathyroid hormone, calcitonin, vitamin D, estrogen and testosterone.

Maintenance of skeletal integrity is a dynamic turnover process of constant bone formation and resorption. At the micro level, periods of bony resorption, mediated by osteoclasts, and bone formation, mediated by osteoblasts, exist in a tightly coupled, finely regulated state of dynamic balance. This turnover allows adaptive responses to changes in force upon bones at particular anatomic sites. However, across the menopause and with reduction in estrogen, a partial uncoupling occurs and bone mineral loss leading to frank osteoporosis through time is common, especially in slender, white women (obesity not only increases gravitational force upon bones but also is associated with higher post-menopausal estrogen (estrone) levels because of aromatization of androgenic adrenal-steroid precursors in adipose tissue). Bone mineral content also declines in aging men, albeit at a slower rate than in women, presumably because the age-related decline in testosterone is more subtle and gradual than the loss of ovarian estrogen across the menopause.

These modulating effects of estrogen and testosterone on bone mineral metabolism have been traced to their impact at the level of cytokines and growth factors. Estrogen decreases IL-1 and TNF α production, in turn reducing IL-6 production by osteoclasts and thereby decreasing osteoclastic bone resorption. Estrogen also stimulates granulocyte-macrophage colony-stimulating factor (GM-CSF), further inhibiting osteoclast formation. Testosterone is thought to cause anabolic bone formation, probably via its effects on TGF- and IGF-1.

Also threatening skeletal integrity in elderly persons is a decrease in cutaneous production of vitamin D_3, diminished 1αhydroxylation of 25-OH vitamin D by the kidney, decreased intestinal calcium absorption, and increased PTH levels. An age-related decline in gastric-acid secretion also diminishes calcium absorption. Moreover, the common advent of lactose intolerance among the elderly tends to cause avoidance of milk products. These various factors that challenge skeletal integrity are listed in Table 2.

Table 2. Factors influencing bone loss in the elderly

Sex hormone deficiency
Estrogen
Testosterone
Vitamin D deficiency
Decreased skin production of vitamin D_3
Decreased α-hydroxylation by the kidney
Calcium malabsorption
Vitamin D deficiency
Hypochlorhydria
Calcium regulatory hormone changes
Increased parathyroid hormone levels
Genetic factors influencing peak bone mass at skeletal maturity
Lifestyle factors
Decreased calcium and vitamin D intake and lactase deficiency
Decreased physical activity (i.e., decreased mechanical loading)
Smoking
Decreased sunlight exposure
Alcohol

Another hormonal change that may contribute to the decline in strength and mobility in the elderly is a decrease in growth hormone levels, especially seen in the frail and most evident during sleep. Trials of recombinant human growth hormone to enhance strength and rebuild lost muscle and bone have been initiated, but clear and consistent beneficial results remain to be reported.

Beyond the fragility of the musculature and skeleton in the elderly, fractures and other untoward effects of loss of mobility and falls threaten independence. Thus a fracture from a fall most often reflects the combination of a fragile skeleton, weakened muscles, and defects in mobility and balance. Whereas many of the features of impaired mobility can be overcome with training, even in the most healthy and fit elderly person, subtle changes that diminish mobility and balance can be demonstrated. These include the results of degeneration of neurons in the frontal cortex, which can lead to Parkinsonian features, and in the cerebellum, causing ataxia. A gradual loss of peripheral sensory proprioception, especially in the large joints, causes a diminished sense of location in space. Furthermore, nerve conduction is retarded, causing slower reflex correction of changes in position and balance. Hence an increase in sway and a decrease in the force required to cause a loss of balance is a common feature. This vulnerability is magnified when the subject's eyes are closed, since elderly persons depend on visual cues to control balance more than do younger persons (the frequent associated loss of visual acuity further exaggerates this vulnerability).

Reproductive Function

Declines in reproductive capacity with advancing age occur in both sexes. However, menopause and its relatively abrupt cessation of menses is confined to women (and menopause is rare in non-human species), and there is little evidence for a male menopause. With advancing age in women between 45 and 55 the ovary becomes less responsive to gonadotropins, plasma levels of 17-estradiol and inhibin decline, and gonadotropin levels rise – FSH more so than LH. As menopause approaches, the intervals between menses lengthen, anovulatory cycles predominate, and ultimately menses cease altogether, most commonly around age 50. Thereafter estrone replaces 17-estradiol as the principal circulating estrogen, as noted above derived importantly from peripheral aromatization of androstenedione in adipose tissue.

In males advancing age is associated with a gradual decrease in testicular size and a decline in Leydig cells (the source of testosterone) and Sertoli cells (the source of spermatozoa and inhibin). As in the female, FSH and LH levels rise with age, with a decline in pulsatile LH secretory amplitude and frequency. The age-related decline in testosterone is subtle, best demonstrated by a decline in afternoon levels. The clinical significance of this decline remains unclear but significant testosterone deficiency is frequent among sick, frail, and declining elderly men. However, the safety and efficacy of its therapeutic administration, of its replacement, or the appropriate pharmacological doses, remain to be demonstrated.

Regulation of the Delivery of Oxygen and Metabolic Substrate to Vital Organs with Advancing Age

All tissues require a continuous supply of oxygen and nutrients and removal of waste products. This requires an efficient circulatory system, with its various components including the blood itself, the vascular tree, the cardiac pump, the lungs, and the chemo- and baroreceptors and neuroendocrine mediators that regulate this complex system. A central force in this system is the blood pressure, which is affected by aging at multiple points of regulation.

Age-Related Changes in Blood Pressure Regulation

Normal human aging is associated with a reduction in baroreflex sensitivity. Thus in elderly humans there is a blunted cardioaccelerator response to assuming the upright posture, nitroprusside infusion, and lower body negative pressure; conversely, phenylephrine produces less bradycardia in elderly than in younger subjects. There is also increased blood pressure variability in the elderly, which can cause untoward hypotension in response to assuming the upright posture or after meals, when blood tends to pool in the intestine. This diminished baroreflex sensitivity is thought to be mediated principally by reduced α-adrenergic receptor sensitivity to agonists as well as to defects in cardiac myocyte post-receptor signal transduction.

This diminished sympathetic sensitivity in the elderly was first suggested by higher resting plasma levels of both epinephrine and, following upright posture and exercise, norepinephrine. Both increased secretion and, to a lesser extent, decreased clearance contribute to these increases. However, in spite of these higher levels, cardiac and vascular responsiveness remain diminished in the elderly. Thus α-adrenegic agonists in the elderly produce smaller increases in heart rate, left ventricular ejection fraction, cardiac output, and vasodilatation than in younger subjects. The mechanism of this reduced responsiveness is traced to a lower affinity of cardiac α-receptors for their agonists, plus reduced G-protein-mediated signal transduction and decreased sarcolemmal calcium channel ionic transport. Since similar changes are induced in experimental animals by chronic exposure of myocardial tissue to α-agonists, it remains to be seen whether these alterations are primary or secondary, attributable in turn to the higher circulating α-agonist levels in older subjects.

This diminished sensitivity to adrenegic stimulation in the elderly appears to extend to their vascular responsiveness, both vasorelaxation with α-agonists and vasoconstriction with α-agonists. This, too, seems secondary to chronic elevations in these agents, since it is reversed through suppression of sympathetic nervous system activity with guanadrel.

Heart rate, too, seems less sensitive to autonomic regulation with advancing age. Specifically, it appears that healthy aging is associated with reductions in both baroreflex and parasympathetic modulation of heart rate. For all these reasons the highly irregular, complex dynamics of heart rate variability characteristic of young persons are diminished with aging. This feature can perhaps be generalized to other physiological systems, which show more regular, less complex regulation with age, in turn rendering the organism less adaptable and hence more vulnerable to perturbations.

Cardiac Ventricular Function

Cardiac output at rest and during exercise tends to decline with advancing age even in the absence of demonstrable coronary disease. This is mediated in part by reduced left ventricular compliance and an element of 'diastolic dysfunction' (aggravated, however, by hypertension when present). This results in slower diastolic left ventricular filling and hence a greater dependence on atrial contraction to complete ventricular filling before systole (and hence a greater vulnerability to the adverse cardiodynamic consequences of atrial fibrillation). Systolic function is reduced principally because of reduced α-adrenegic responsiveness and increased afterload. The latter increases progressively with aging, attributable to aortic stiffening and diminished peripheral arterial compliance. Thus maximum cardiac output during exercise is reduced with aging. In the absence of ventricular systolic dysfunction (usually a consequence of coronary artery disease), this, however, is principally attributable to a diminished heart rate response to exercise, with greater dependence than in younger subjects on the Frank-Starling mechanism to maintain output through increased stroke volume [12]. Hence elderly persons harbor less cardiac reserve before decline and clinical heart failure supervene.

Intravascular volume regulation is also affected by aging, which is associated with progressive declines in plasma renin, angiotensin II, and aldosterone and an increase in atrial natriuretic peptide, all of which promote kidney salt and water loss. Moreover, elderly persons are less aware of dehydration during water deprivation and hence less likely to drink fluids in such circumstances. Thus dehydration and its devastating sequelae of orthostatic hypotension, falls, and delirium presents a grave risk in the elderly. These and other changes in renal physiology and salt and water metabolism are further detailed elsewhere in this series.

Regulation of organ blood flow is also accomplished at the local level, where, for instance, it appears that aging is associated with a reduced vasodilatory response to acetylcholine – a measure of endothelium-dependent vasoregulation. Local regulation of cerebral blood flow may also be impaired with advancing age, rendering older individuals especially vulnerable to the untoward effects of orthostatic hypotension.

Respiratory Control

Aging is associated with a progressive albeit modest decline in pO_2, principally attributable to ventilation-perfusion mismatch in dependent areas of the lung, this proceeding in turn from a reduction in lung compliance causing premature airway closure at higher lung volumes. With advancing age, there occurs a decline in sensitivity of brain-stem respiratory chemoreceptors to both oxygen and carbon dioxide. Thus older persons may be more vulnerable to ischemia during stresses such as surgery, pneumonia, or high altitudes.

Closing Comment

From this preview a cardinal principle of geriatrics should emerge: Given the multiple layers of complexity and redundancy of homeodynamics that define normal physiology, and given the long plateau of robust physiological regulation that characterizes human survival until advanced old age, no disease state should be attributed to 'just old age', and old age *per se* as the cause of disease and dysfunction is thus at most a 'diagnosis' of exclusion. Moreover, whereas 'natural death' may legitimately occur, proceeding from the simultaneous collapse of multiple physiological systems (and perhaps become the norm in a Utopian society in which all premature death has been prevented, part of the attraction of the thesis of Fries [5]), at this juncture assigning diseases, dysfunction, or death to 'just old age' is rarely justified. Therefore, an exhaustive search for etiology and, especially potential treatment of disease and dysfunction is equally justified and imperative in the elderly as in the younger patient.

Note

1. Reflecting another principle of the physiology of aging: the time required to return to baseline following a given stimulus increases with advancing age.

References

1. Rowe JW, Kahn RL. Human aging: usual and successful: a review. Science 1987; 237: 143–149.
2. Rowe JW, Kahn RL. Successful Aging. New York: Pantheon Books, 1998.
3. Hazzard WR. Preventive gerontology: strategies for healthy aging. Postgrad Med 1983; 74: 279–287.

4. Hazzard WR. Successful aging: ways to make 'usual' and 'successful' aging synonymous. Western J Med 1997; 167(4): 206–215.
5. Fries JF. Aging, natural death, and the compression of morbidity. N Engl J Med 1980; 303: 130–135.
6. Harper DW, et al. Aging, health risks, and cumulative disability. N Engl J Med 1998; 339: 481.
7. Hazzard WR, Blass JP, Ettinger WH, Halter JB, Ouslander JG. Principles of Geriatric Medicine and Gerontology, 4th ed. New York: McGraw-Hill, 1999.
8. Lipsitz LA. Clinical physiology of aging. In: Kelley WN, editor. Textbook of Internal Medicine, 3rd edition. Philadelphia: Lippincott-Raven, 1997; 110–119.
9. Hazzard WR, Ettinger WH. Aging and atherosclerosis: changing considerations in cardiovascular disease prevention as the barrier to immortality is approached in old age. Amer J Geriatr Cardiol 1995; 4: 16–36, 41.
10. Noel M, Smith T, Ettinger W. Characteristics and outcomes of hospitalized older patients who develop hypocholesterolemia. J Am Geriatr Soc 1991; 39: 455–461.
11. Fiatarone MA, et al. Exercise training and nutritional suppplementation for physical frailty in very elderly people. N Engl J Med 1994; 330: 1769.
12. Rodeheffer RJ, et al. Exercise cardiac output is maintained with advancing age in healthy human subjects: cardiac dilatation and increased stroke volume compensate for a diminished heart rate. Circulation 1984; 69: 203.

Aging Kidneys in an Aging Population: How Does This Impact Nephrology and Nephrologists?

WILLIAM R. HAZZARD
J. Paul Sticht Center on Aging, Wake Forest University School of Medicine, Winston-Salem, NC 27157-1207, U.S.A.

Of all of the forces that will impinge upon the daily professional lives of nephrologists in the 21st century, none will be more powerful than the progressive aging of the population. Thus a strategy to integrate nephrology with gerontology and geriatrics will assist both disciplines in adapting to this phenomenon, the 'demographic imperative' that will drive health and health care on a global basis at all levels from individual patients to populations and systems of health care. Thus just as we did at the recent Geriatric Education Retreat (GER) in Nephrology, we shall begin with a review of that demographic imperative.

Its dimensions can be framed by comparing the distribution of the population by age in a developing nation e.g., Mexico in the early 1970s (Fig. 1) with that of a developed, industrialized nation, notably one of northern Europe, illustrated here by Sweden. Thus the changes that come with economic development and societal maturation produce a 'rectangularization' of the population distribution by age, as opposed to the triangular or pyramidal distribution in developing nations. These changes include improved nutrition, housing, transportation, public health and sanitation, education, and communication. At the same time, with the tendency toward urbanization that tends to parallel economic development, the traditional pressures that drive high reproductive rates in rural nations diminish, birth rates decline, and family size decreases. Hence, a smaller number of infants are born but a higher proportion survive childhood and enter young and middle adulthood, and, increasingly, old age. This pattern, which has been reproduced in all nations that have undergone industrialization and maturation to date, may be expected to be replicated in the third-world nations of today in the 21st century. In 1970 (Fig. 1) the United States was still a population in flux, with post-World War II 'baby boomers' in childhood and adolescence outnumbering those of middle and old age who preceded them. However, by the year 2030, the United States will approach a steady state, with relatively equal proportions of its population in each five-year-age group from five to 75+ years of age.

However, perhaps unique to the present epoch, those baby-boomers will be followed by the 'baby-bust' generation, producing a special challenge to

Oreopoulos et al. (eds.), Nephrology and Geriatrics Integrated, 17–26.

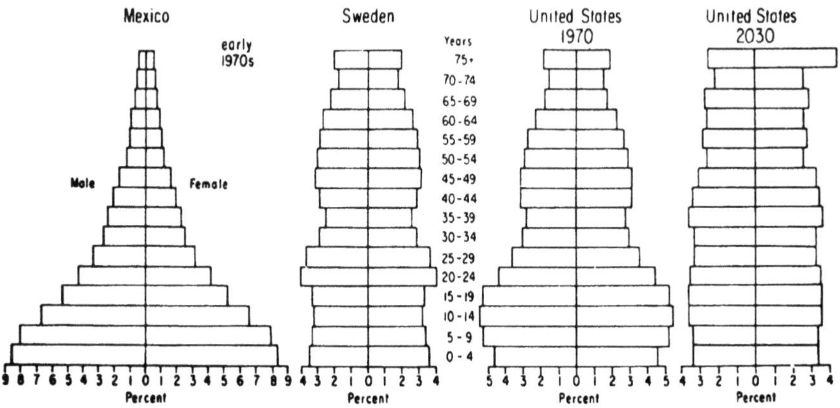

Figure 1. Age distribution by sex in Mexico and Sweden in the early 1970s and in the United States in 1970 and 2030. (Source: Somers, A: The high cost of health care for the elderly: Diagnosis, prognosis, and some suggestions for therapy. J Health Politics, Policy, and Law 1978; 3: 168).

those successors to support their parents in their post-retirement years while providing for their children's welfare and their own future economic requirements when they leave the workforce. An important byproduct of this progressive maturation of society is also illustrated in Fig. 1 as it applies to the United States; namely, because of the lower mortality rates of females than males at all points in the lifespan beyond conception, with advancing age there is a progressive shift in the oldest cohorts toward a predominance of women. This predominance is especially evident in long-term care institutions, where the combination of living to the stage of infirmity and dependency and having outlived their spouses causes a concentration of elderly women in nursing homes and other assisted living facilities for the elderly.

These trends are inexorable and the results inevitable. Indeed, the percentage of the population over age 85 will grow more than any other, and the numbers of those over 85, who are at greatest risk to frailty, dependency and long term institutional care, will rise exponentially well into the middle of the 21st century. In absolute terms, while the numbers of those 65 years of age and older will grow progressively through 2050, disproportionate growth will take place in the oldest old – those over 85 years of age. However, these are only estimates, and the predictions of various researchers and the Census Bureau reflect a wide variation in the predicted size of the oldest old cohort. Perhaps most optimistic (but also most challenging) the estimates of demographer Ken Manton [1] suggest that as many as 48.7 million Americans will be age 85 and over by the 2050. His figure is based upon research that demonstrates a progressive decline in mortality rates among those over age 85 in recent decades. Perhaps most encouraging, his research also reports a decreased use of the health-care system among that oldest old cohort, who appear to be increasingly robust as survivors of the 20th century [2].

This demographic imperative is not confined to the United States. Indeed, all portions of the globe will show progressive increases in the average age of their populations in the 21st century, and the percentage of the population age 60 and over will grow substantially as all portions of the world proceed to industrialization and development. Perhaps at the extreme of this 21st-century demographic shift is the projected growth in the population of Americans age 100 years and over between 1900–2050 (Fig. 2). Thus, in spite of the 'barrier to immortality' described by Fries and the perhaps fixed *average* upper limit of the human lifespan in the steady state at 85 years [3], anything that increases the number of persons surviving beyond age 85 will extend the tail of the curve of the distribution to include increasing numbers of centenarians. This increased possibility of living to 100 years of age is capturing the attention of American baby boomers as they pass through the middle of middle age. However, even as they have an increased probability of living to be 100 years of age, they also have an increased probability of becoming frail, dependent, and financially precarious in advanced old age. In anticipation of the former, increasingly travel, hotel and leisure businesses are adapting to the needs of older and older customers, as are the housing, transportation, and other related industries catering to those who will enjoy increased leisure and discretionary time. However, reflecting the darker but very real alternative, more and more middle-aged persons (especially women) are spending more and more time caring for their own aging parents just as their children (though generally fewer in number) will be called upon to provide support for them when they enter advanced old age.

Winston-Salem artist Ruth Newman has captured the reality of this dual philosophical approach to old age in a pair of bookends sculpted to become

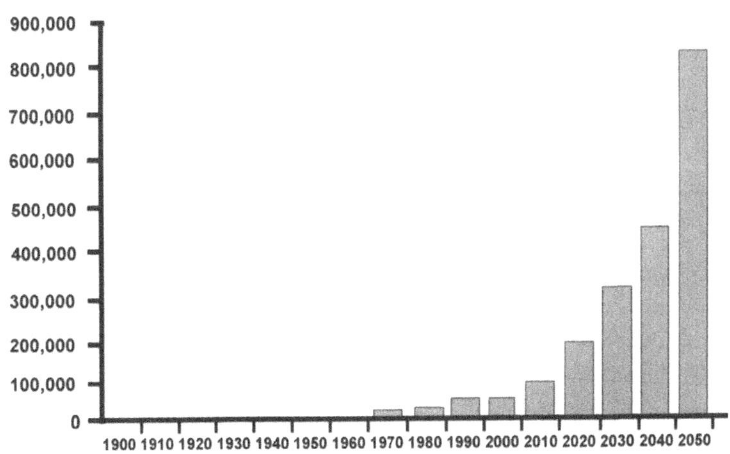

Figure 2. Population 100 years and over 1900–2000.

the symbols of the comprehensive program in gerontology and geriatrics under development at the Wake Forest University School of Medicine under the umbrella of the J. Paul Sticht Center on Aging (Fig. 3). On the one hand, as represented by the senior runner, an increasing number of elderly will be vigorous, fit, exercising actively, independent, and participating fully in the social and intellectual activities of their communities. However, the other bookend, depicting a frail, gloomy old man, represents the increasing proportion of older persons, who will become disabled, discouraged, depressed, and require support from both formal and informal health and social-care systems. One cannot focus solely on the optimistic 'bookend' if one seeks to realistically address the social and physical consequences of progressive aging. Of course, physicians – notably nephrologists – will focus their professional efforts on the frail, needy, and dependent end of this dichotomy.

The challenge to health-care practitioners, both generalists and subspecialists, therefore is to deal squarely with these realities. This will require them to recognize and effectively manage the complexities and burdens presented by the health problems of old age, especially the chronic diseases so clearly associated with aging and so prevalent in advanced old age (impaired renal function and indeed end-stage-renal disease being a prime example). The 20th century has seen a dramatic shift from those acute diseases and causes of death that are characteristic of a young, developing population. Those disorders associated with underdevelopment are principally infections and other

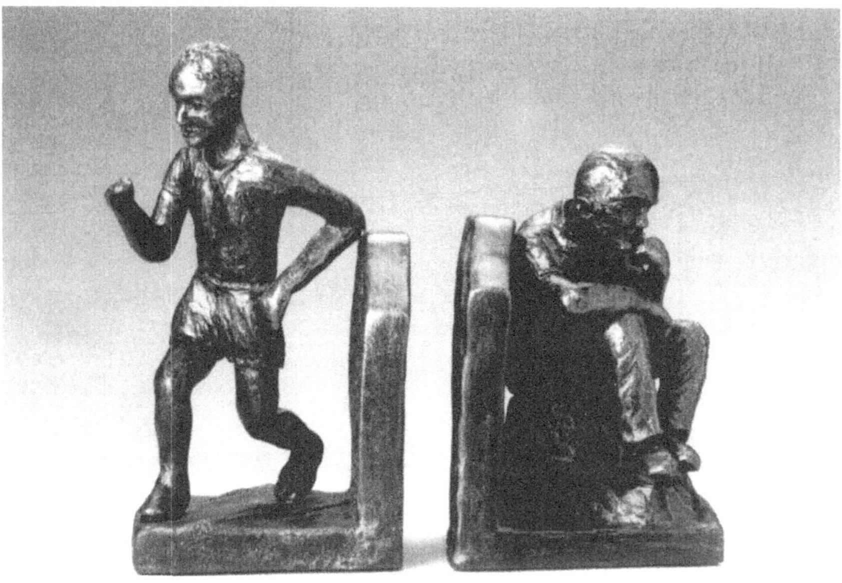

Figure 3. The 'book-ends' of the dual challenges and commitments to geriatric health and health care at the J. Paul Sticht Center on Aging of Wake Forest University.

consequences of poverty, such as lack of education, malnutrition, poor housing, and poor sanitation. With economic and social development these shift to the chronic, progressive diseases of aging and old age which are typical of advanced, generally affluent societies. Table 1 is a short list of those disabling but non-fatal diseases of old age. Thus all internists, both generalists and subspecialists alike, must seek to diagnose and manage these chronic diseases. Among the latter, nephrologists will become responsible for the principal care of the elderly patient at risk of or with end-stage renal disease.

During the same time frame, there will be a progressive decline in acute hospital-bed capacity and an explosion in long-term-care beds in the nursing-home industry (Table 2). Of course, health-care expenditures, especially those borne by public sources, will grow exponentially, reflecting the dominance of health resource consumption by Medicare beneficiaries. Already the American health care system is the most expensive in the world (Fig. 4), consuming the highest proportion of gross domestic product even though we are a relatively young nation compared to our counterparts in Western Europe. Thus the challenge will be great to contain further growth of health-care expenditures, even as we deal with our progressively aging and ultimately frail and dependent population. This conundrum frames the current debate over the future of Medicare and the anxiety of younger cohorts in our population, who face the prospect of escalating health care expenditures for their parents, grandparents, and ultimately themselves. Already such expenditures by older Americans are high, many Medicare beneficiaries have limited incomes and hence spend a high proportion of their fixed and limited resources on out-

Table 1. Examples of common diseases in elderly patients that are chronic and generally produce impairments or disabilities well before death

Chronic Disabling but Non-Fatal Diseases of Advanced Age
• Arthritis
• Hearing impairment
• Visual impairment
• Osteoporosis fractures
• Dementia
• Diabetes
• Depression
• Parkinson's disease

Table 2. Estimated numbers of acute hospital and nursing home beds in the U.S. in 1993 and 2040

	1993	2040
Acute Hospital Beds	1,000,000	500,000
Nursing Home Beds	1,500,000	5,000,000

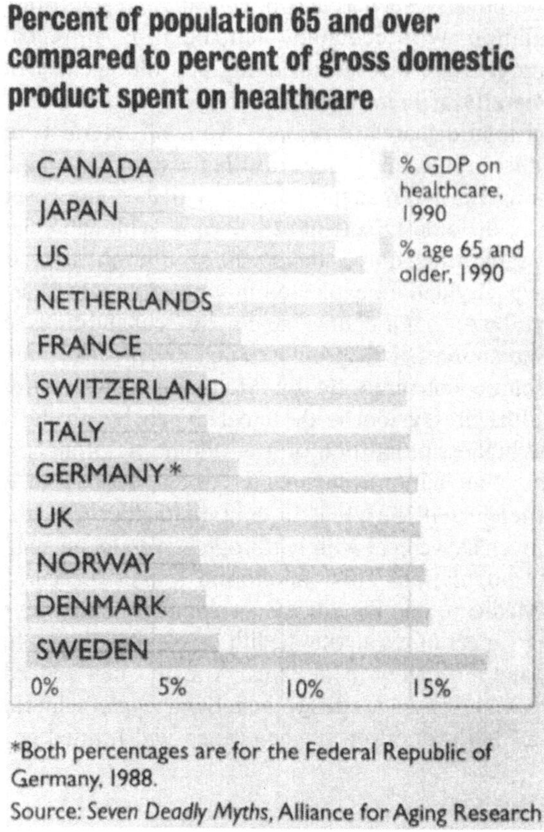

Figure 4. Percent of population 65 and over compared to percent of gross domestic product spent on healthcare.

of-pocket, health-care costs, especially those poor and near poor clustered at the lower end of the economic spectrum. With respect to the proportion of the population age 65 and older in need of long-term care, those over 85 years of age represent over one-half of the population requiring long-term care services (Fig. 5). In 1990 nearly one-quarter of Americans over age 85 were in nursing homes, of whom approximately one-half had lengths of stay less than three months but the other one-half distributed into stays of from three months to over five years.

In no medical subspecialty is the imperative of this challenge to deliver better, more informed, more thoughtful, more evidence-based, and yet more efficient and effective care more evident than nephrology: Aging is associated with progressive loss of physiologic renal reserve; the prevalence of the chronic diseases that accompany aging, notably hypertension and diabetes, rises exponentially with age increasing the predicted incidence and complexity

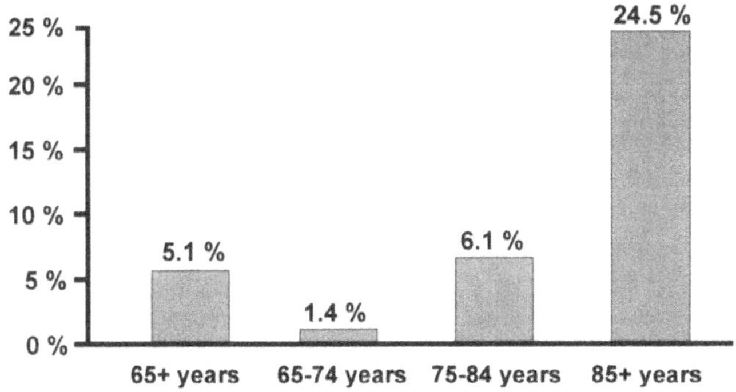

Figure 5. Proportion of elderly persons who reside in nursing homes: by age, 1990.

of end stage renal disease (ESRD) as the population ages; and the economic burden of caring for the burgeoning population of elderly ESRD patients with their limited life expectancy and array of co-morbidities (and potential for iatrogenesis), threatens to overwhelm the capabilities of the nephrology community, bankrupt the Medicare resources that finance ESRD care, and paralyze rational decision-making in such care by ethical dilemmas in the allocation of resources and the struggle to balance quality with quantity of life in ESRD patients and patient populations.

Thus the charge to the nephrology community is clear and dramatic: while the inevitability of increased health-care expenditures associated with the progressive aging of the population is clear, how, where, and by whom that care will be provided (and how it will be financed) frames our present deliberations. In our conceptualization at Wake Forest (which appears to be shared by most health-care providers and medical educators in the United States), primary health care for the elderly will be delivered mainly by internists and family practitioners, with geriatricians providing direct care for only a small fraction of the oldest, frailest, and most complex patients (Fig. 6). (Such board-certified geriatricians will be internists or family practitioners with at least one year of full-time clinical training in an accredited geriatric fellowship program.) This relatively small role of the formally-trained geriatrician in the direct provision of clinical services in the U.S. health care system proceeds from the assumption that primary-care practitioners will continue to dominate the provision of health-care services to the elderly, at least until those patients become frail and likely transfer their residence to continuing care retirement communities or nursing homes. Moreover, in this model, that limited number of geriatricians will be clustered in practices serving such communities or in university health centers where, when additionally trained during advanced fellowship years in the academic aspects of gerontology and geriatrics, they will serve as researchers and teachers for the generalists and specialists within those centers. This projection is also based upon the small number of geriatricians recruited to the field thus far and the substan-

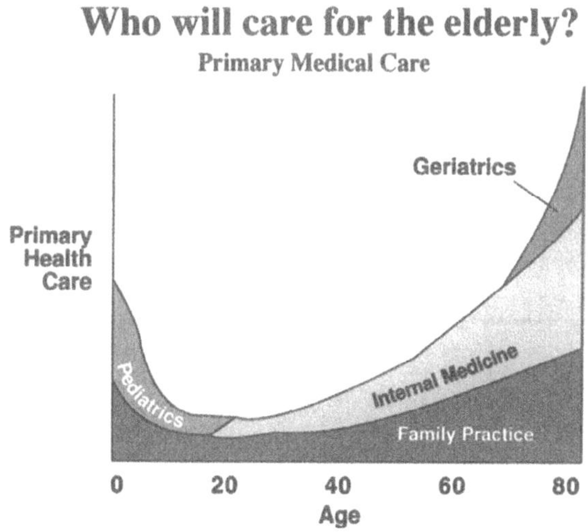

Figure 6. A conceptual estimate of the relative contributions of the primary care specialties to aggregate primary care across the lifespan. Note it is predicted that internists and family physicians without additional, fellowship level training in geriatrics will deliver the bulk of primary care of elderly patients.

tial and very real overlap between their capabilities and those of well-trained professionals equally competent in the care of the non-elderly with similar problems. Another view describes the provision of geriatric medical care as a series of overlapping circles in a Venn diagram (Fig. 7). In this model medical care of the elderly will be dominated by general internal medicine, neurology, psychiatry, rehabilitation, surgery and surgical subspecialties, and family practice, with geriatrics overlapping with all four, plus importantly, and the focus of this series of Geriatric Educational Retreat (GER), the subspecialists of internal medicine (in this instance nephrologists). This important overlap is reinforced by the typical complexity of the medical problems of older patients, many of which will require the sophistication and depth of knowledge and practice that define the medical subspecialist.

This conceptualization underlies the American Geriatrics Society/Wake Forest University School of Medicine/John A. Hartford Foundation project, entitled 'Integrating Geriatrics into the Subspecialties of Internal Medicine' [4]. This project is founded upon the hypothesis that: (1) internal medicine is and will continue to be the largest specialty in medicine; (2) internists (and family physicians) generally will be the primary-care physicians of choice for the burgeoning numbers of elderly Americans; (3) however (at least until very recently), most physicians completing residencies in internal medicine pursued training in the medical subspecialties, the largest and best compensated of which captured a disproportionate share of the 'best and the brightest'; (4) therefore, to best serve the medical needs of older Americans, the training

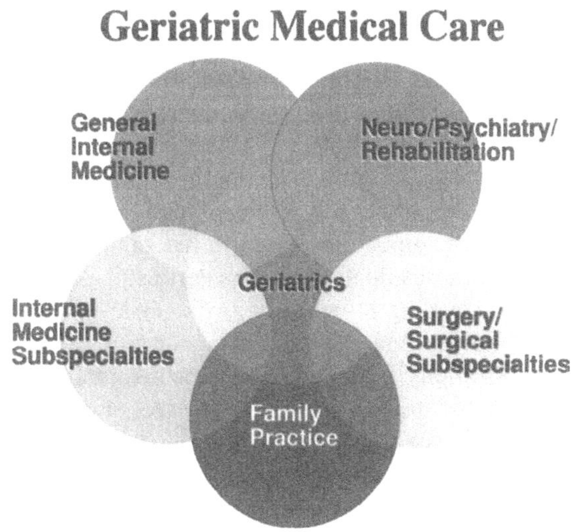

Figure 7. A Venn diagram of the medical and surgical disciplines that will contribute to geriatric health care in the 21st century.

of medical subspecialists must be enriched in the gerontological and geriatric aspects of their disciplines.

Thus the purpose of this initiative is to capture the interest and support of subspecialists through development of clinical practice, research and teaching agendas and identification of funding opportunities to support those efforts to bring forth the interest and commitment of the subspecialist. The strategy includes the following goals: (1) to incorporate geriatric content into the training of fellows in each subspecialty; (2) to 'gerontologize' present and future faculty in each subspecialty to provide that training (while simultaneously teaching medical students and residents); (3) to enrich American Board of Internal Medicine (ABIM) subspecialty examinations and Residency Review Committee – Internal Medicine (RRC-IM) training requirements in geriatric content; (4) to disseminate concepts and experiences at regional and national conclaves of subspecialists (as well as in reverse fashion, to enrich the education of generalists, e.g., at meetings of the Society of General Internal Medicine, American College of Physicians, etc., including geriatricians, in the subspecialty aspects of geriatric care; e.g., American Geriatrics Society).

The principal vehicle to initiate this intense collaboration between geriatrics and the subspecialties has been the Geriatric Educational Retreat (GER). The 'recipe' for a successful GER combines one part academic geriatricians, one part subspecialists turned geriatricians (the 'converted'), and several parts subspecialist 'movers and shakers' as yet to become involved in geriatrics (the 'unconverted'). We mix these elements in a crucible of intense review and creative discussion, a total immersion experience in a pleasant destination resort for a combination of didactic/Socratic, formal/informal, professional/social, and intellectual/extracurricular interaction. And at the end, *voilà*, 'gerontologized' subspecialty leaders emerge. The GER for Nephrology was the sixth such conclave, previous GER's having been held in Endocrinology, Diabetes, and Metabolism (1995); Cardiology (1996); Medical Oncology (1997); Rheumatology/Infectious Diseases/Immunology (1997); and Pulmonary/Critical Care (1998); that in Gastroenterology and, as a capstone, in General Internal Medicine will complete the cycle in the summer of 1999.

Thus far, by informal evaluation, this experiment seems to have worked in each subspecialty, leading to an ambitious agenda of follow-up activities which embed gerontology and geriatrics into each subspecialty through time and led by the subspecialty leaders themselves 'gerontologized' through this exercise. It was with this strategy in mind that leaders in nephrology convened at Jasper Park Lodge in the Canadian Rockies in August of 1998, a five-day, intensive exercise of intellectual and social interaction, the specific content of which is elaborated in this and other papers in this series.

References

1. Manton KG, Vaupel SW. Survival after the age of 80 in the United States, Sweden, France, England, and Japan. N Engl J Med 1995; 333: 1232–1235.
2. Manton KG, Corder L, Stallard E. Chronic disability trends in elderly United States populations. Proc Natl Acad Sci USA 1997; 94: 2593–2598.
3. Fries JF. The compression of morbidity: near or far. Milbank Q 1989; 67: 208–232.
4. Hazzard WR, Woolard N, Regenstreif DI. Integrating geriatrics into the subspecialties of internal medicine: the Hartford Foundation/American Geriatrics Society/Wake Forest University Bowman Gray School of Medicine initiative. JAGS 1997; 45: 638–640.

The Aging Kidney

SARBJIT V. JASSAL[1] and DIMITRIOS G. OREOPOULOS[2]
[1] *Department of Geriatric Medicine, University of Liverpool, Liverpool L69 3GA, U.K.;*
[2] *University of Toronto, The Toronto Western Hospital, Toronto, Ontario, Canada*

Aging is an inevitable consequence of life. Despite increased knowledge of the molecular and biological changes seen with aging, the underlying processes remain incompletely understood. A considerable literature on the histological and physiological changes in the kidney has been compiled over the past four decades. Initial reports showed consistent sclerotic features with generalized progressive deterioration in function. However, longitudinal studies suggest that normal aging is considerably more varied and often produces less dramatic alterations in both renal function and structure than initially reported. Recently, using laboratory data, workers have generated further hypotheses about the implications of and the reasons for the pathophysiological changes seen at maturity. This review summarizes current knowledge of the histological and physiological processes of aging in the kidney and, where appropriate, discusses some of these hypotheses.

Structural Changes

Renal size and weight decrease steadily with age, declining between 10 to 43% by the age of 80 years [1–4]. The accuracy of estimates of the total reduction in size is poor despite many such studies, in part because it is difficult to separate changes due to old age from those associated with subclinical disease. However the inaccuracy of these estimates also illustrates methodological differences [3].

Microscopically, the number of glomeruli and proximal tubules decrease in parallel to the total renal mass. The greatest reduction is in the cortex [5]. The glomeruli change in a gradual sequence, with initial folding and thickening of the glomerular basement membrane (GBM), followed by hyaline deposition and eventual degeneration of the glomerulus [6]. The eventual appearance is similar to that of chronic renal disease, with marked glomerulosclerosis and interstitial fibrosis predominantly in the cortex [7–9]. In addition, increased age appears to be associated with a larger number of columnar epithelial cells in Bowman's capsule [10]. Glomerular basement

Oreopoulos et al. (eds.), Nephrology and Geriatrics Integrated, 27–36.

membrane thickening results in a loss of lobulation of the glomerular tuft and a decrease in the effective filtering surface. Despite GBM thickening, glomerular permeability and filtration characteristics show no change [1]. In addition, aging appears to be associated with an increased number of columnar epithelial cells in the Bowman's capsule [10]. Overall, the total number of nuclei per glomerulus is unchanged. However there is a progressive increase in the number of mesangial cells with a reciprocal decrease in the number of epithelial cells [11]. With the increase in the number of mesangial cells, there is an overall expansion of mesangial tissue – an increase from 8% of total glomerular volume at age 45 years to nearly 12% by age 70 years [12, 13]. Because of glomerulosclerosis and mesangial expansion the number of nephron units becomes significantly decreased per unit tissue mass. Factors known to ameliorate sclerosis include sodium restriction, normoglycemia, female gender, castration, adrenalectomy and hypophysectomy [4, 14, 15].

In addition to a decline in the absolute number of proximal tubules, the length of each tubule shortens with increasing age. Tubular structures appear sparsely scattered with marked interstitial fibrosis [16]; this change in the number of tubules correlates well to the total renal mass [16]. Microscopically the tubular basement membrane becomes thickened with focal loss of the brush border, apical vesicles and heterophagic vacuoles [10, 13]. Although the cells of the distal tubule are not affected, both the distal tubule and the collecting duct system develop small diverticuli of unknown significance. It has not been decided whether these diverticuli play a part in the production of pyelonephritis (through harboring organisms and causing and maintaining recurrence of renal infection) [5].

The kidney displays distinct vascular changes [17–20]. The arcuate arteries become angulated and irregular; the large interlobar vessels show an increased tortuosity that eventually produces a spiraled appearance; and smaller vessels show an increased propensity to lipid deposition. Interstitial sclerosis is also common. These changes are independent of hypertension and other renal disease but are augmented if hypertension is present. Smaller vessels appear to be spared; fewer than 20% of senescent kidneys from non-hypertensive individuals display arteriolar changes. In areas that show marked glomerulosclerosis, a high percentage of afferent and efferent arterioles communicate directly with one another, diverting blood from the cortex to the relatively well-preserved juxtamedullary glomeruli. Sometimes this appearance is referred to as 'aglomerular arterioles' [4].

Abrass and colleagues surmise that aging may result from distinct changes in collagen metabolism. Such changes may include either a disordered synthetic pathway which has become activated with maturity, or the accumulation of unique isoforms of laminin over a prolonged period of time [21]. Although complex, and described in detail elsewhere, three points are of interest [21]: The first relates to the thickening of the GBM. Increased sulphation of the glycosaminoglycans was reported as early as 1983 [22]. However, Abrass et al. have shown a relative increase in laminin, particularly β_1 laminin, compared to collagen IV or fibronectin [21]. Because β_1 laminin is seen more commonly during fetal growth and development, this finding is unexpected. Although this is unexplained, Abrass and colleagues surmise that aging may reflect either a disordered synthetic pathway that has become activated with maturity, or the accumulation of unique isoforms of laminin over a prolonged period [21]. The second important observation is of an increased, extracellular, matrix-protein deposition in the renal interstitium [21], which appears to be due mainly to fibronectin and thrombospondin deposition with a noted absence of certain types of proteins – for example, collagen IV and laminin. In fact, the authors comment on the general paucity of collagen throughout the interstitium. Furthermore, the accumulation of extracellular matrix appears to predate both the glomerulosclerosis and the tubular atrophy. Although a possible link between interstitial fibrosis and angiogenesis is proposed, there is as yet no evidence to support it. Lastly, areas of focal tubular atrophy and interstitial scarring are seen, which are distinct from generalized changes of tubular atrophy and are associated with significant tubular basement membrane collapse. Future findings may elucidate the mechanisms underlying these interesting observations.

Functional Changes of Aging

Renal blood flow falls progressively with age, at an approximate rate of 10% per decade between the age of 30 and 60. Although some decrease in renal blood flow results from reduced renal size, Hollenberg and colleagues have demonstrated a constant decrease in renal blood flow with age, even after correction for reduced renal mass [20]. Most of the change occurs in the cortex with a relative increase in blood flow to the juxtamedullary region. These changes may account for the patchy cortical defects commonly seen on renal scans in healthy older adults. Furthermore, the redistribution of blood flow through the juxtamedullary region may explain the increase in the filtration fraction of sodium seen with advancing age.

Glomerular filtration is fundamental to renal function and, in the clinical setting, rapid alterations in the glomerular filtration rate (GFR) may be seen in an elevation in the serum creatinine. With aging, the glomerular filtration rate decreases gradually over time. However, because this decline is accompanied by a gradual loss of muscle mass, less creatinine is generated. Therefore deterioration in renal function may not result in an increase in serum creatinine [2–4, 10]. As numerous investigators have demonstrated, GFR declines with age and, in their landmark paper, Rowe and colleagues report a mean estimated fall of 8.0 mL/min per 1.73 m^2/decade [23]. However, the longitudinal follow up of individual subjects shows that the rate of decline is unique to each person [23]. Interestingly, a small proportion of patients showed an increase in GFR over time. The use of the Cockcroft-Gault equation, which has been used to estimate the GFR at different ages, though common, is not recommended [24]. Other formulae and bedside tests have been proposed, and although initial tests appeared promising, recent studies show measurement errors of between 33 mL/min underestimation to overestimation by 18 mL/min [25–28]. Unfortunately we have no ideal bedside test that accurately measures glomerular filtration rate and hence the most accurate clinical estimate remains the 24-hour creatinine clearance. Particularly in older subjects, caution must be used even with the creatinine clearance because inadequate urine collections may lead to misleadingly low estimates of GFR [29]. Alternatively, short timed-urine collections (for example, over a six-hour collection) are acceptable when clinical circumstances demand more rapid results or where 24-hour collections are impractical.

Renal functional reserve is a measure of the ability of the kidney to increase GFR above baseline values. Physiological maneuvres that elicit the reserve include an increased protein load (ingested or infused amino acids), dopamine or pregnancy. It has been proposed that, as renal function diminishes (regardless of cause), the kidney defends the GFR by using the reserve capacity and ultimately the kidney filters on maximal capacity even under normal unstressed conditions. Thus the functional reserve has been used as an alternative measure of renal function. In a small cross-sectional study, 10 elderly patients had measurements of residual reserve under controlled conditions [30]. After an amino-acid infusion, the GFR, as measured by inulin clearance, rose in all but one subject. The renal plasma flow (measured by the clearance of para-amino hippurate) increased in four, decreased in three and remained the same in the remaining three subjects. From these results, the authors concluded that renal reserve was preserved with age [30]. In a subsequent study of 18 elderly patients, approximately 50% showed diminished renal reserve, despite normal initial creatinine clearance studies (personal communication, Dr. S. Donnelly). The renal reserve measurements in all patients were assessed in three ways – using dopamine stimulation, amino acid infusion and a combined amino-acid and dopamine challenge. Long-term follow-up studies are underway to assess the relationship between renal reserve and long-term outcome in patients undergoing unilateral nephrectomy.

Regulation of plasma volume and osmolality also is altered with age and older persons are more vulnerable to rapid fluctuations in blood volume and electrolyte balance [3, 4, 31, 32]. The explanations for this are complex, however tubular secretion of diodrast and para-amino-hippuric acid in the elderly is decreased, particularly when the patient is placed under stress. In keeping with this, sodium balance is well maintained in older patients providing the total intake of sodium remains stable over time [33–36]. Under experimental conditions, however, older patients deprived of dietary sodium take longer to adjust their renal excretion rate to a lower maintenance level (31 hours compared with 18 hours in old and young subjects respectively) [34]. Thus, patients become increasingly prone to sodium and hence volume depletion with maturity. If an acute load of sodium is administered, for example as an intravenous solution, older subjects are unable to excrete sodium as effectively as younger persons [37]. Kirkland et al. found that older patients have altered diurnal variation with maximal renal excretion of sodium and potassium overnight [38].

The renal excretion of potassium has not been well studied in older human subjects; however, clinical experience suggests that potassium metabolism also is affected with increasing age. Failure to excrete large loads of potassium and subsequent hyperkalemia are partially explained by the decreased GFR and low basal levels of aldosterone. Furthermore, an overall reduction in total body potassium (by around 20%) predisposes the individual to hypokalemia [39]. Preliminary experimental work has shown that aged animals have a tendency to develop hyperkalemia when given an acute load of potassium [2, 3, 40].

With maturity the renal medulla and countercurrent system become less efficient at urinary concentration and dilution. In a study of 98 active community volunteers, older subjects could not raise their urine osmolality in response to dehydration, despite a similar dietary intake and total solute excretion to that before fluid restriction [34]. It seems unlikely that the reduction in GFR seen with aging would explain this observation because, in this study, the measured urinary osmolality, did not correlate with creatinine clearance. One may speculate that the relative increase in blood flow through the medulla may cause medullary 'washout' and thus defective sodium and water resorption. However one cannot exclude defective solute reabsorption as an explanation. Studies examining the secretion and effectiveness of antidiuretic hormone (ADH) release in aged persons show conflicting results. Although most workers found little difference in basal ADH levels in the young and old, some have reported lower serum concentrations in the elderly [32, 33, 35, 36, 41]. In older patients, ADH release is greater in response to volume depletion or increased tonicity, and available data suggests increased osmoreceptor sensitivity but decreased renal responsiveness. Because stimulation with exogenous ADH (given as 4 μg DDAVP) does not achieve as high urine osmolality in older persons as in younger controls (mean maximum urinary concentration 982 mOsm/kg vs. 823 mOsm/kg for 20- and 80-year-old subjects, respectively) it is likely that increased age results in partial nephrogenic diabetes insipidus [36]. Furthermore, animal studies suggest that renal Na-K-ATPase activity decreases with age, although this has not been confirmed in humans [40]. Few studies have measured the kidney's ability to respond appropriately to water loading, however, several workers have noted an appropriate fall in plasma ADH levels with water loading [42, 43].

As mentioned previously, intrarenal vascular tone increases with age. Vasoactive factors may contribute to this increased tone although the data describing this change are both complex and contradictory. For example, high basal levels of renal nerve activity, angiotensin II, and endogenous endothelin contribute to vasopressor activity but endothelin, endothelin-derived, relaxing-factor blockers (L-NAME and L-NMME) and angiotensin II all produce an exaggerated vasopressor response in aged rats [43–46]. The data for basal renin and angiotensin levels remain confusing, e.g. studies report both normal and low levels of renin and angiotensin in unstressed aged rats compared to younger controls [47–51]. A blunted renin response to stimulation with artificial stressors, upright posture or sodium depletion, consistently noted, suggests that age does affect vascular reactivity under physiological conditions. However other data show that vasodilators, including angiotensin-converting-enzyme inhibitors and angiotensin-II blockers, have similar effects regardless of age [47]. Consequently, one may only surmise that a relative increase in endogenous EDRF activity preserves renal blood flow and GFR but reduces the vasodilatory reserve and adaptation to superimposed hemodynamic insults.

Mechanisms of Age-related Reductions in Renal Function

The cause of age-related changes in the kidney remain unknown [52]. Among the two hypotheses most favored are (1) that an imbalance between synthesis and degradation of matrix proteins causes the glomerulosclerosis described previously and (2) that altered glomerular hemodynamics are responsible (the hyperfiltration theory and reduced nephron mass) [13, 45, 52]. The former hypothesis for which we have only minimal data is still under investigation. The second hypothesis – altered glomerular hemodynamics – is more important and will be discussed in more detail below.

The hyperfiltration hypothesis proposes that, in a kidney with a reduced number of glomeruli, there is increased capillary blood flow through each glomerular capillary bed and thus a correspondingly high intracapillary pressure [15, 53]. Within the glomerulus, capillary blood flow rate and intracapillary hydraulic pressures are maintained at a stable level using a fine balance of vasodilatory and vasoconstrictor substances. Thus, as the kidney ages and becomes more sclerotic, the total network of vessels is reduced producing an increase in the filtration rate across the basement membrane of each individual nephron – termed the single-nephron, glomerular filtration rate, (SNGFR) [54]. Systemic pressures remain unchanged. This high SNGFR pressure results in local endothelial cell damage and glomerular injury. The sequence of events start with small increases in blood flow, associated with increased SNGFR. In turn, this leads to disproportionate increases in glomerular pressure, endothelial cell damage, platelet aggregation and thrombin production [15, 55, 56]. The activation of platelets releases growth factors including platelet-derived growth factor (PDGF), epidermal growth factor (EGF), fibroblast growth factor (FGF) and tumor necrosis factor beta (TNF_{β}), all of which are associated with increased fibroblast collagen production and mesangial-cell sclerosis [57]. At the same time, shear stresses disrupt the ion exchange, change cell-membrane voltage and alter protein transcription within the endothelial cells. Alterations in the endothelin-derived relaxing factor (EDRF)/endothelin axis upset vascular hemodynamics and increase angiotensin

II secretion. As the glomeruli become sclerosed, the volume of blood flow that is directed to each of the remaining nephrons increases, further increasing the damage.

Dietary protein intake affects the rate of renal decline [8, 53, 58–61]. As early as 1935, it was shown that rats fed a protein-restricted diet had an increased survival. Subsequent animal studies confirmed that high protein intake accelerates glomerular deterioration. In humans, dietary protein intake correlates both with the total creatinine excretion and with the 24-hour creatinine clearance [29]. This observation is important for two reasons: firstly, it suggests that GFR is likely to vary over time; secondly, it supports the theory that renal damage results from single nephron glomerular hyperfiltration [53]. In fact, in patients with impaired creatinine clearance, dietary manipulation can prolong the time to doubling of serum creatinine [53]. Similarly, drugs that reduce single nephron GFR (e.g. ACE inhibitors and angiotensin II blockers) reduce glomerular injury more than those that solely control systemic blood pressure [62]. Unfortunately it is still unclear whether the protective effects of ACE inhibitors or dietary manipulation alter glomerular hemodynamics and thus prevent renal damage or if they act through altered signaling pathways. The latter argument holds that angiotensin II acts as a growth factor *in vitro* and directly induces mesangial hypercellularity and sclerosis. Thus any decrease in angiotensin II production may produce a change in cellular characteristics regardless of glomerular pressure.

Furthermore, reduced nephron mass at the time of birth is believed to contribute to the natural progression of renal disease [53, 63]. Animals subjected to renal ablation and hence a reduction in the number of functioning nephron units develop single-nephron hyperfiltration, progressive systemic hypertension, proteinuria, and renal failure associated with glomerular sclerosis. Similarly patients with congenital, unilateral renal agenesis show focal and segmental glomerulosclerosis on biopsy, consistent with chronic hyperfiltration from birth [64]. From these observations one may surmise that individuals born with reduced nephron mass have an increased tendency to hyperfiltrate and thus have a faster rate of renal decline. This theory may explain chronic transplant failure where a low nephron mass results in nonimmunogenic graft failure. Animal studies support this hypothesis. For example, pregnant rats fed a restricted protein diet have offspring with fewer glomeruli and tubular structures and increased connective tissue. Unfortunately this is difficult to confirm in humans. Conflicting clinical data come from the long-term follow-up of kidney transplant donors who, despite a higher incidence of hypertension and proteinuria, rarely have impaired renal function even 20 years after nephrectomy [65].

Conclusion

Although all aspects of renal function appear to decline with age, in most cases such function remains sufficient to maintain a steady state. In both experimental and observational studies, external stresses on the kidney however cause abnormal responses, which in the clinical setting may result in disease. Only with a greater understanding of the fundamental mechanisms of aging can we design methods of prevention.

References

1. Artursen G, Groth T, Grotte G. Human glomerular membrane porosity and filtration pressure: dextran clearance data analyzed by theoretical models. Clin Sci 1971; 40: 137–158.
2. Beck LH. Changes in renal function with aging. Clinics in Geriatric Medicine 1998; 11: 199–209.
3. Epstein M. Aging and the kidney. J Am Soc Nephrol 1996; 7: 1106–1102.
4. Jassal V, Fillit H, Oreopoulos DG. Aging of the urinary tract. In: Brocklehurst JC, Tallis RC, Fillet H, editors. Brocklehurst's Textbook of Geriatric Medicine and Gerontology. New York: Churchill Livingstone, 1997.
5. McLachlan MS. The ageing kidney. Lancet 1978; 2: 143–145.
6. Anderson S, Brenner BM. Effects of aging on the renal glomerulus. Am J Med 1986; 80: 435–442.
7. Kaplan C, Pasternack B, Shah H, Gallo G. Age-related incidence of sclerotic glomeruli in human kidneys. Am J Pathol 1975; 80: 227–234.
8. Bolton WK, Sturgill BC. Spontaneous glomerular sclerosis in aging Sprague-Dawley rats. II. Ultrastructural studies. Am J Pathol 1980; 98: 339–356.
9. Anand SK, Landing BH, Heuser ET, Olson DL, Grushkin CM, Lieberman E. Changes in glomerular basement membrane antigen(s) with age. J Pediatrics 1978; 92: 952–953.
10. Haley DP, Bulger RE. The aging male rat: structure and function of the kidney. Am J Anat 1983; 167: 1–13.
11. McDermott GF, Ingram A, Scholey J, Kirkland JL, Whiteside CI. Glomerular dysfunction in the aging Fischer 344 rat is associated with excessive growth and normal mesangial cell function. J Gerontology 1996; Series A, Biological Sciences & Medical Sciences 51: M80–M85.
12. Sorenson FH. Quantitative studies of the renal corpuscles. I. Intraglomerular, interglomerular and interfocal variation in the normal kidney. Acta Pathol Microbiol Scand 1972; 80: 115–124.
13. Baylis C, Corman B. The aging kidney: insights from experimental studies. J Am Soc Nephrol 1998; 9: 699–709.
14. Baylis C. Age-dependent glomerular damage in the rat. Dissociation between glomerular injury and both glomerular hypertension and hypertrophy. Male gender as a primary risk factor. J Clinical Investigation 1994; 94: 1823–1829.
15. Neuringer JR, Brenner BM. Haemodynamic theory of progressive renal disease: a 10 year update in brief review. Am J Kidney Dis 1993; 22: 98–104.
16. Darmady EM, Offer J, Woodhouse MA. The parameters of the aging kidney. J Pathol 1973; 109: 195–207.
17. Davidson AJ, Talner LB, Downs WM. A study of the angiographic appearance of the kidney in an aging normotensive population. Radiology 1969; 92: 975–983.
18. Takazakura E, Sawabu N, Handa A, Takasa A, Shinoda A, Takeuchi J. Intrarenal vascular changes with age and disease. Kidney Int 1972; 2: 224–230.

19. Ljungqvist A, Lagerggen C. Normal intrarenal arterial pattern in adult and aging human kidney. J Anat 1962; 96: 285.
20. Hollenberg NK, Adams DF, Solomon HS, Rashid A, Abrams HL, Merrill JP. Senescence and the renal vasculature in normal man. Circulation Research 1974; 34: 309–316.
21. Abrass CK, Adcox MJ, Raugi GJ. Aging-associated changes in renal extracellular matrix. Am J Pathol 1995; 146: 742–752.
22. Cohen MR, Kin L. Age-related changes in sulfation of basement membrane glycosaminoglycans. Exp Gerontol 1983; 1983: 461–469.
23. Rowe JW, Andres A, Tobin JD, Norris AH, Shock NW. The effect of age on creatinine clearance in men: a cross-sectional and longitudinal study. J Gerontol 1976; 32: 155–163.
24. Cockcroft DW, Gault MH. Prediction of creatinine clearance from serum creatinine. Nephron 1976; 16: 31–41.
25. Rolin HA, Hall PM, Wei R. Inaccuracy of estimated creatinine clearance for prediction of iothalamate glomerular filtration rate. Am J Kidney Dis 1984; 4: 48–54.
26. Reichley RM, Ritchie DJ, Bailey TC. Analysis of various creatinine clearance formulas in predicting gentamicin elimination in patients with low serum creatinine. Pharmacotherapy 1995; 15: 625–630.
27. Bloor GK, Welsh KR, Goodall S, Shah MV. Comparison of predicted with measured creatinine clearance in cardiac surgical patients. J Cardiothoracic & Vascular Anesthesia 1996; 10: 899–902.
28. Malmrose LC, Gray SL, Pieper CF, et al. Measured versus estimated creatinine clearance in a highly functioning elderly sample: MacArtur Foundation study of a successful aging. J Am Geriatr Soc 1993; 41: 715–721.
29. Lew SQ, Bosch JP. Effect of diet on creatinine clearance and excretion in young and elderly healthy subjects and in patients with renal disease. J Am Soc Nephrol 1991; 2: 856–865.
30. Fliser D, Zeler M, Nowack R, Ritz E. Renal functional reserve in healthy elderly subjects. J Am Soc Nephrol 1993; 3: 1371–1377.
31. Faubert PF, Porush JG. Disorders of water, sodium, and divalent-ion metabolism. In: Jacobson HR, Striker GE, Klahr S, editors. The Principles and Practices of Nephrology. St. Louis: Mosby, 1995; 515–518.
32. Miller M. Fluid and electrolyte balance in the elderly. Geriatrics 1971; 42: 65–68.
33. Faull CM, Holmes C, Baylis PH. Water balance in elderly people: is there a deficiency of vasopressin? Age & Ageing 1993; 22: 114–120.
34. Epstein M, Hollenberg NK. Age as a determinant of renal sodium conservation in normal man. J Lab & Clinical Medicine 1976; 87: 411–417.
35. Os I, Kjeldsen SE, Westheim A, et al. Aging and urinary vasopressin excretion in healthy men. Scand J Urology & Nephrology 1987; 21: 235–239.
36. Tryding N, Berg B, Ekman S, Nilsson JE, Sterner G, Harris A. DDAVP test for renal concentration capacity. Age-related reference intervals. Scand J Urology & Nephrology 1988; 22: 141–145.
37. Helderman JH, Vestal RE, Rowe JW, Tobin JD, Andres R, Robertson GL. The response of arginine vasopressin to intravenous ethanol and hypertonic saline in man: the impact of aging. J Gerontol 1978; 33: 39–47.
38. Kirkland JL, Lye M, Levy DW, Banerjee AK. Patterns of urine flow and electrolyte excretion in healthy elderly people. BMJ (Clin Research Ed) 1983; 3: 1665–1667.
39. Cox JR, Shalaby WA. Potassium changes with age. Gerontology 1981; 27: 340–344.
40. Benegle HH, Perkins JH, McNamara ER, Alexander EA. Impaired renal and extrarenal potassium adaptation in old rats. Kidney Int 1983; 23: 684–690.
41. Ledingham JG, Crowe MJ, Forsling ML, Phillips PA, Rolls BJ. Effects of aging on vasopressin secretion, water excretion, and thirst in man. Kidney Int (Suppl) 1987; 21: S90–S92.
42. Davis PJ, Davis FB. Water excretion in the elderly. Endocrinology & Metabolism Clinics of North America 1987; 16: 867–875.

43. Crowe MJ, Forsling ML, Rolls BJ, Phillips PA, Ledingham JG, Smith RF. Altered water excretion in healthy elderly men. Age & Ageing 1987; 16: 285–293.
44. Greenfeld Z, Engels K, Samsell I, Baylis C. The role of endothelin in the age dependent increase in renal vascular resistance in the rat kidney. Mech Ageing Dev 1998; 101: 145–152.
45. Baylis C, Schmidt R. The aging glomerulus. Seminars in Nephrology 1996; 16: 265–276.
46. Baylis C, Engels K, Beierwaltes WH. Beta-adrenoreceptor-stimulated renin release is blunted in old rats. J Am Soc Nephrol 1998; 9: 1318–1320.
47. Zoja C, Remuzzi A, Corna D, Perico N, Bertani T, Remuzzi G. Renal protective effect of angiotensin-converting enzyme inhibition in aging rats. Am J Med 1992; 92: 60S–63S.
48. Zhang XZ, Qiu C, Baylis C. Sensitivity of the segmental renal arterioles to angiotensin II in the aging rat. Mechanisms of Ageing & Development 1997; 97: 183–192.
49. Crane MG, Harris JJ. Effect of aging on renin activity and aldosterone excretion. J Lab Clin Med 1976; 87: 947–959.
50. Weidmann P, De Myttenaere-Bursztein S, Maxwell MH, de Lima J. Effect on aging on plasma renin and aldosterone in normal man. Kidney Int 1975; 8: 325–333.
51. Baylis C, Engels K, Hymel A, Navar LG. Plasma renin activity and metabolic clearance rate of angiotensin II in the unstressed aging rat. Mechanisms of Ageing & Development 1997; 97: 163–172.
52. Viig J, Wei JY. Understanding the biology of aging: the key to prevention and therapy. J Am Geriatr Soc 1995; 43: 426–434.
53. Brenner BM, Meyer TW, Hostetter TH. Dietary protein intake and the progressive nature of kidney disease: the role of hemodynamically mediated glomerular injury in the pathogenesis of progressive glomerular sclerosis in aging, renal ablation, and intrinsic renal disease. New Eng J Med 1982; 307: 652–659.
54. Reckelhoff JF, Samsell L, Dey R, Racusen L, Baylis C. The effect of aging on glomerular hemodynamics in the rat. Am J Kidney Dis 1992; 20: 70–75.
55. Hostetter TH, Olson JL, Rennke HG, Venkatachalam MA, Brenner BM. Hyperfiltration in remnant nephrons: a potentially adverse response to renal ablation. Am J Physiol 1981; 241: F85–F93.
56. Brenner BM. Nephron adaptation to renal injury or ablation. Am J Physiol 1985; 249: F324–F337.
57. Wardle EN. Cellular biology of glomerulosclerosis. Nephron 1992; 61: 125–128.
58. Blum M, Averbuch M, Wolman Y, Aviram A. Protein intake and kidney function in humans: its effect on 'normal aging'. Arch Intern Med 1989; 149: 211–212.
59. Iwasaki K, Gleiser CA, Masoro EJ, McMahan CA, Seo EJ, Yu BP. The influence of dietary protein source on longevity and age-related disease processes of Fischer rats. J Gerontol 1988; 43: B5–12.
60. Iwasaki K, Gleiser CA, Masoro EJ, McMahan CA, Seo EJ, Yu BP. Influence of the restriction of individual dietary components on longevity and age-related disease of Fischer rats: the fat component and the mineral component. J Gerontol 1988; 43: B13–B21.
61. Tucker SM, Mason RL, Beauchene RE. Influence of diet and feed restriction on kidney function of aging male rats. J Gerontol 1976; 31: 264–270.
62. Zucchelli P, Zuccala A, Borghi M, Fusaroli M, Sanna G, Gaggi R. Long-term comparison between captopril and nifedipine in the progression of renal insufficiency. Kidney Int 1992; 42: 452–458.
63. Brenner BM, Mackenzie H. Nephron mass as a risk factor for progression of renal disease. Kidney Int 1997; 63: S124–S127.
64. Weinstein T, Zevin D, Gafter U, Ben-Bassat M, Levi J. Proteinuria and chronic renal failure associated with unilateral renal agenesis. Isr J Med Sci 1985; 21: 919–921.
65. Holdaas H, Hartmann A, Fauchald P, et al. Twenty-three years follow-up of living donors. J Am Soc Nephrol 1997; 8: 685A.

Aging: Its Influence on Drug Disposition and Effect

DARRELL R. ABERNETHY
Division of Clinical Pharmacology, Georgetown University School of Medicine, Washington, DC, U.S.A.

Frequently older patients suffer from multiple concurrent illnesses, which are best treated with different medications. The accepted standard of care is therapy targeted to specific illness for which there is a clear likelihood of patient benefit. However, as has been clear for some time, the incidence of adverse drug reactions is substantially increased in older patients. Epidemiological and surveillance data indicate a clear relationship between the frequency of occurrence of adverse drug reaction and number of medications to which the patient is exposed concurrently. Thus the 'therapeutic burden' is likely to co-vary with the 'disease burden.' In aged patients, clinical presentation of the adverse drug reaction is marked by non-specific signs and symptoms, in particular central nervous system symptoms of impaired cognition and confusional states. In addition, a final common pathway for adverse drug affect in the aged is postural hypotension. In some cases the increased incidence of adverse drug reactions is due to increased drug exposure (pharmacokinetic), in others it is due to altered drug effect at a fixed drug exposure (pharmacodynamic), and more commonly it is a combination of the two. Consistent age-related pathophysiologic changes such as decreased renal glomerular filtration with decreased drug renal clearance and modest decreases in hepatic drug oxidation result in increased drug exposure. The oxidative pathways best studied are the cytochrome P450 (CYP) 3A isoenzymes. The most clearly defined pharmacodynamic changes are β-adrenoceptor dysfunction, baroreflex dysfunction, and impaired vascular endothelial function. The combination of increased risk from multiple drug therapies and a pathophysiologic basis that explains the source of increased risk in some cases and the need to limit both dose and number of drugs administered.

Therapeutic Burden

Although one might expect older and frail individuals to be more susceptible to adverse drug reactions, from a given time exposure, however that is not the case. Instead when the analysis includes a number of concurrent

Oreopoulos et al. (eds.), Nephrology and Geriatrics Integrated, 37–43.

medications, irrespective of indication, age no longer contributes significantly to risk of adverse drug reaction [1–5] (Fig. 1). In all of these studies, which include inpatient, outpatient, and recently discharged outpatients, those concurrently receiving five or more drugs have an exponential increase in likelihood of adverse drug reaction, irrespective of the therapeutic classes of the prescribed drugs. In addition to the number of drugs prescribed, compliance to therapy is a component of therapeutic burden. Erratic compliance may subject the patient to variable drug effects, which are magnified in the presence of concurrent therapies. Compliance to therapy is also a function of the number of drugs prescribed; again the expectation that older patients are less compliant with the doctor's instructions concerning drug therapy than younger patients is not supported when data are controlled for number of medications prescribed [6, 7]. Instead, the older patient may be less compliant to the therapy simply because they are prescribed larger numbers of concurrent medications. Finally, drug-drug interactions (when the patient has been prescribed multiple drugs) make a contribution to the therapeutic burden that has not been studied completely. Available data suggest that interactions and clinical adverse drug reactions are most common with cardiovascular and psychotropic drugs [8–12] (Table 1). Such drug reactions most commonly are non-specific, central-nervous-system impairment, hypotension, and renal failure associated with volume depletion (Table 2).

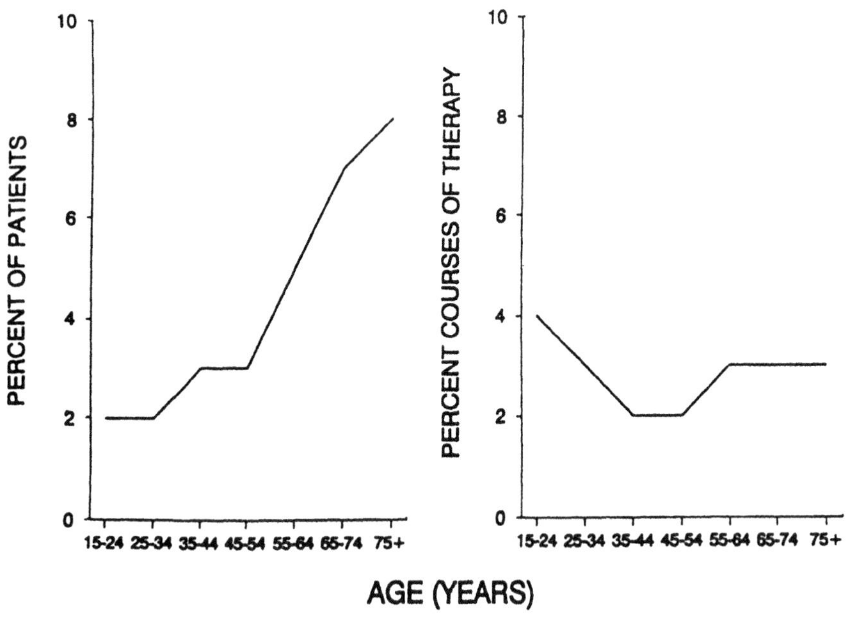

Figure 1. The relationship of increasing age and likelihood of adverse drug reactions (left) and the relationship of increasing age and adverse drug reaction when corrected for number of drugs per patient (right). Adapted from [5].

Table 1. Prevalence of main classes of drugs, drug-drug interactions (DDI) and side effects among 894 older patients (mean age 83 years) prescribed two or more drugs

	Percent Patients Prescribed Drug	Percent Patients with Potential DDI	Percent Patients with DDI Side Effects
Cardiovascular drugs			
Diuretics	50.6	43.8	7.0
Nitrates	36.4	18.5	1.9
Ca antagonists	34.0	15.9	1.9
Angiotesin converting enzymes inhibitors	27.5	19.0	3.9
cardiac glycoside	18.8	11.3	1.0
Psychotropic drugs			
Benzodiazepines	43.8	21.0	6.8
Neuroleptics	25.4	16.6	3.7
Antidepressants	20.5	11.4	2.9

Adapted from [12].

Table 2. ADR associated with DDI in older patients

Clinical Presentation	Percent of Total
CNS depression/cognitive impairment	44.1
Hypotension	21.8
Acute renal failure associated with volume depletion	15.7
Hypo/hyperkalemia	5.6
Heart arrhythmia	4.5
Anticholinergic toxicity	3.3
Other	5.0

Pathophysiologic Changes of Aging that Relate to Altered Drug Response

Pharmacokinetic

Decreased renal function is the most predictable age-related change that relates to increase in drug exposure due to reduced clearance of drugs that are eliminated in a pharmacologically active form [13, 14]. If one selects drugs with a narrow therapeutic index, the dose should be adjusted downward based on calculated creatinine clearance (Table 3) [15]: In patients with stable renal function the Cockcroft-Gault equation is a widely accepted approach [16].

$$\text{Creatinine clearance} = \frac{(140 - \text{age}) \times \text{weight (kg)}}{72 \times \text{serum creatinine (mg/dl)}} \times 0.85 \text{ for females}$$

In drugs that undergo oxidative (phase I) biotransformation via CYP3A iso-

Table 3. Examples of narrow therapeutic index drugs which undergo renal clearance

aminoglycosides	vancomycin
Digoxin	Lithium

enzymes, their clearance is moderately decreased in aged individuals because of a decreased activity of those enzymes [17]. Drugs that are predominantly cleared by CYP3A oxidation include triazolam and midazolam; in older individuals both have markedly decreased oral and intravenous clearance because of substantially increased drug exposure at a given dose [18, 19]. Other benzodiazepines, such as diazepam and flurazepam, which undergo CYP-mediated oxidation via several isoenzymes, also show decreased clearance in older individuals [20, 21]. The pharmacodynamic consequences of the increased exposure is excessive benzodiazepine-mediated sedation, particularly for long-acting agents in this class. The clinical consequences are increased sedation and risk of hip fracture [21–23]. Other pathways of metabolic biotransformation, such as glucuronidation, sulfation, and acetylation do not change significantly with advancing age.

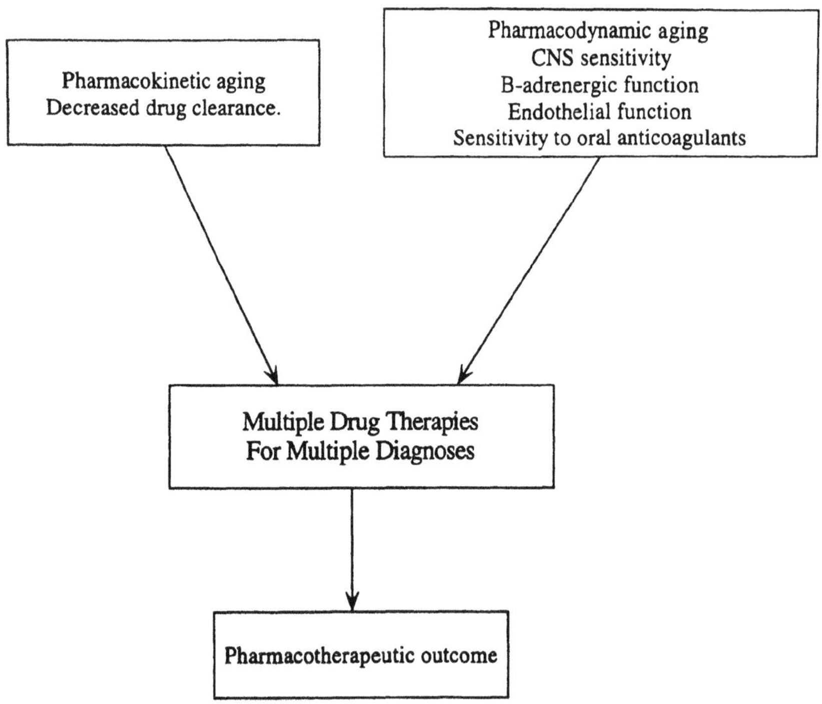

Figure 2. The convergence of pharmacokinetic changes, pharmacodynamic changes, and multiple therapies may lead to adverse as well as beneficial outcome in the aged patients.

Pharmacodynamic

Central nervous system depression with exposure to sedative hypnotics, anxiolytics, and anticholinergics is more severe in older individuals than in younger, even when the doses and length of drug exposure are corrected for the pharmacokinetic changes noted above [24–26]. Mechanisms for these observations are not well understood; the clinical observations are consistent, however.

Oral anticoagulant effect also is increased in the elderly, even when the dose and drug concentrations are adjusted [18, 27]. When one makes the appropriate dose adjustment, there is no longer evidence of increased adverse drug reaction, suggesting that, at least in the case of oral anticoagulant therapy, when the narrow therapeutic index of the drug is well understood, complications from that therapy can be averted [19, 28].

Cardiovascular changes of aging that result in altered drug response are perhaps the most extensively characterized; β-adrenoceptor function, both β_1-cardiac and β_2-vascular, is impaired in aged healthy individuals [30, 31]. The mechanism(s) for this finding is (are) not conclusively established; however, impaired adenylyl-cyclase function and impaired cAMP-dependent protein kinase activity contribute to the dysfunction [32–34]. Alpha-adrenergic function is maintained with aging [31]. This combination may result in particularly marked hypotensive response from alpha-adrenergic blockade and alpha-beta blockade [35]. Because of the widespread treatment of benign prostatic hypertrophy by α_1-adrenergic blockade, we must emphasize the clinical evaluation for orthostatic hypotension when considering patients for this therapy.

Impaired endothelial function has recently been demonstrated in elderly subjects who are normotensive, normocholesterolemic, and nonsmoking [36, 37]. This has been documented in both the coronary and the systemic circulation [38]. This loss of vasodilating response to acetylcholine may be due to decreased endothelial elaboration of nitric oxide or increased breakdown of nitric oxide; however, the elderly still maintain their vascular-smooth-muscle relaxation to exogenous nitric oxide (administered as sodium nitroprusside) [36]. In addition, as women approach menopause, they develop impaired endothelium-mediated vasorelaxation, which is reversed by estrogen replacement [39, 40]. Current research aims to determine how this impairment in endothelial function may alter drug response in aged patients.

Summary and Conclusion

We do not completely understand the relationship between pathophysiological changes of aging and altered drug responses. The examples presented here demonstrate that we can optimize pharmacotherapy in aged patients through an increased understanding of these relationships.

References

1. Hutchinson TA, Flegel KM, Kramer MS, Leduc DG, Kong HH. Frequency, severity, and risk factors for adverse drug reactions in adult outpatients: a prospective study. J Chronic Disease 1986; 39: 533–542.
2. Williamson J, Chopin JM. Adverse reactions to prescribed drugs in the elderly: a multicentre investigation. Age Ageing 1980; 9: 73–80.
3. Kellaway GS, McCrae E. Intensive monitoring for adverse drug effects in patients discharged from acute medical wards. New Zealand Med J 1973; 78: 525–528.
4. Smith JW, Seidl LG, Cluff LE. Studies on the epidemiology of adverse drug reactions V. Clinical factors influencing susceptibility. Ann Int Med 1966; 65: 629–640.
5. Gurwitz JH, Avorn J. The ambiguous relation between aging and adverse drug reactions. Ann Int Med 1991; 114: 956–966.
6. Darnell JC, Murray MD, Martz BL, Weinberger M. Medication use by ambulatory elderly. An in-home survey. J Am Geriatr Soc 1986; 34: 1–4.
7. Spagnoli A, Ostino G, Borga AD, et al. Drug compliance and unreported drugs in the elderly. J Am Geriatr Soc 1989; 37: 619–624.
8. Mitchell GW, Stanaszek WF, Nichols NB. Documenting drug-drug interactions in ambulatory patients. Am J Hosp Pharm 1979; 36: 653–657.
9. Armstrong WA, Driever CW, Hays RL. Analysis of drug-drug interactions in a geriatric population. Am J Hosp Pharm 1980; 37: 385–387.
10. Cadieux RJ. Drug interactions in the elderly. How multiple drug use increases risk exponentially. Post-grad Med 1989; 86: 179–186.
11. Costa AJ. Potential drug interactions in an ambulatory geriatric population. Fam Pract 1991; 8: 234–236.
12. Doucet J, Chassagne P, Trivalle C, Landrin I, Pauty MD, Kadri N, Menard JF, Bercott E. Drug-drug interactions related to hospital admissions in older adults: a prospective study of 1000 patients. J Am Geriatr Soc 1996; 44: 944–948.
13. Davies DF, Shock NW. Age changes in glomerular filtration rate, effective renal plasma flow, and tubular excretory capacity in adult males. J Clin Invest 1950; 29: 496–507.
14. Lindeman RD, Tobin J, Shock NW. Longitudinal studies on the rate of decline in renal function with age. J Am Geriatr Soc 1985; 33: 278–285.
15. Cusack B, Kelly J, O'Malley K, Noel J, Lavan J, Horgan J. Digoxin in the elderly: pharmacokinetic consequences of old age. Clin Pharmacol Ther 1979; 25: 772–776.
16. Cockcroft DW, Gault MH. Prediction of creatinine clearance from serum creatinine. Nephron 1976; 16: 31–41.
17. George J, Byth K, Farrell GC. Age but not gender selectively affects expression of individual cytochrome P-450 proteins in human liver. Biochem Pharmacol 1995; 50: 727–730.
18. Greenblatt DJ, Divoll M, Abernethy DR, Moschitto LJ, Smith RB, Shader RI. Reduced clearance of triazolam in old age: relation to antipyrine oxidizing capacity. Brit J Clin Pharmacol 1983; 15: 303–309.
19. Greenblatt DJ, Abernethy DR, Locniskar A, Harmatz JS, Limjuco RA, Shader RI. Effect of age, gender, and obesity on midazolam kinetics. Anesthesiology 1984; 61: 27–35.
20. Greenblatt DJ, Shader RI, Abernethy DR. Drug therapy: current status of benzodiazepines. N Engl J Med 1983; 309: 354–358, 410–416.
21. Greenblatt DJ, Allen MD, Shader RI. Toxicity of high-dose flurazepam in the elderly. Clin Pharmacol Ther 1977; 21: 355–361.
22. Ray WA, Griffin MR, Schaffaer W, Baugh DK, Melton LJ. Psychotropic drug use and the risk of hip fracture. N Engl J Med 1987; 316: 363–369.
23. Ray WA, Griffin MR, Downey W. Benzodiazepines of long and short elimination half-life and the risk of hip fracture. J Am Med Assoc 1989; 262: 3303–3307.
24. Reidenberg MM, Levy M, Warner H, et al. Relationship between diazepam dose, plasma level, age, and central nervous system depression. Clin Pharmacol Ther 1978; 23: 371–374.

25. Smith JM, Baldessarini RJ. Changes in prevalence, severity, and recovery in tardive dyskinesia with age. Arch Gen Psychiatry 1980; 37: 1368–1373.
26. Moleman P, Janzen G, von Bargen BA, Kappers EJ, Pepplinkhuizen L, Schmitz PIM. Relationship between age and incidence of parkinsonism in psychiatric patients treated with haloperidol. Am J Psychiatry 1986; 143: 232–234.
27. Shepherd AM, Hewick DS, Moreland TA, et al. Age as a determinant of sensitivity to warfarin. Br J Clin Pharmacol 1977; 4: 315–320.
28. Gurwitz JH, Goldberg RJ, Holden A, Knapic N, Ansell J. Age-related risks of long-term oral anticoagulant therapy. Arch Int Med 1988; 148: 1733–1736.
29. Petitti DB, Strom BL, Melmon KL. Duration of warfarin anticoagulant therapy and the probabilities of recurrent thromboembolism and hemorrhage. Am J Med 1986; 81: 255–259.
30. Vestal RE, Wood AJJ, Shand DG. Reduced beta-adrenoceptor sensitivity in the elderly. Clin Pharmacol Ther 1979; 26: 181–186.
31. Pan HYM, Hoffman BB, Porshe RA, Blaschke TF. Decline in beta-adrenergic receptor-mediated vascular relaxation with aging in man. J Pharmacol Exp Ther 1986; 239: 802–807.
32. Scarpace PJ. Decreased -adrenergic responsiveness during senescense. Fed Proc 1986; 45: 51–54.
33. Montamat SC, Davies AO. Physiological response to isoproterenol and coupling of beta-adrenergic receptors in young and elderly human subjects. J Gerontol 1989; 44: M100–M105.
34. White M, Roden R, Minobe W, Khan MF, Larrabee P, Wollmering M, Port JD, Anderson F, Campbell D, Feldman AM, Bristow MR. Age-related changes in β-adrenergic neuroeffector systems in the human heart. Circulation 1994; 90: 1225–1238.
35. Abernethy DR, Schwartz JB, Plachetka JR, Todd EL, Egan JM. Comparison in young and elderly patients of pharmacodynamics and disposition of labetalol in systemic hypertension. Am J Cardiol 1987; 60: 697–702.
36. Taddei S, Virdis A, Mattei P, Ghiadoni L, Gennari A, Fasolo CB, Sudano I, Salvetti A. Aging and endothelial function in normotensive subjects and patients with essential hypertension. Circulation 1995; 91: 1981–1987.
37. Jones D, Andrawis NS, Abernethy DR. Aging is associated with altered vascular reactivity to angiotensin II (AII) and acetylcholine (ACH). (abstract) Clin Pharmacol Ther 1998; 63: 174.
38. Zeiher AM, Drexter H, Saurbier B, Just H. Endothelium-mediated coronary blood flow modulation in humans: effects of age, atherosclerosis, hypercholesterolemia, and hypertension. J Clin Invest 1993; 92: 652–662.
39. Herrington DM, Braden GA, Williams JK, Morgan TM. Endothelium-dependent coronary vasomotor responsiveness in post-menopausal women with and without estrogen replacement therapy. Am J Cardiol 1994; 73: 951–952.
40. Reis SE, Gloth ST, Blumenthal RS, Resar JR, Zacur HA, Gerstenblith G, Brinker JA. Estradiol acutely attenuates coronary vasomotor responses to acetylcholine in postmenopausal women. Circulation 1994; 89: 52–60.

Drug-Related Renal Dysfunction in the Elderly

WILLIAM M. BENNETT
Division of Nephrology, Hypertension and Clinical Pharmacology, Oregon Health Sciences University, Portland, Oregon, U.S.A.

The kidney is particularly vulnerable to various nephrotoxic drugs and chemicals because of its high blood flow relative to its mass [1]. It is estimated that the kidneys receive 20 to 25% of the cardiac output per minute, and this results in an increased delivery of drugs and chemicals to the renal parenchyma. Because of the countercurrent concentrating system the renal cells are exposed to local drug concentrations far in excess of those achieved in blood. Thus, compounds that are not injurious at blood concentrations may cause renal damage because of urinary concentration. Many do not appreciate that the kidney also has the capacity for drug metabolism, and thus the kidneys can metabolize drugs and chemicals to toxic or reactive metabolites. Furthermore, the kidney has a large endothelial surface area relative to its weight and also has various mechanisms for releasing drugs from their binding plasma proteins. Finally, renal function declines with age; thus the various co-morbidities that affect elderly patients with multiple drug administration may magnify the potential for adverse drug interactions.

In 2000 the clinically relevant nephrotoxins include antimicrobial agents such as aminoglycoside antibiotics, amphotericin B, antiviral drugs (protease inhibitors, and intravenous acyclovir), pentamidine, and foscarnet. Particularly important in the elderly are the renal effects of non-steroidal anti-inflammatory drugs and other analgesics. In patients with predisposing co-morbid conditions, angiotensin-converting-enzyme inhibitors and angiotensin receptor blockers may produce hemodynamically relevant renal dysfunction. Drugs used to treat neoplasms in the elderly, such as cisplatinum, methotrexate, mitomycin C, nitrosoureas, and biologicals such as interleukin 2, can produce renal dysfunction. Some immunosuppressive drugs, e.g. cyclosporine and tacrolimus, produce renal dysfunction as their major toxic side effect. Finally, miscellaneous compounds such as radiographic contrast media, lithium, gold, penicillamine, and numerous other compounds can produce renal dysfunction for individual patients.

Oreopoulos et al. (eds.), Nephrology and Geriatrics Integrated, 45–50.

Clinical Presentation of Nephrotoxicity

Most of the clinical syndromes in nephrology can be reproduced by drugs and chemicals by a variety of pathophysiologic mechanisms. Some individual toxins may produce more than one clinical picture depending on the dose, host factors, and the duration of therapy. Usually, we think of drug nephrotoxicity as acute renal dysfunction, generally defined by a rise in serum creatinine of 0.5 mg/dl in a patient with previously normal renal function or a rise of 1 mg/dl in a patient with some pre-existing renal disease.

Acute renal dysfunction secondary to nephrotoxic drugs can be a direct result of drug-induced renal injury. The prototypical classes of drugs causing this type of renal dysfunction are the aminoglycoside antibiotics and the chemotherapeutic agent, cisplatinum.

Other drugs compromise renal function by causing decrements in renal blood flow, particularly in individuals predisposed by co-morbid conditions. Drugs in this category include non-steroidal anti-inflammatory drugs, angiotensin-converting-enzyme inhibitors, and immunosuppressive drugs such as cyclosporine and tacrolimus.

Acute renal dysfunction also can be caused by obstructive uropathy and acute interstitial nephritis. Often the latter is due to hypersensitivity, idiosyncratic reaction to agents such as sulfonamides, penicillins, and miscellaneous other compounds. Since these phenomena are idiosyncratic rather than dose-related, the mechanisms involving their occurrence, which usually is uncommon, is unclear. Non-oliguric acute renal failure with recovery upon withdrawal of the offending drug is typical for these agents.

Drugs and chemicals may also produce chronic renal insufficiency, even if the attending physician does not detect acute renal dysfunction. In the past few years, attention has been drawn once again to the preventable syndrome of analgesic-associated nephropathy. Elseviers and colleagues have developed objective criteria for making this diagnosis [2]. A variable percentage of those now undergoing treatment for end stage renal disease with dialysis or transplantation have analgesic abuse as their major lesion. The epidemiologic studies have made it clear that the renal disease is due to the abuse of combined complex analgesics rather than a single ingredient preparation [3]. Since these compounds are available over the counter, often it is not possible to quantify the intake of an individual patient. Abundant prescription and non-prescription combination analgesics are available in the United States that contain, in addition to acetaminophen and/or salicylate, various combinations of caffeine, barbiturates or other opioid analgesics. At the present time, it is unclear whether chronic non-steroidal anti-inflammatory drug use alone will lead to chronic renal failure, but some data suggest that this is possible.

Specific Drug Issues and Toxins for Elderly Patients

NSAIDs

A variety of renal syndromes are associated with non-steroidal anti-inflammatory drugs [4]. They include acute renal dysfunction, which usually is functional and reversible and is most commonly seen in patients with defined risk factors. More rarely, one may see, as an idiosyncratic or immunologic reaction, interstitial nephritis with variable proteinuria. This occurs in very few patients relative to the large number of doses of these drugs taken with and without prescription. Non-steroidal anti-inflammatory drugs can also produce renal papillary necrosis, hyporeninemic hypoaldosteronism with hyperkalemia, worsening hypertension, and renal sodium retention with edema [5]. The pathogenesis of this functional acute renal failure probably reflects blockade of normal physiologic prostaglandin responses to renal stimuli in predisposed patients. An example of this pathophysiology is shown in Fig. 1.

Analgesic-associated nephropathy has a worldwide incidence of 2–20% for new cases of end-stage renal disease. In the United States, probably less than five percent of all patients have this as an etiology, most prominently in the southeastern portion of the United States. Cases seem to be clustered where the analgesic products are manufactured. The general threshold requirement is 3–5 kg of cumulative combination analgesic products. The characteristic renal lesion is papillary necrosis, which may be hard to recognize radiographically, especially if the papilla stays *in situ*. Clinical features are non-specific, but the new CT scan radiology criteria, defined by DeBroe and colleagues [2, 3], require evidence of irregular kidney outlines, small

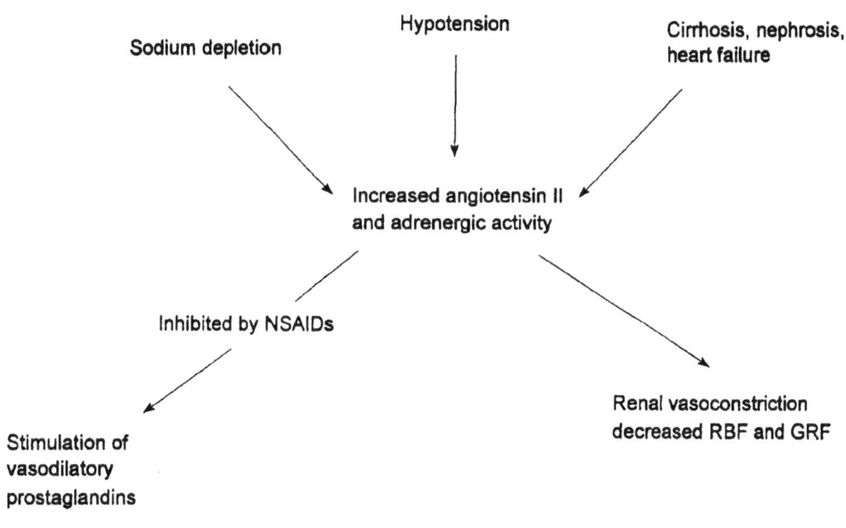

Figure 1. Pathophysiology of acute renal dysfunction with NSAIDs.

kidneys, and corticomedullary calcifications. These radiologic signs are relatively sensitive and specific in making this diagnosis.

Reasonable steps in prevention includes limitation of combination analgesic compounds to prescription medication only, and widespread education concerning the potential nephropathy associated with the excessive use of combination analgesic products. Obviously it is much easier to prevent renal disease than to treat it when it occurs.

Angiotensin-Converting-Enzyme Inhibitors/Angiotensin Blockers

These enzyme inhibitors can cause acute renal dysfunction in predisposed patients such as those with bilateral renal-artery stenosis in the course of generalized atherosclerotic vascular disease, renal-artery stenosis in a solitary functional kidney, renal transplant, and severe congestive heart failure in which the glomerular filtration rate depends upon angiotensin II mediated efferent arteriolar vasoconstriction. Under these circumstances blockade of the renin angiotensin system by angiotensin converting enzyme inhibitors or angiotensin II receptor blockers can reduce the efferent arteriolar tone and decrease the GFR. Usually this is reversible, although if the pressure drops dramatically, this may precipitate renal artery thrombosis.

These important drugs are used to treat hypertension and heart failure in elderly patients. Certain patients, whose renal perfusion and glomerular filtration depend on an activated angiotensin II system, may suffer acute reductions in glomerular filtration rate if the renin angiotensin suffers significant pharmacologic blockade. In patients with critical stenoses of upstream renal arteries, this can lead to renal vascular thrombosis. It is a good practice to check a chemistry panel seven to 14 days after institution of ACE inhibitor or angiotensin II receptor blockade therapy.

Aminogycloside Antibiotics

These antibiotics produce acute renal dysfunction in approximately 10 to 15% of therapeutic courses. These drugs are cationic and have molecular weights of approximately 500. They are totally excreted by the kidney and have no metabolites. The clearance of aminoglycosides is virtually identical with the inulin clearance. Despite this, a small proportion of drug is filtered and becomes bound to anionic phospholipid receptors in the lumenal membrane of the proximal tubule. The drug receptor complex then is internalized into the cell. There gentamicin interferes with the endocytosis recycling pathways of the cell. The drugs themselves inhibit phospholipases, producing an accumulation of phospholipids in the lysosomes [6, 7]. The clinical features of aminoglycoside nephrotoxicity include non-oliguric acute renal failure with an early vasopressin-resistant concentrating deficit. Humans show a patchy proximal tubular necrosis on light microscopy and characteristic myeloid bodies or myelin figures are visible under electronmicroscopy in renal tissue and urine. As a rule the GFR recovers if the drug is discontinued promptly; these patients rarely need dialysis. In diseases such as cystic fibrosis repeated courses of aminoglycosides can induce chronic tubulointerstitial renal disease. Blood level monitoring is controversial, although adequate peak concentration is necessary for bacteriocidal effects, and thus the peak level is used to assess antibacterial efficacy. Aminoglycosides kill bacteria by concentration-dependent killing, and thus, the height of the peak of the serum level is an important determinant of drug efficacy [8, 9]. Trough serum concentrations rise as a result of the decreased GFR and gentamicin trough levels are actually better filtration monitors than the serum creatinine. The many risk factors for aminoglycoside nephrotoxicity include extracellular fluid volume depletion, potassium depletion, calcium/magnesium deficiency, increased dose frequency, and probably preexisting renal dysfunction.

Immunosuppressive Drugs

Increasingly agents such as cyclosporine and tacrolimus are used to treat older renal transplant patients and other solid-organ transplant recipients. In addition, these drugs are effective in low doses for the management of autoimmune diseases such as psoriasis, inflammatory bowel disease, and rheumatoid arthritis. The major toxic effect of cyclosporine and tacrolimus is on the kidney, particularly with the use of cyclosporine, renal vasoconstriction contributes to hypertension. These drugs, which are highly metabolized by the liver through the hepatic P450 enzyme system, have many important drug interactions with medications used by older individuals, such as amiodarone, anticonvulsants, diltiazem, verapamil, and erythromycin antibiotics.

The clinical features of cyclosporine and tacrolimus nephrotoxicity are non-specific elevations in BUN and creatinine without any abnormal urinary sediment. Patients tend to be hyperkalemic and hyperchloremic with a mild metabolic acidosis. New hypertension is common, particularly in cardiac transplant recipients. Rarely, such patients develop hemolytic uremic syndrome, either *de novo* or as a recurrence of an original diagnosis. The differential diagnosis between nephrotoxicity and transplant rejection is usually made retrospectively when decreasing the dosage results in an increased GFR. Blood level monitoring is useful because levels correlate in general with toxicity or the risk of rejection. However, trough blood level monitoring involves such overlap that a solitary level in the individual patient should be used only as part of the overall database for making the distinction between rejection and toxicity, not as a target level and of itself. Renal biopsy in acute cyclosporine nephrotoxicity is usually relatively normal.

Chronic immunosuppression with cyclosporine or tacrolimus often produces fibrosis, tubular atrophy, and glomerular sclerosis without any changes in the incidence of vascular rejection [10]. Some patients, including approximately 8–10% of cardiac transplant patients who survive more than 5 years, progress to end-stage renal disease. It is important to recognize that a patient may have abnormal renal morphology even when his/her serum creatinine is normal, particularly in those patients with autoimmune disease.

Conclusion

This short paper emphasizes problems of renal dysfunction, both acute and chronic in elderly patients receiving medications and who are prone to multiple drug interactions. By understanding the mechanisms of these toxic injuries, we may gain insights unto renal disease of other etiologies.

References

1. Bennett WM, Finn WF. Drug and chemical-induced nephropathy. In: Stein J, editor. Internal Medicine. St. Louis: Mosby, 1998; 866–871.
2. Elseviers MM, De Schepper A, Corthouts R, Bosmans JL, Cosyn L, Lins RL, et al. High diagnostic performance of CT scan for analgesic nephropathy in patients with incipient to severe renal failure. Kidney Int 1995; 48: 1316–1323.
3. Elseviers MM, De Broe ME. A long-term prospective controlled study of analgesic abuse in Belgium. Kidney Int 1995; 48: 1912–1919.
4. Bennett WM, Henrich WL, Stoff JS. The renal effects of non-steroidal anti-inflammatory drugs: Summary and recommendations. Am J Kidney Dis 1996; 28: 556–562.
5. Henrich WL, Agodoa LE, Barrett B, Bennett WM, Blantz RC, Buckalew VM, et al. Analgesics and the kidney: summary and recommendations to the Scientific Advisory Board of the National Kidney Foundation from an Ad Hoc Committee of the National Kidney Foundation. Am J Kidney Dis 1996; 27: 162–165.
6. Sundin DP, Meyer C, Dahl R, Geerdes A, Sandoval R, Molitoris BA. Cellular mechanism of aminoglycoside tolerance in long-term gentamicin treatment. Am J Physiol 1997; 272: C1309–C1318.
7. Moestrup SK, Cui S, Vorum H, Bregengard C, Bjorn SE, Norris K, et al. Evidence that epithelial glycoprotein 330/megalin mediates uptake of polybasic drugs. J Clin Invest 1995; 96: 1404–1413.
8. Nicolau DP, Freeman CD, Belliveau PP, Nightingale CH, Ross JW, Quintiliani R. Experience with a once-daily aminoglycoside program administered to 2,184 adult patients. Antimicrob Agents Chemother 1995; 39: 650–655.
9. Bennett WM. Mechanisms of aminoglycoside nephrotoxicity. Clin Exp Pharmacol Physiol 1989; 16: 1–6.
10. Bennett WM, DeMattos A, Meyer MM, Andoh T, Barry JM. Chronic cyclosporine nephropathy: The Achilles' heel of immunosuppressive therapy. Kidney Int 1996; 50: 1089–1100.

Fluid and Electrolyte Balance in the Elderly

LAURENCE H. BECK
Department of Internal Medicine, Cleveland Clinic Florida, 3000 W. Cypress Creek R.D., Ft. Lauderdale, FL 33309, U.S.A.

This article reviews physiologic and pathophysiologic changes in the metabolism of water, sodium, and potassium in elderly individuals. In each case, these changes are related to common clinical syndromes, and areas that are ripe for clinical investigation are highlighted.

Water Metabolism

Total body water decreases with age, in absolute and in relative terms, so that the proportion of body weight that is water falls from 60–65% in early middle age to about 50% by age 75, with a greater proportionate decrease in women [1]. This means that water shifts in the elderly will be reflected by a greater change in body osmolality than in younger individuals with the same absolute water loss or gain.

The aging individual is vulnerable to water deprivation because of predictable physiologic changes that render him or her susceptible to hypertonic dehydration. This is particularly true among frail elderly during the course of other disease processes.

One of the best known physiologic changes with increasing age is the decreasing ability to concentrate the urine. Despite an appropriate hypertonic stimulus, the aging kidney achieves urine osmolalities only one-half that of younger individuals, resulting in an enhanced loss of body water. The mechanism is *not* due to a defect in ADH (antidiuretic hormone) secretion, because most investigators have shown that circulating vasopressin levels are increased in elderly individuals, both in the basal and the stimulated state [2]. Despite these normal to *increased* levels of ADH, urinary osmolatity does not achieve the high levels typical of younger individuals. It is not known, in humans at least, whether the concentrating 'defect' is due to failure to establish a steep medullary concentration gradient, or whether the response of the collecting tubule cells to vasopressin is diminished, at the receptor or postreceptor level. This area would be appropriate for investigation.

Superimposed on the urinary concentrating defect, elderly individuals are

Oreopoulos et al. (eds.), Nephrology and Geriatrics Integrated, 51–55.

hampered by a diminished to absent thirst mechanism. Phillips and colleagues at Oxford [3] showed this most elegantly when they compared the responses of normal young and older men to 24 hours of fluid deprivation, measuring plasma and urine osmolality, and using a self-reported Likert scale to assess thirst. As expected, after water deprivation in the older subjects, the plasma osmolality was higher, and the urine osmolality lower. Furthermore, when given access to water after 24 hours, the younger subjects quickly drank enough to restore body-fluid osmolality, whereas the normal older subjects had not fully corrected themselves even two hours later. This raises another research question: given the *supra normal* vasopressin response, why does another hypothalamic response (thirst) deteriorate with age?

In patients with Alzheimer's type dementia, it appears that all three arms of the water conservation system are defective. Albert and colleagues [4] restricted overnight fluid intake in nine patients with Alzheimer's disease and compared their physiologic responses to nine age-matched controls. Those subjects with Alzheimer's developed more severe dehydration, and this was associated with a subnormal vasopressin response; eight of the nine had vasopressin levels that were below expected levels for their serum osmolalities. Therefore, in addition to the urinary concentrating defect and decreased thirst (confirmed in the Albert study), these demented patients apparently have defective osmotic stimulation of vasopressin release, rendering them at even greater risk of hypertonic dehydration than are non-demented elderly individuals.

Fewer studies of water load responses have been done in aging individuals. Those that exist indicate that, when compared to younger subjects, older individuals require more time to excrete a standard water load [5]. Maximal rates of free water clearance, even when adjusted for decreased GFR, are depressed in normal elderly individuals. Clark and colleagues administered water loads, before and after hydrochlorothiazide, to older and younger subjects [6]. The maximal free water clearance in the older individuals was less than 50% that achieved in younger ones. After hydrochlorothiazide, free-water clearance was abolished in the older subjects. Once again, the mechanism is unknown: is there a failure to suppress ADH adequately, or is the sluggish response due to altered tubular physiology e.g. increased vasopressin-independent 'back-leak' of water in the collecting tubules?

Altered water metabolism can have severe clinical consequences in the elderly. Hypernatremia is one of the most common electrolyte abnormalities in hospitalized elderly, particularly among older nursing-home residents requiring hospitalization, in whom the prevalence is over 30% [7]. In these individuals, there is an associated mortality of 42% [8]. Although the high mortality most likely is related to underlying disease, the hypertonic dehydration may well contribute. There has been little clinical investigation of this state specifically in elderly patients. It is not known, for example, if *hypernatremic* hypertonicity generates 'idiogenic osmols' similar to those demonstrated in hyperglycemic hypertonicity. Nor is it clear what is the proper and safe rate of correction of hypertonicity in the very old.

An interesting and useful clinical research study would be to test the effect of *doubling* the fluid intake of nursing-home patients, either by increasing the volume of their gastrostomy water boluses or by instituting a timed water-drinking schedule, comparing that intervention to 'usual care'. My hypothesis is that this maneuver would *markedly* diminish the number of hospitalizations for change of mental status due to hypertonic dehydration, and there would *not* be any undue side effects such as unintended hyponatremia.

*Hypo*natremia is an even more common electrolyte disturbance in 'healthy' elderly (about 8% prevalence) and institutionalized elderly, where it is 15–18% [9]. The multiple causes include true volume depletion with water replacement, end-organ disease (e.g. congestive heart failure) with secondary hemodynamic and vasopressin-stimulated water retention, or conditions associated with the syndrome of inappropriate antidiuretic hormone secretion (SIADH). Of those elders with SIADH, a significant proportion have no apparent underlying illness, and may represent 'idiopathic SIADH of the elderly' [10, 11].

Management of hyponatremia is similar to that in younger individuals. However, the always-controversial topic of the 'osmotic disequilibrium syndrome' (ODS) has not been specifically addressed in the elderly, and its relative risk in such aged individuals is not known. Therefore, research is needed to evaluate the proper rate of correction of hyponatremia. It is likely that vasopressin receptor antagonists soon will be clinically available and will play an important role in the management of hyponatremic states. It will be important to investigate whether pharmacologic response to these agents in the elderly is similar to that in younger individuals.

Sodium metabolism

Evidence, both clinical and experimental, show that elderly patients do not adapt to low sodium intake with a reduction in urinary sodium excretion as rapidly as their younger counterparts, thus placing them at risk for hypovolemia. Over 20 years ago, Epstein and Hollenberg showed that the half-time for reduction of urinary sodium is almost doubled in elderly subjects compared to younger [12]. More recently, the mechanism, which has been partially elucidated, appears to be due to a sluggish or blunted renin-angiotensin-aldosterone response. Weidmann and colleagues demonstrated that plasma renin and plasma aldosterone do not rise to levels characteristic of younger individuals, when both are placed on the same low sodium intake [13]. Superimposed on these changes, atrial natriuretic peptide (ANP) metabolism is altered in aging. Baseline ANP levels are higher in older individuals, and the ANP is not completely suppressed under the stimulus of hypovolemia, as it is in younger individuals. Furthermore, Heim and colleagues have shown that the renal response to a bolus of intravenous ANP is exaggerated in older individuals, measured either as plasma cyclic GMP (cGMP) or as the rate of renal sodium excretion [14]. On the other hand, when Ohashi and colleagues gave a saline load to older and younger subjects, both plasma ANP levels and plasma cGMP concentrations were higher in the elderly [2].

These several changes in the body's sodium homeostatic systems contribute to relative 'salt-wasting' in *normal* elderly, and increase the risk of hypovolemia during an intercurrent illness, particularly in the presence of another cause of salt loss, such as in diarrheal states. A research question in this area is whether the altered renal ANP response is a pharmacokinetic or a pharmacodynamic phenomenon.

Potassium Homeostasis

Hyperkalemia is another common electrolyte abnormality in elderly patients. The Boston Drug Surveillance Program has shown a clear relationship between age and the likelihood of drug-induced hyperkalemia [15]. One report from that database examined the relationship between age and assorted side effects of oral potassium supplements. Whereas the frequency of non-specific adverse side effects was the same across the ages, the probability of hyperkalemia rose progressively with increasing age, reaching 5% in those over 75.

Hyperkalemia may develop through an interaction of physiologic, pathophysiologic, and iatrogenic factors. The physiologic reasons include: decreased renal mass and renal blood flow which limits the availability of potassium at potassium secretory sites, and the sluggish renin-angiotensin-aldosterone system (described before). Recently Mulkerrin and colleagues [16] studied the *direct* aldosterone response to hyperkalemia, comparing younger and older subjects' plasma aldosterone levels after potassium infusion. The older subjects had a slower rise and a decreased maximum level of aldosterone, compared to younger subjects. No published studies have compared the *tubular response* to aldosterone in older and younger individuals.

Given the narrowed homeostatic capability for potassium excretion, it is not surprising that disease-related or drug-related stresses more easily induce dangerous hyperkalemia in older patients. This is seen commonly in clinical

Table 1. Causes of hyperkalemia in elderly

I. Decreased delivery of filtrate to potassium secretory sites
   a. Hypovolemia
   b. Congestive heart failure

II. Drug-induced hyperkalemia
   a. Potassium supplements
   b. Potassium-sparing diuretics
   c. Nonsteroidal anti-inflammatory agents (NSAID's)
   d. ACE inhibitors
   e. Beta-blocker
   f. Heparin (rare)
   g. Trimethoprim-sulfa (rare)

conditions that lead to decreased delivery of tubular urine to the distal potassium secretory sites (CHF, hypovolemia) or, more commonly, with a wide variety of drugs that interfere with individual components of the potassium homeostatic system. These are shown in Table 1. Drugs commonly implicated include potassium supplements, 'potassium-sparing' diuretics, NSAID's, ACE inhibitors, and, rarely, beta blockers. The clinician, who is aware of the underlying homeostatic constraints of the aged should appreciate the risk of age-enhanced side effects and should be prepared to avoid them.

References

1. Beck LH. Changes in renal function with aging. Clin Geriatr Med 1998; 14: 199–209.
2. Ohashi M, Fujio N, Nawata H, et al. High plasma concentrations of human atrial natriuretic peptide in aged men. J Clin Endo Metab 1987; 64: 81–85.
3. Phillips PA, Rolls BJ, Ledingham JGG, et al. Reduced thirst after water deprivation in healthy elderly men. N Engl J Med 1984; 311: 753–759.
4. Albert SG, Nakra BRS, Grossberg GT, et al. Vasopressin response to dehydration in Alzheimer's disease. J Amer Geriatr Soc 1989; 37: 843–847.
5. Meyer BR. Renal function in aging. J Amer Geriatr Soc 1989; 37: 791–800.
6. Clark BA, Shannon RP, Rosa RM, et al. Increased susceptibility to thiazide-induced hyponatremia in the elderly. J Am Soc Nephrol 1994; 5: 1106–1111.
7. Beck LH, Lavizzo-Mourey RJ. Geriatric hypernatremia. Ann Intern Med 1987; 107: 768.
8. Snyder NA, Feigal DW, Arieff AI. Hypernatremia in elderly patients. Ann Intern Med 1987; 107: 309–319.
9. Miller M. Fluid and electrolyte balance in the elderly. Geriatrics 1987; 42: 65–76.
10. Miller M, Hecker MS, Friedlander DA, et al. Apparent idiopathic hyponatremia in an ambulatory geriatric population. J Amer Geriatr Soc 1996; 44: 404–408.
11. Hirshberg B, Ben-Yehuda A. The syndrome of inappropriate antidiuretic hormone secretion in the elderly. Am J Med 1997; 103: 270–273.
12. Epstein M. Hollenberg NK. Age as a determinant of renal sodium conservation in normal man. J Lab Clin Med 1976; 87: 411–417.
13. Weidmann P, De Myttenaere-Bursztein S, Maxwell MH, et al. Effect of aging on plasma renin and aldosterone in normal man. Kidney Internat 1975; 8: 325–333.
14. Heim JM, Gottmann K, Weil J, et al. Effects of a bolus dose of atrial natriuretic factor in young and elderly volunteers. Eur J Clin Invest 1989; 19: 265–271.
15. Lawson DH. Adverse reactions to potassium chloride. Quart J Med 1974; 63: 433–440.
16. Mulkerrin E, Epstein FH, Clark BA. Aldosterone responses to hyperkalemia in healthy elderly humans. J Amer Soc Nephrol 1995; 6: 1459–1462.

Glomerular Disease in the Elderly Population

RICHARD J. GLASSOCK
Department of Internal Medicine, University of Kentucky, Lexington, KY 40536, U.S.A.

Introduction

As the second millennium dawns, it has become increasingly apparent that the elderly population will constitute an increasing fraction of the total disease burden of society. In the last decade of the 20th Century, approximately one in every 15 individuals was over the age of 65 and as the 'baby boomers' reach maturity, this fraction was expected to increase. Renal disease, in general, becomes increasingly common with aging, particularly those diseases related to urinary-tract obstruction and infection and to atherosclerosis. However, glomerular disease also is quite prevalent. The types of glomerular disease observed in the elderly generally reflect those seen in the population as a whole, however, certain disorders may have an increased prevalence among them. For example, renal complications of type 2 non-insulin dependent diabetes are seen with increasing frequency in the aging population. Amyloidosis, renal paraneoplastic syndromes and adverse effects of therapeutic agents are examples of renal and glomerular disorders also seen with increased frequency in older patients. This paper discusses glomerular disease in the elderly, focusing on specific issues of geriatric care that need to be embraced by practicing nephrologists.

Clinical Presentation

The clinical presentation of glomerular disease in the elderly is similar to that in the population as a whole. The abnormal clinical and laboratory features can be aggregated into five common syndromes; namely, the acute nephritic syndrome, rapidly-progressive glomerulonephritis, nephrotic syndrome, asymptomatic hematuria and/or hematuria, and chronic progressive glomerulonephritis.

Each of these syndromes can be due to underlying primary glomerular diseases, in which the glomeruli are the sole or predominant tissue involved and in which the outward clinical manifestations are primarily the consequence

Oreopoulos et al. (eds.), Nephrology and Geriatrics Integrated, 57–66.

of glomerular abnormalities. Glomerular diseases secondary to systemic disease processes, such as diabetes mellitus or amyloidosis, also occur frequently in the elderly, and give rise to specific clinical features.

The dissection of these clinical presentations into specific clinical pathologic entities has been materially advanced by the application of percutaneous renal biopsy and the analysis of tissue by sophisticated pathologic techniques of light, immunofluorescence, and electron microscopy.

The indications for renal biopsy in the elderly are similar to those for younger patients, although renal biopsies appear to be used more frequently for acute nephritis or acute renal failure and somewhat less frequently for asymptomatic urinary abnormalities (Table 1). Overall, renal biopsy findings in the elderly reveal primary glomerular disease in about 70% and a secondary glomerular disease in approximately 30%. Of course, some disorders are underrepresented in surveys that analyze renal biopsy findings, because the clinical diagnosis, e.g. diabetes mellitus and acute infectious disease, often renders renal biopsy unnecessary.

Acute Nephritic Syndrome

The acute nephritic syndrome arises most often in the presence a soft-tissue infection – pharyngitis, wound or cellulitis with a nephritogenic strain of a group A beta hemolytic streptococci. In the elderly, cutaneous infections are far more common than pharyngeal infections as a cause of acute post-streptococcal glomerulonephritis. As in younger patients, acute nephritis follows the streptococcal infection after a latent period of between seven and 21 days. Latent periods are somewhat longer in patients with cutaneous infections. The typical presentation includes the abrupt onset of hematuria – gross or microscopic, proteinuria, hypertension and fluid retention. In elderly patients, the urinary abnormalities may be trivial and the predominant findings are related to hypertension and/or fluid retention. Another common presentation

Table 1. Glomerular disease in the elderly. Indications for renal biopsy

Clinical Presentation	Age	
	< 60 year (%)	> 60 year (%)
Nephrotic syndrome	24	31
Acute nephritis/ARF	12	26
Chronic renal disease	12	25
Asymptomatic urine abnormality	35	8
Hypertension	2	1
Unknown	15	9

* Davison A and Johnston P. Neph., Dialysis, Transplant; 1996 [Supplement 9: 34–37])

in the elderly is that of an acute exacerbation of congestive heart failure with pulmonary edema or unexplained acute renal failure accompanied by hypertension and pulmonary edema.

With rare exceptions, the urinalysis will be abnormal and reveal dysmorphic hematuria and modest proteinuria. Heavy proteinuria, with nephrotic syndrome, is distinctly uncommon. The patient will show marked sodium retention with very low fractional excretion of sodium and calcium, low plasma aldosterone levels, low plasma renin activity and often a type IV renal tubular acidosis – hyperkalemic, hyperchloremic metabolic acidosis. The C3 component of complement is profoundly depressed whereas the C4 component of complement is normal. The depression of C3 levels is transient, and levels will return to normal within eight to 10 weeks in most patients. Often serologic investigations for a previous streptococcal infection are positive. The antistreptolysin O titer, however, will be normal in these patients who have had a previous *cutaneous* streptococcal infection, whereas such patients often will have elevated anti-DNAase or anti-NAD antibodies. Early treatment with penicillin or other antimicrobials may suppress the serological response to the streptococcal organism and thereby confuse the diagnosis. Such treatment has only a marginal effect on the risk of developing nephritis. In patients, who have not previously received antimicrobials, throat or skin lesions may be positive for beta-hemolytic streptococci.

The clinical course of acute poststreptococcal glomerulonephritis in the elderly is similar to that in the general population, although there may be a somewhat increased likelihood of developing superimposed crescents and rapidly-progressive glomerulonephritis (see below). Some patients may show prolonged persistence of hematuria and/or proteinuria, but progression to chronic renal insufficiency is unusual. The acute nephritic syndrome also can be a presenting feature of other non-poststreptococcal disorders, such as IgA nephropathy and membranoproliferative glomerulonephritis. However, these two entities are relatively uncommon in the elderly.

In the elderly acute poststreptococcal glomerulonephritis is treated in a manner similar to that in younger patients, although those who develop acute symptomatic congestive heart failure may require marked sodium restriction and aggressive use of loop-acting diuretics (e.g. furosemide). Digitalis and other inotropic agents are of limited utility, since the predominant problem is volume expansion rather than abnormalities of myocardial contractility. Hypertension, if present, needs to be treated aggressively with loop-acting diuretics, hydralazine (or other vasodilators), or angiotensin-converting-enzyme inhibitors. Because of the hyporeninemic state that frequently accompanies acute poststreptococcal glomerulonephritis, one would expect inhibitors of angiotensin-converting enzyme or angiotensin 1 receptor antagonist to be less effective, particularly if diuretics are not used concomitantly. Severe hyperkalemia and/or oliguric acute renal failure may require dialysis.

Rapidly Progressive Glomerulonephritis

This syndrome consists of clinical evidence of glomerulonephritis (dysmorphic hematuria and proteinuria) accompanied by rapid and progressive decline in glomerular filtration rate. As such, it is a common presenting feature in glomerular disease in the elderly and most frequently, is due to underlying microscopic polyangiitis. The clinical presentations of this form includes *Henoch-Schönlein* or anaphylactoid purpura, Wegener's syndrome, Goodpasture's syndrome, and organ-limited disease (also known as pauci-immune crescentic glomerulonephritis). *Henoch-Schönlein* purpura is characterized by episodes of palpable purpura, often predominantly involving the lower extremities, abdominal pain, arthralgias, and glomerulonephritis. Wegener's syndrome consists of upper and lower respiratory disease (otitis media, rhinitis, sinusitis) and lower respiratory disease (necrotizing pneumonia, tracheitis) and glomerulonephritis; Goodpasture's syndrome consists of alveolar hemorrhage and glomerulonephritis. Organ-limited disease, refers to forms of microscopic polyangiitis that selectively affect the renal glomeruli in the absence of extrarenal manifestations.

Antineutrophil cytoplasmic autoantibodies (ANCA) are found in 75–80% of elderly patients with the syndrome of rapidly progressive glomerulonephritis due to underlying microscopic polyangiitis or pauci-immune crescentic glomerulonephritis. Most of these autoantibodies react with myeloperoxidase. Anti-neutrophil cytoplasmic autoantibodies also are found in Wegener's syndrome. Approximately 95% of patients with Wegener's syndrome, who have not been treated previously, will demonstrate elevated antineutrophil cytoplasmic autoantibodies, predominantly directed to proteinase 3. Goodpasture's syndrome (alveolar hemorrhage and glomerulonephritis) may be due to a wide variety of pathological lesions, including both microscopic polyangiitis due to antineutrophil cytoplasmic autoantibodies and to antiglomerular basement-membrane antibody-induced disease. Approximately 10–15% of elderly patients presenting with rapidly progressive glomerulonephritis will have autoantibodies to glomerular-basement-membrane antigens. In these cases the male/female ratio is approximately one, unlike the male predominance of antiglomerular basement-membrane, antibody-associated disease in younger patients. Approximately 10–15% of patients will have neither anti-neutrophil cytoplasmic autoantibody nor antiglomerular basement membrane antibodies. Such patients often are referred to as 'idiopathic' rapidly progressive glomerulonephritis although, in some circumstances, these serological findings may be associated with an underlying immune complex-mediated glomerulonephritis – such as IgA nephropathy, infective endocarditis, etc. In addition, approximately 10% of patients may have both antiglomerular basement membrane autoantibodies and antineutrophil cytoplasmic autoantibodies. These patients appear to have a rapidly progressive and treatment-resistant form of disease.

In the absence of treatment, the prognosis of rapidly-progressive glomerulonephritis due to underlying microscopic polyangiitis and/or pauci-immune crescentic glomerulonephritis is very poor. Aggressive management with intravenous high-dose methylprednisolone, oral or intravenous cyclophosphamide will improve renal function in most patients. Nevertheless, elderly patients, who tolerate these medications poorly, have a high risk of potential side effects, including lethal infections. The addition of intensive plasma exchange (plasmapheresis) does not appear to materially improve the outcome, although some studies have demonstrated a more complete recovery of renal function when plasma exchange is added to the treatment of rapidly-progressive glomerulonephritis which has advanced to dialysis dependency. Plasma exchange appears to offer no advantage in those who have not progressed to dialysis dependency, at least among patients with non-antiglomerular basement membrane, antibody related disease. On the other hand, patients with antiglomerular basement membrane antibody disease, who have not progressed to dialysis probably benefit when plasma exchange is added to an immunosuppressive regimen. Patients with anti-GBM antibody disease, who have already advanced to dialysis, derive little additional benefit from the combination of plasma exchange and immunosuppression.

Nephrotic Syndrome

This syndrome consists of heavy proteinuria, usually > 3.5 g/d accompanied by hypoalbuminemia and variably by edema and hyperlipidemia. As mentioned previously, nephrotic syndrome is the most common indication for percutaneous renal biopsy in an elderly patient.

Approximately 15–18% of newly-diagnosed adult nephrotic syndrome patients are over the age of 60 – a fraction that is similar to that of individuals over the age of 60 in the general population. Nevertheless, nephrotic syndrome probably is under-reported in patients over the age of 80 and, as mentioned previously, patients with diabetes mellitus and nephrotic syndrome undergo renal biopsy less frequently than expected and, therefore, are under-represented in retrospective reviews that tabulate the patterns of renal disease in the elderly.

Retrospective surveys of renal biopsy findings among elderly patients presenting with nephrotic syndrome indicate that approximately 60% will have either membranous glomerulonephritis, minimal change disease, or amyloidosis. The leading renal pathologic finding in nephrotic syndrome in the elderly, membranous glomerulonephritis, accounts for between 35–40% of these cases (Table 2). Proliferative glomerulonephritis, including the crescentic and membranoproliferative forms underlies the nephrotic syndrome in about 15%.

Table 2. Glomerular disease in the elderly. Renal biopsy findings in nephrotic syndrome in the elderly[1]

	n	%
Membranous GN	416	37.3
Minimal Change	140	12.6
Amyloidosis	151	11.8
Other[2]	427	38.3
	1114	100%

[1] 12 published series 1980–1993. Modified from Cameron J, Seminars in Nephrology, 1996; 16: 319–329.
[2] FSGS, proliferative, diabetes, MPGN.

Membranous Glomerulonephritis

In the elderly membranous glomerulonephritis most often is idiopathic; however, it may also occur in association with other diseases most notably malignant neoplasia, or following exposure to certain drugs. Malignancies that underlie membranous glomerulonephritis, include: carcinoma of the lung, stomach, breast, and colon, and less commonly, lymphomas, melanoma, prostatic carcinoma and bladder carcinoma. In collected series, approximately 6–7% of patients found to have membranous glomerulonephritis on renal biopsy will have an underlying malignant neoplasia. When one considers only patients over the age of 60, approximately 13% of those diagnosed as membranous glomerulonephritis will have underlying neoplasia. In large epidemiologic surveys, the concurrence of malignancy and membranous glomerulonephritis was not greatly different from that in an age-matched control population; therefore, the association of these two disease states may largely be the consequence of their frequency in an aging population. Nevertheless, it is well known that the nephrotic syndrome may undergo remission with the removal or successful treatment of malignancy and may relapse with the recurrence of neoplasia. In addition, tumor neoantigens may be localized to the capillary deposits of membranous glomerulonephritis.

Because of the association of malignancy and membranous glomerulonephritis, all elderly patients with nephrotic syndrome due to membranous glomerulonephritis should undergo a careful and complete physical examination with special attention to the breast, lymph nodes, skin and prostate. Stools should be examined for occult blood on three occasions, a standard chest X-ray (or computerized tomography of the chest) done and a mammogram in females. A prostatic surface antigen should be measured in males. Additional diagnostic studies are not indicated unless the preliminary evaluation raises the examiner's suspicions. Overall, in approximately one-third of those patients with associated malignancy and membranous glomerulonephritis the neoplasia will be recognized before the onset of nephrotic syndrome; in about one third the two diagnoses will be simultaneous, and in about one-third, the malignancy will be recognized after the discovery of nephrotic syndrome. The morphologic appearance of membranous glomerulonephritis associated with malignancy is similar to that found in the idiopathic disorder.

Drugs frequently prescribed for elderly patients that may be associated with nephrotic syndrome, including membranous glomerulonephritis, include non-steroidal anti-inflammatory drugs, oral or parenteral gold compounds, oral, topical or parenteral mercurial compounds, probenecid, penicillamine and anti-convulsants. Hence one must keep these drugs in mind when analyzing the development of nephrotic syndrome in older patients. The use of non-steroidal anti-inflammatory drugs may be associated with the abrupt onset of nephrotic syndrome, accompanied by renal insufficiency. In such patients, renal biopsy may reveal minimal change disease complicated by an acute interstitial nephritis.

Minimal Change Disease

Minimal change disease is the second most common histopathological finding in the renal biopsy of elderly patients with the nephrotic syndrome, accounting for between 15 and 20% of them. Because of the concomitant presence of nephroangiosclerosis, a definitive diagnosis of minimal change disease may be difficult. Elderly patients frequently have globally sclerotic glomeruli and tubulointerstitial pathology. Thus, in the elderly patient minimal change disease often is superimposed on other renal pathological findings. Hypertension is more frequent in the elderly patient with minimal change disease than in younger patients. The most striking difference in minimal change disease between the elderly and younger patients is the very high risk of acute renal failure in the former. In a retrospective survey, Nolasco and colleagues found that, overall, 23% of patients with minimal change disease over the age of 60 had acute renal failure [14]. Such patients tended to have more severe proteinuria and more profound reduction in serum albumin levels but otherwise could not be differentiated from other patients. Elderly patients with minimal change disease may respond to steroid therapy. However, they may require longer periods of treatment to induce the first remission. Relapses of nephrotic syndrome appear to be less common among elderly adults than among children and young adults. Cyclophosphamide and other alkylating agents have been used to prolong the remission in frequently relapsing minimal change disease in the elderly. These drugs may be associated with an increased risk of infection, particularly herpes zoster.

Amyloidosis

Systemic amyloidosis, usually of the AL or primary type, is found frequently in elderly persons with the nephrotic syndrome. Most series have found this lesion in approximately 10–12% of patients over the age of 60 years who present with nephrotic syndrome. These patients may lack the extrarenal manifestations of amyloidosis, such as carpal tunnel syndrome, restrictive cardiomyopathy, postural hypotension, easy bruising, diarrhea and gastroparesis. A paraproteinemia or paraproteinuria (abnormal light-chain excretion) may be found in 33–70% of patients with primary amyloidosis presenting with the nephrotic syndrome. Another presenting feature of amyloidosis in the elderly is mild proteinuria unaccompanied by urinary sediment abnormalities. As noted above, the amyloidosis usually is of the AL type, although elderly patients with rheumatoid arthritis or chronic infectious diseases – such as tuberculosis or osteomyelitis may, at times, develop the AA or secondary type.

In the elderly the prognosis of primary or AL amyloidosis is poor because in most of these patients, the nephrotic syndrome will worsen and they will develop progressive renal insufficiency. Treatment with melphalan and prednisone may delay the onset of end-stage renal failure. All elderly patients, who present with unexplained proteinuria or the nephrotic syndrome, should undergo serum and urinary electrophoresis and/or immunofixation for serum monoclonal paraproteins or monoclonal urinary light-chain excretion. Those with abnormal findings should undergo bone marrow aspiration or biopsy, to exclude an underlying multiple myeloma. Abdominal fat-pad aspiration examined with Congo red stain also may be used to detect primary amyloidosis. When renal biopsies are done in the elderly, the material should be stained routinely with Congo red and examined under electron microscopy at high magnification for the typical fibrillar lesions.

Other Causes

Other causes of nephrotic syndrome in the elderly include diabetic nephropathy (type 2) non-insulin dependent diabetes mellitus, fibrillary glomerulonephritis, light-chain disease, focal and segmental glomerulosclerosis and membranoproliferative glomerulonephritis. Mesangial proliferative glomerulonephritis, crescentic glomerulonephritis, and focal necrotizing glomerulonephritis also may produce nephrotic syndrome, but generally these lesions relate to underlying systemic diseases such as polyangiitis. Systemic lupus erythematosus complicated by nephritis is an uncommon disorder in the elderly. Only 2% of patients with SLE present after the age of 60. In the elderly most positive fluorescent anti-nuclear antibody tests are false positives.

Asymptomatic Hematuria and/or Proteinuria

An abnormal urinalysis, with microscopic hematuria and/or non-nephrotic proteinuria often prompts a nephrology consultation. However, these abnormal findings seldom justify a renal biopsy. Hematuria in the elderly usually arises from the urinary tract – renal carcinoma, bladder cancer, stones and prostatic disease. Such hematuria usually is normo or isomorphic rather than dysmorphic. Dysmorphic erythrocytes (small, poorly hemoglobinized and of distorted shape) are best recognized by phase-contrast microscopy of a freshly-voided urinary sediment. Nevertheless, dysmorphic hematuria, particularly if accompanied by proteinuria, should raise the suspicion of an underlying glomerular disease, such as IgA nephropathy, IgM nephropathy, thin basement membrane disease, fibrillary or immunotactoid glomerulonephritis and membranoproliferative glomerulonephritis. For reasons that are not well understood, IgA nephropathy is uncommon in persons over the age of 65. Fibrillary glomerulonephritis also may present with nephrotic syndrome and progressive renal insufficiency. Often membranoproliferative glomerulonephritis can be traced to an underlying chronic viral infection, particularly hepatitis C virus. Any elderly patient given the diagnosis of membranoproliferative glomerulonephritis should be studied serologically for the presence of these chronic viral infections. Amyloidosis may produce isomorphic hematuria, largely the consequence of bladder involvement.

Summary

This brief review of glomerular disease in the elderly contains several lessons for the geriatric nephrologist. Remember the atypical presentation of acute nephritis in older individuals. Remember the common causes of nephrotic syndrome in the elderly; namely, membranous glomerulonephritis, minimal change disease, proliferative glomerulonephritis and amyloidosis. Remember the special risks of cytotoxic drug therapy of glomerular disease. Remember the importance of pauci-immune crescentic glomerulonephritis and polyangiitis associated with antineutrophil cytoplasmic antibody in the aging population. Remember the value of and use of urinary erythrocyte dysmorphism in the differential diagnosis of hematuria in the elderly.

References

1. Cameron JS. Nephrotic syndrome in the elderly. Semin Neprol 1996; 16: 319–329.
2. Davison AM, Johnston PA. Glomerulonephritis in the elderly. Neph Dialysis Transplant, 1996 (Supplement); 11: 534–537.
3. Kincaid-Smith P. Renal disease in the elderly in hypertension and renal disease in the elderly. In: Martinez-Maldando M, editor. Hypertension and Renal disease in the Elderly. Oxford: Blackwell Scientific , 1992; 200–210.
4. Glassock RJ. Glomerular disease in the elderly. In: Martinez-Maldando M, editor. Hypertension and Renal Disease in the Elderly. Oxford: Blackwell Scientific, 1992; 211–224.
5. Glassock RJ. Secondary membranous glomerulonephritis. Neph Dialys Transp 1992 (Supplement); 1: 564–571.
6. Johnston PA, Brown JS, Davison AM. The nephrotic syndrome in the elderly. Clinicopathological correlations in 37 patients. Geriatric Neph Urol 1993; 2: 85–90.
7. Moorthy RV and Zimmerman SW. Renal diseases in the elderly. Clinico-pathological analyses of renal disease in 115 patients. Clin Nephrol 1980; 14: 223–229.

8. Bolton WR. Nephrotic syndrome in the aged. In: Cameron S, Glassock R, editors. The Nephrotic Syndrome. New York: Marell Dekker, 1988; 523–553.
9. Eagen JW, Lewis E. Glomerulonephritis of neoplasia. Kidney Int 1977; 11: 297–306.
10. Rameriz G, Saba N. Primary glomerulonephritis in the elderly. In: Zawada E, Sica P, editors. Geriatric Nephrology and Biology. Littleton: PSG Publishing Co, 1985; 49–66.
11. Abrass CK. Glomerulonephritis in the elderly. Am J Nephrol 1985; 5: 409–418.
12. Murray B, Raij L. Glomerular disease in the aged. In: Nunes JFM, Cameron JS, editors. Renal Function and Disease in the Elderly. London: Butterworths, 1987; 298–320.
13. Serra-Cardus A, Cameron JS. Renal vasculitis in the aged. In: Nunes JFM, Cameron JS, editors. Renal Function and Disease in the Elderly. London: Butterworths, 1987; 321–347.
14. Nolasco F, Cameron J, Heywood E, et al. Adult onset minimal change nephrotic syndrome: a long-term follow-up. Kidney International 1986; 29: 1215–1225.
15. Jennette J, Falk R. The pathology of vasculitis involving the kidney. Amer J Kid Disease 1994; 24F: 130–141.

Renal Artery Disease in the Elderly

WILLIAM L. HENRICH
University of Maryland Hospital, Baltimore, MD 21201, U.S.A.

Atherosclerosis is common in the elderly population, and therefore it is not surprising that atherosclerosis involving the renal artery is being recognized with increasing frequency. The following review summarizes several key features of the presentation, diagnosis and management of this disorder with a focus on the elderly population. The reader is referred to several excellent reviews that discuss the pathophysiology of this condition and the extant literature in detail [1–5]. This review is divided into seven brief discussions designed to provide an overview of this subject.

Clinical Presentations of Renal Artery Stenosis

Atherosclerotic disease of the renal artery in the elderly has two main presentations: The first, hypertension, is suspected in those who develop new onset hypertension over the age of 60, or in previously hypertensive patients whose blood pressure becomes difficult to control. Hence, in this age group, a sudden change in blood pressure should warrant consideration of this diagnosis. A third category in whom we should consider this diagnosis are those patients with difficult-to-treat hypertension. Thus, those requiring three or four medicines and who require a high dose of anti-hypertensive medicines should be considered for evaluation for renal-artery stenosis. Obviously, other causes of an exacerbation of blood pressure should be considered such as non-compliance, the recent ingestion of non-steroidal anti-inflammatory drugs or a decline in renal function from another cause. Also the possibility of renal artery stenosis is suggested by the presence of atherosclerosis in other locations, for example, a patient with a prior history of transient ischemic attacks, coronary artery disease or peripheral vascular disease requiring an intervention or a bypass operation would be a candidate for atherosclerosis of the renal arteries. In patients suspected of having renal artery stenosis, one should seek risk factors associated with atherosclerosis in all vascular beds including a history of hyperlipidemia or cigarette smoking.

The second major mode of presentation of renal artery atherosclerosis is

Oreopoulos et al. (eds.), Nephrology and Geriatrics Integrated, 67–75.

renal insufficiency, which may present as a slow, insidious decline in renal function over time or may develop rapidly after one has achieved tight blood pressure control after a period of poor control. In this connection, Textor and colleagues demonstrated that the decrease in blood pressure in individuals with high-grade, bilateral renal-artery stenosis or unilateral renal-artery stenosis to a single functioning kidney resulted in a decline in renal function [6]. Ying and colleagues [7] also reported similar results. In recent years, atherosclerosis of the renal arteries has been detected with increasing frequency following therapy with angiotensin-converting enzyme inhibitors [8, 9]. These drugs unmask the disorder in those patients who have significant ($\geq$ 70%) stenosis of both renal arteries (two functioning kidneys), or of a single renal artery (a single functioning kidney). In this clinical presentation, angiotensin II seems to produce efferent arteriolar vasoconstriction at a time when the renal perfusion pressure is diminished by renal artery stenosis. The angiotensin II-driven, efferent-arteriolar vasoconstriction maintains the hydrostatic filtration pressure (P_{GC}) constant during periods of underperfusion. In this context, when the patient is given an angiotensin converting enzyme inhibitor, there is efferent arteriolar vasodilatation and, as a consequence, there is a decrease in the decrement in the hydrostatic glomerular pressure. As a result the filtration pressure (P_{GC}) falls and GFR declines. This event is signalled by a rise in the serum creatinine concentration and thus comes to the attention of clinicians. A key feature of this form of pathophysiology is that it develops in those patients who have ischemia of the entire renal mass. Hence, when the patient has unilateral ischemia but a patent contralateral artery, the administration of an angiotensin-converting-enzyme inhibitor will produce some decline in glomerular filtration on the stenotic side but some increase in filtration on the side with the patent artery. The net result is that the whole-body glomerular filtration usually is unchanged and is not marked by an increase in the serum creatinine concentration [10]. In contrast, when the patient has ischemia to the entire renal mass (bilateral renal artery stenosis or stenosis to a solitary functioning kidney), the fall in filtration pressure produces a fall in overall glomerular filtration rate and a rise in the serum creatinine concentration.

While we believe the lesion of proximal renal artery stenosis produces an insidious decline in renal function when the disease is progressive, there are other explanations for a gradual decline in renal function. In this connection, Zucchelli and Zuccala [11] recently have postulated that many patients with atherosclerosis of the aorta and renal arteries have atheromatous vascular disease. They point out that many patients suspected of having renal failure due to hypertensive nephrosclerosis may instead have atheromatous disease as the cause, presumably from embolization of microatheromata from lesions in the aorta or renal arteries. Further studies are needed to clarify this point.

Incidence of Renal Artery Stenosis

It has been proposed that renal artery stenosis is a common cause of secondary hypertension, but the overall prevalence is estimated to be at about 1% in the general population with hypertension [12, 13]. With regard to presentations as renal failure, the overall incidence and prevalence are unknown. Figure 1 shows the frequency of renal artery stenosis in over 1200 patients who had coronary angiograms in one center [14]. In this series, the incidence of significant bilateral renal artery stenosis was 4% and the incidence of significant unilateral renal artery stenosis was 11%. Taken together, approximately one of seven patients, who underwent a coronary arteriogram had significant renal artery stenosis; in this study, this condition was defined as significant if the lesion occupied ≥ 50% of the lumen. This group of patients does not represent the general population, because they already had some manifestations of atherosclerosis in order to be candidates for coronary angiography. Thus, we would expect the overall incidence and prevalence of the disorder to be lower in the asymptomatic general population; in the elderly, the incidence of the disorder would be approximately 10%. Future prospective studies will be needed to establish the precise incidence of this disorder and to determine the relative frequencies of unilateral vs. bilateral disease.

Recently Hansen et al. [15] studied the presentations of renal artery atherosclerosis in an elderly cohort (patients over 60 years old) over an eight-year period; they identified 153 patients between the ages of 70–79, and 70 patients were between the ages of 80–89. Remarkably, seven patients were over the age of 90. Their study included 117 men and 113 women; the mean blood pressure in this group was 202/102 mm Hg. Seventy-eight per cent of the cohort had renal insufficiency, as defined by a serum creatinine concentration ≥ 2.0 mg/dl. Interestingly, 93% had some evidence of cardiac disease and 33% had

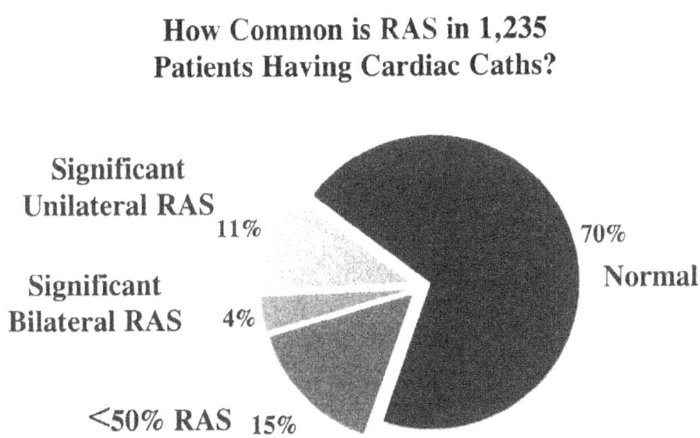

Figure 1. Incidence of renal artery stenosis in 1235 patients who had cardiac catheterization. From Ref. [14].

evidence of cerebrovascular disease, confirming that the disease develops in patients with manifestations of atherosclerosis in other locations. Of note, 78% of the cohort had aortoiliac disease.

The Current Approach to Patients Suspected of Having Renal Artery Stenosis Secondary to Atherosclerosis

It is not clear whether the true incidence of renal artery stenosis secondary to atherosclerosis is changing or whether physicians now make this diagnosis more easily than in previous years. Moreover, the approach to renal artery stenosis has changed in the last five to 10 years. Until five years ago, the primary remedy for atherosclerotic renal artery stenosis was bypass surgery: either aortorenal, splenorenal or hepatorenal bypasses to circumvent atherosclerosis in proximal locations of the renal artery. Because such patients often have atherosclerosis in many vascular beds and thus are poor operative risks, they require an extensive preoperative work-up to ensure that the bypass operation would give significant clinical benefit. In this regard, the indicators for this operation are critical renal-artery stenosis with a clear decline in renal function or moderate to severe renal insufficiency, difficult-to-treat hypertension and anatomic evidence of tight renal artery stenosis. In addition, preoperative evaluation often included renal vein renins and captopril scintigraphy.

Recently, the widespread availability of percutaneous transluminal angioplasty (PTLA) with intravascular stent deployment has brought more of a 'find it, fix it' approach to the disorder. Now many centers do not perform extensive preoperative work-ups routinely; the usual preoperative assessment includes a measurement of serial serum creatinines and a careful blood pressure record. This new approach to renal artery disease is aided by the fact that many of the new diagnostic tests for the disorder are more accurate than before. Many series have asserted that renal scintigraphy with captopril challenge has a sensitivity and specificity of about 90% [8, 16, 17]. In one study, the use of furosemide helped to differentiate patients with significant renal artery obstruction from those with patent arteries [16]. It should be pointed out that some patients with underperfusion of the renal mass because of heart failure, or those who have distal small-blood-vessel disease ('arterial pruning') may have false positive renal scintigrams; such patients do not have main renal artery disease [18]. Of the newer angiographic techniques, magnetic resonance angiography [19] is reported to have sensitivities and specificities in the 90% range; the technique is expensive and still requires local expertise and experience, which is not universally available. Digital subtraction angiography using an intra-arterial injection has the advantage of not requiring aortic access and has a reduced contrast requirement compared to standard angiography; however, the resolution of the renal artery may not be as explicit as with an intra-renal injection. Spiral computerized tomography with intravenous contrast requires more contrast than other techniques and is somewhat less helpful in renal failure. Some are concerned about the use of contrast because of the possibility of contrast-associated renal failure in this patient cohort, whose members often have underlying renal insufficiency. Carbon-dioxide digital angiography using intra-arterial carbon dioxide has the advantage of not using contrast but has not achieved good resolution, at least in some centers [20]. This promising technique may prove more useful as more experience is gained [5]. Also we can now study renal artery anatomy with duplex scanning using color doppler ultrasound; this technique can be useful in selected patients, particularly those who have not had prior abdominal surgery or who are obese [21]. Finally, the application of magnetic resonance technology using gadolinium is favored in some centers. Resolution of anatomic detail is improving with each of these new techniques.

Treatment of Renal Artery Stenosis

As mentioned above, the widespread availability of percutaneous transluminal angioplasty (PTLA) has made the approach to and treatment of renal artery atherosclerosis routine in many centers. However the newer studies using PTLA usually have been done on unselected patients with a short follow-up. Moreover, these studies have not established with certainty the association between a patent artery and a salutary result. Thus, the fact that blood pressure improves following a procedure does not mean that the artery that was treated has remained patent during the follow-up period. This also holds true for those individuals who have some decrease in serum creatinine concentration following manipulation of the renal artery. Despite these limitations, the treatment of atherosclerotic renal arteries has improved dramatically, at least from a technical standpoint. In this connection, Blum et al. [22] recently documented the value of invasive angiography in treating ostial renal artery disease; this represented a genuine advance because 50% of atherosclerotic lesions are ostial. These investigators placed 74 stents in 68 patients with ostial lesions (defined as lesions within 5 mm of the aorta), and followed the patients for a mean of 27 months with duplex sonography, blood pressure measurements, serum creatinine concentrations, and, in some cases, repeat angiography. They showed that the use of stents and PTLA resulted in a sharp decline in blood pressure, which lasted for four to five years in most patients. This study showed that stent placement was feasible even in ostial lesions and therefore that ostial lesions are no longer a contraindication to PTLA and stent placement. The study referred to earlier [15], followed the elderly cohort for a mean of 28 months and observed that 77% of them were improved and 9% were cured of their hypertension. Recently Harden et al. set out to determine whether PTLA could improve renal function [23]; they placed 33 stents in 32 patients and followed the $1/S_{CR}$ concentration as a surrogate for renal function. In this study renal artery narrowing was defined as $\geq 50\%$. These investigators focused on patients with renal artery narrowing and renal insufficiency defined as a serum creatinine concentration between 2.2 and 4.4 mg/dl. Three of the 32 patients in this study were dialysis dependent. Initially, placement of the stents achieved a 100% technical success rate. There were several complications and 21 of the patients had follow-up angiography at six months. Six patients died before angiography could be repeated; these deaths were attributed to complications of atherosclerosis, two died of myocardial infarction, two died of peripheral vascular disease, one died of renal failure, and one patient died after a gastrointestinal bleed. The main finding from this study (Fig. 2) is that in this patient cohort the placement of stents resulted in some leveling of renal function and slowed its decline. However as shown in Fig. 3, the survival curve for the 32 patients undergoing stent placement generally was poor; at 24-month follow-up, approximately 40% of the patients were alive. Although other recent studies of this patient population have emphasized the high morbidity rate associated with revascularization [24, 25], the studies are hopeful in that those patients who achieve a lower blood pressure or some reduction in the serum creatinine concentration can expect to benefit from the procedure. After another large retrospective study, Bonelli et al. [25] suggested that the most predictable beneficial effect from a successful angioplasty is improvement in blood pressure [26].

Patient Selection for Renal Artery Procedures

In the elderly patient population one commonly encounters renal artery stenosis as a diagnostic possibility. Those who can be considered for an angiogram

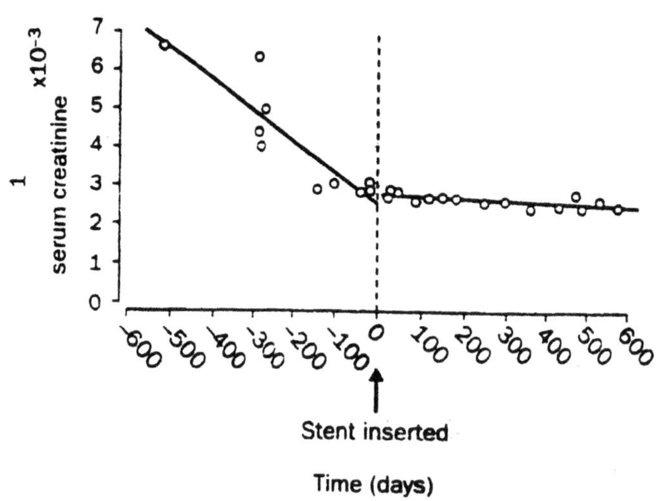

Figure 2. Role of reciprocal serum creatinine plot (y) in one patient, before and after stent placement. From Ref. [23].

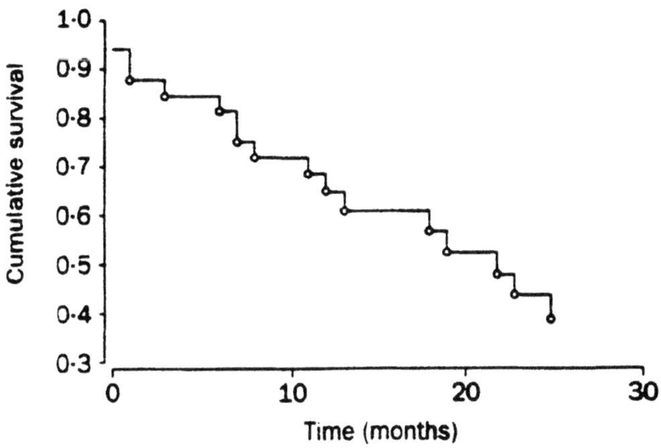

Figure 3. Survival curve of 32 patients after insertion of renal artery stent. From Ref. [23].

and possible intervention are individuals with severe hypertension with retinopathy, and those with difficult-to-treat hypertension. In addition, patients with the abrupt onset of hypertension, those with a loss of blood pressure control, and those who have an unexpected decline in renal function with or without provocation by an angiotensin-converting-enzyme inhibitor should also be considered for diagnostic evaluation. The presence of associated vascular disease increases the likelihood of renal artery atherosclerosis. On physical examination one should seek a systolic/diastolic murmur over the aorta and the area of the renal arteries. Renal artery disease also may be signalled by recurrent sudden pulmonary edema. Patients with marginal left ventricular function may decompensate and develop pulmonary edema rapidly when they experience a sudden increase in blood pressure. Elderly patients who have atherosclerosis in other locations but do not have hypertension or renal insufficiency should not have incidental renal arteriograms because the main benefit of PTLA *plus* stent insertion is some lowering in blood pressure and a decrease in the serum creatinine concentration. If the patient has neither hypertension nor renal insufficiency it is unlikely that the correction of renal artery stenosis will bring any measurable clinical improvement. In addition, the procedure runs the risk of producing atheroembolic renal disease, as a complication.

In the future, more studies are needed to clarify our approach to these patients, particularly those who are elderly. Recently Zuccala and Zucchelli [27] have emphasized that angioplasty is less than ideal in that it inflicts endothelial damage and intimal proliferation, thus we need a prospective and randomized study of carefully selected patients with a medical limb and a PTLA (plus or minus stent deployment) limb. In addition, angiographic follow-up is needed with measured patency of vessels in the untreated vs. treated groups so that we can have some link between clinical 'success' or 'failure' and the actual anatomy in the renal artery. It is possible that the increased expertise and resolution obtained with newer diagnostic techniques, such as CO_2 angiography and magnetic resonance angiography, will provide us with alternatives to the more invasive renal-artery angiography. Until such prospective and randomized studies have been done, clinicians should continue to include renal artery atherosclerosis in the differential diagnosis of the populations described above. They should approach potential candidates for PTLA and stent deployment with the clear understanding that the cohort has only limited overall survival and that the main benefit of the procedure is some decrease in blood pressure. These guidelines presented above provide a rational approach to the management of these complicated individuals.

References

1. Rimmer JM, Gennari FJ. Atherosclerotic renovascular disease and progressive renal failure. Ann Intern Med 1993; 118: 712–719.
2. Jacobsen HR. Ischemic renal disease: an overlooked clinical entity? Kidney Int 1988; 34: 729–743.
3. Libertino JA, Bosco PJ, Ying CY, Breslin DJ, Wood BO, Tsapatsaris NP, et al. Renal revascularization to preserve and restore renal function. J Urol 1992; 147: 1485–1487.
4. Henrich, WL. Functional and organic ischemic renal disease. In: Seldin D, Giebisch G, editors. The Kidney, second edition. New York: Raven Press, 1992; 3289–3304.
5. Reiser IW, Spitalewitz S. Screening for renovascular hypertension: which patients – what approach? J Crit Illness 1998; 13(5): 301–308.
6. Textor SC, Novick AC, Tarazi RC, Klimas V, Vidt DG, Pohl M. Critical perfusion pressure for renal function in patients with bilateral atherosclerotic renal vascular disease. Ann Intern Med 1985; 102: 308–314.
7. Ying CY, Tifft CP, Gavras H, Chobanian AV. Renal Revascularization in the azotemic hypertensive patient resistant to therapy. N Engl J Med 1984; 311: 1070–1075.
8. Van de Ven PJG, Beutler JJ, Kaatee R, Beek FJA, Mali WPTM, Koomans HA. Angiotensin converting enzyme inhibitor-induced renal dysfunction in atherosclerotic renovascular disease. Kid Int 1998; 53: 986–993.
9. Cuocolo A, Esposito S, Volpe M. Renal artery stenosis detection by combined Gates' technique and captopril test in hypertensive patients. J Nucl Med 1989; 30: 51–56.
10. Johnston CI, Jackson B. Overview: Angiotensin converting enzyme inhibition in renovascular hypertension. Kidney Int 1987; 31: S154–S156.
11. Zucchelli P, Zuccalà A. Recent data on hypertension and progressive renal disease. J Hum Hypertens 1996; 10: 679–682.
12. Mann SJ, Pickering TG. Detection of renovascular hypertension: state of the art: 1992. Ann Intern Med 1992; 117: 845–853.
13. Derkx FHM, Schalekamp MADH. Renal artery stenosis and hypertension. Lancet 1994; 344: 237–239.
14. Harding MB, Smith LR, Himmelstein SI, Harrison K, Phillips HR, Schwab SJ, Hermiller JB, Davidson CJ, Bashore TM. Renal artery stenosis: prevalence and associated risk factors in patients undergoing routine cardiac catheterization. J Am Soc Nephrol 1992; 2(11): 1608–1616.
15. Hansen KJ, Benjamin ME, Appel RG, Craven TE, Dean RH. Renovascular hypertension in the elderly: results of surgical management. Geriatric Nephrology and Urology 1996; 6: 3–11.
16. Erbslöh-Möller B, Dumas A, Roth D, Sfakianakis GN, Bourgoignie JJ. Furosemide-^{131}

I-hippuran renography after angiotensin-converting enzyme inhibition for the diagnosis of renovascular hypertension. Am J Med 1991; 90: 23–29.
17. Wilcox CS. Use of angiotensin-converting-enzyme inhibitors for diagnosing renovascular hypertension. Kidney Int 1993; 44: 1379–1390.
18. Cristol L, Walker B, Henrich WL. Distal vessel atherosclerosis as a cause for false-positive renal scintigraphy. Renal Failure 1996; 18(6): 923–930.
19. Farrugia E, King BF, Larson TS. Magnetic resonance angiography and detection of renal artery stenosis in a patient with impaired renal function. Mayo Clin Proc 1993; 68: 157–160.
20. Weaver FA, Pentecost MJ, Yellin AE, Davis S, Finck E, Teitelbaum G. Clinical applications of carbon dioxide/digital subtraction arteriography. J Vasc Surg 1991; 13: 272–273.
21. Ilélénon O, Rody FE, Correas JM, Melki P, Chauveau D, Chrétien Y, Moreau JF. Color doppler US of renovascular disease in native kidneys. Radiographics 1995; 15: 833–854.
22. Blum U, Krumme B, Flügel P, Gabelmann A, Lehnert T, Buitrago-Tellez C, Schollmeyer P, Langer M. Treatment of ostial renal-artery stenoses with vascular endoprostheses after unsuccessful balloon angioplasty. NEJM 1997; 336(7): 459–465.
23. Harden PN, MacLeod MJ, Rodger RSC, Baxter GM, Connell JMC, Dominiczak AF, Junor BJR, Briggs JD, Moss JG. Effect of renal-artery stenting on progression of renovascular renal failure. Lancet 1997; 349: 1133–1136.
24. Van Damme H, Jeusette F, Pans A, Defraigne JO, Creemers E, Albert A, Limet R. The impact of renal revascularisation on renal dysfunction. Eur J Vasc Endovasc Surg 1995; 10: 330–337.
25. Bonelli FS, McKusick MA, Textor SC, Kos PB, Stanson AW, Johnson CM, Sheedy II PF, Welch TJ, Schirger A. Renal artery angioplasty; technical results and clinical outcome in 320 patients. Mayo Clin Proc 1995; 70: 1041–1052.
26. Tegtmeyer CJ. Percutaneous renal revascularization. Mayo Clin Proc 1995; 70: 1127–1129.
27. Zuccalà A, Zucchelli P. Atherosclerotic renal artery stenosis – when is intervention by PTA or surgery justified? Nephrol Dial Transplant 1995; 10: 585–600.

Diabetic Nephropathy in Patients with Type II Diabetes

JULIA LEWIS
Division of Nephrology, Vanderbilt University, Medical Center, Nashville, TN, U.S.A.

Diabetic nephropathy is the single most common cause of end-stage renal disease (ESRD) in the United States. Patients with diabetes account for 35% of all those enrolled in the Medicare ESRD Program and, at current rates of increase, patients with diabetes will soon account for 50% of all ESRD patients [1]. Most of these patients have Type II diabetes and are elderly [2]. In 1992 the cost of caring for these patients' renal disease alone exceeded 2 billion dollars per year in the United States [1]. Similarly, European registry data reveal a dramatic increase in the incidence of ESRD due to diabetic nephropathy [2]. In European renal replacement programs, the relative increase in acceptance rates has been considerably greater for patients classed as having Type II diabetes than for those with Type I diabetes. This dramatic increase in Type II diabetes and diabetic nephropathy in both Europe and the United States reflects the epidemic of Type II diabetes worldwide [4]. Also it may reflect the increased survival of patients with Type II diabetes and proteinuria. In Germany the survival rate, five years after the onset of proteinuria, for a patient with Type II diabetes was 35% in the period 1966 to 1975, but rose to 75% from 1976 to 1985 [5].

Despite the increased survival in patients with Type II diabetes and diabetic nephropathy, a discrepancy persists between the incidence of early renal failure, as detected by elevated serum creatinine, and the incidence of ESRD in patients with Type II diabetes. The incidence of elevated serum creatinine is 176 per million per year and the incidence of ESRD is 95 per million per year [6]. This striking difference is due to attrition primarily from death from atherosclerotic cardiovascular disease.

Risk Factors for the Development of Renal Disease

The variety of risk factors for the development of renal disease in patients with Type II diabetes are shown in Table 1. Race is an important risk factor; compared to Caucasian populations, a dramatically higher incidence of renal disease related to Type II diabetes is reported among a variety of minority

Dimitrios G. Oreopoulos (ed.), Nephrology and Geriatrics Integrated, 77–89.

Table 1.

Risk Factors for Development of Renal Disease in Type II Diabetes
○ Race: African Americans, Native Americans, Polynesians, Maori, Mexican Americans
○ Gender: African American males at greater risk than African American females
○ Family history
○ Smoking
○ Hypertension
○ Hyperglycemia

populations including Australian Aborigines, Polynesians, Maori, African-Americans, Mexican-Americans, and Native Americans [7–11]. It is unclear whether the susceptibility to diabetic nephropathy in these populations with Type II diabetes is due to genetic factors, socioeconomic factors or environmental exposures. Patients with Type II diabetes, who have either one or two parents with diabetes and proteinuria, are at much greater risk of developing proteinuria themselves [12]. Although these data suggest a shared genetic susceptibility, the influence of common environmental factors has not been evaluated. In Pima Indians in the United States in whom the prevalence of Type II diabetes is nearly 50% at age 35, the cumulative incidence of diabetic nephropathy is 50% after diabetes of 20 years duration [13]. Because of the high prevalence and early age of onset of Type II diabetes, many Pima families have diabetes in two generations and, among them, familial clustering of diabetic nephropathy has been demonstrated.

Hypertension is common among patients with Type II diabetes and often precedes the onset of their illness [14]. Several studies suggest that elevated blood pressure is a risk factor for the subsequent development of diabetic nephropathy. Hypertension is more prevalent in patients with Type II diabetes, who have renal disease, than among those with Type II diabetes and no evidence of renal involvement [15]. Patients with diabetes who subsequently develop proteinuria are more likely to be hypertensive and more severely hypertensive before the development of diabetic nephropathy than those matched for age, gender and duration of diabetes, who never go on to develop nephropathy. Two of four studies in patients with Type II diabetes found increased sodium-lithium countertransport rates that suggest a genetic predisposition to hypertension in those with Type II diabetes and diabetic kidney disease [16–19].

Hyperglycemia may itself be a risk factor for the development of diabetic nephropathy in patients with Type II diabetes. Cross-sectional cohort studies, seeking a relationship between glycemic control and the development of nephropathy have given variable results [20]. The recent United Kingdom Prospective Diabetes Study (UKPDS) showed that more stringent blood glucose control slowed the progression of diabetic microvascular but not macrovascular disease; this suggests that higher blood sugars are a risk factor for the complications of diabetes including renal disease [21].

Lastly, cigarette smoking is a strong predictor of renal disease in patients with Type II diabetes [22] but the mechanism by which smoking increases the risk of subsequent nephropathy is unclear. However, tobacco smoking has been shown to cause vasoconstriction, impaired platelet function, and abnormalities of coagulation [23–24].

Natural History of Type II Diabetic Nephropathy

In contrast to Type I diabetes, it is often difficult to determine the time of onset of Type II diabetes. Thus studies of the natural history of Type II diabetic nephropathy are more difficult because the duration of diabetes is often unknown (Fig. 1). However, careful studies of its natural history, done in the Pima Indians in Arizona, among whom the onset of Type II diabetes is identified by frequent glucose tolerance testing, show that the natural history of diabetic nephropathy is similar to that in Type I diabetes [25]. Although

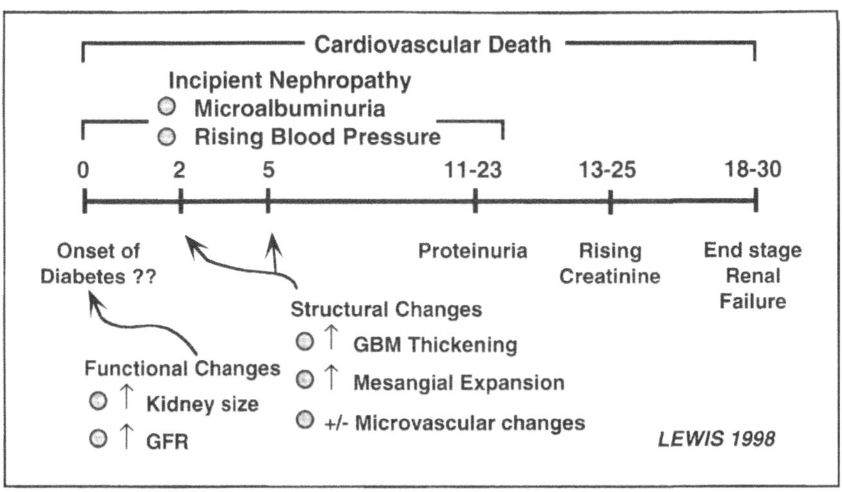

Figure 1.

much controversy surrounds the data reported in Caucasian patients with Type II diabetes at least some of these natural history studies suggest a course similar to that in Type I diabetes [26].

Functional Changes

Patients in whom the onset of Type II diabetes is clearly identified, such as the Pima Indians, have glomerular hyperfiltration at the onset of diabetes [27, 28]. The average GFR iothalamate clearance in Pima Indians is 15% higher than in non-diabetic controls [29]. The findings in Caucasian populations show some variability, which may reflect differences in the time at which the measurement of GFR was made in relation to the onset of diabetes. No one has examined early increases in glomerular filtration rate in patients with Type II diabetes, to see whether they correlate with later progression to overt diabetic nephropathy, as has been reported in patients with Type I diabetes.

Similarly, reports have been variable concerning the presence of renal hypertrophy and reversible microalbuminuria at the onset of Type II diabetes [30]. Although there is evidence for impaired glomerular charge selectivity in patients with Type II diabetes [29], the extent of renal hypertrophy may be limited in those with uncomplicated Type II disease. In fact, kidney size may perhaps be reduced in these patients because of superimposed hypertensive and atherosclerotic microvascular disease.

Structural Changes

Within a few years after the onset of Type II diabetes and the early functional changes described above, one can detect structural or morphologic changes on renal biopsy. The characteristic histologic changes of diabetic nephropathy include glomerular basement membrane thickening – a sensitive measure of the presence of diabetes, mesangial expansion, diffuse or nodular glomerulosclerosis and microvascular changes, including arteriolar hyperplasia and hyalinosis. From renal biopsy studies it appears that the morphological lesions of diabetic nephropathy in Type II diabetes is indistinguishable from those in with Type I diabetes [31]. However, two recent reports suggest that this may not be true, at least in a subset of patients with Type II disease [32, 33]. These reports describe two distinct patterns of glomerular pathology in Type II diabetes and nephropathy. In one instance, the classical glomerular lesion of nodular glomerulosclerosis (Kimmelstiel-Wilson lesion) is prominent, while in the other, there is mesangial or nephroangiosclerosis without nodular changes. The lesion in non-nodular glomerular mesangial sclerosis appears to be less commonly associated with diabetic retinopathy than does the classical Kimmelstiel-Wilson lesion. These lesions also may have prognostic differences.

Microalbuminuria

In careful studies of natural history, microalbuminuria and elevations in mean arterial blood pressure appear anywhere from five to 15 years after the onset of Type II diabetes. However, because in most patients the time of onset of diabetes is unknown, it is possible that microalbuminuria is present at the time of diagnosis. Current guidelines recommend that all patients with Type II diabetes be tested for microalbuminuria at the time of diagnosis and yearly thereafter. If microalbuminuria excretion is elevated, the test should be repeated to confirm the presence of persistent microalbuminuria and to rule out other transient causes of increased albumin excretion, including uncontrolled hypertension, uncontrolled congestive heart failure, increased physical exercise and hyperglycemia. Before the diagnosis is established, one should have collected two of three abnormal specimens over a period of three to six months. Urine dipsticks that screen for microalbuminuria rather than protein excretion are adequate for the screening of large populations [34].

In recent cross-sectional studies of patients with newly diagnosed Type II diabetes, the prevalence of microalbuminuria varies between 10 and 40% [5, 35–38]. The Appropriate Blood Pressure Control and Diabetes Trial, a large prospective randomized clinical trial, was designed to compare the effects of moderate versus intensive hypertensive control on the frequency of diabetic complications [39]. This trial found that 29% of the 933 patients in baseline had microalbuminuria – defined as a urinary albumin excretion between 20 and 200 micrograms per minute.

Several longitudinal studies suggest that, once microalbuminuria appears, it progresses to proteinuria in 22–50% of patients over five to 10 years [14, 40–44]. In some studies this rate of progression is slower than it is in patients with Type I diabetes. In part this slower progression reflects the many factors contributing to microalbuminuria in some patients with Type II diabetes. Elevated urinary albumin excretion may be due to hypertension or other underlying renal diseases. Also fewer patients progress from microalbuminuria to proteinuria and end-stage renal disease because of the attrition in these patients due to cardiovascular deaths. Microalbuminuria is a major risk factor for death in patients with Type II diabetes. Of 503 patients with Type II diabetes, who were followed for 10 years, only 3% died from uremia but 58% died of cardiovascular causes [45]. Those with microalbuminuria were at much greater risk of cardiovascular death than those with normal urinary albumin excretion. Indeed, in a retrospective study of Type II diabetes, microalbuminuria was second only to hypercholesterolemia as a risk factor for mortality and was an independent predictor of all causes (chiefly cardiovascular) mortality [46]. This association of microalbuminuria and increased risk of cardiovascular death accounts at least partly for a reduction in the number of patients with established microalbuminuria, who progress to proteinuria and ESRD.

Proteinuria and Declining Renal Function

In these patients, one must exclude important causes of renal insufficiency and proteinuria other than diabetic nephropathy. Many patients with Type II diabetes are elderly and have risk factors for other renal diseases. Retrospective series and prospective biopsy studies have found that renal diseases other than diabetic nephropathy range from 8 to 23% [47–50]. A recent prospective study, in which renal biopsies were performed on 30 patients, found only 10% with a diagnosis other than diabetic nephropathy [32].

Renal diseases reported to be coincident with diabetes include glomerulopathies such as IgA nephropathy, polycystic kidney disease, ischemic nephropathy and analgesic nephropathy. However it is likely that the vast majority of patients with proteinuria and Type II diabetes have diabetic nephropathy. In those with Type I diabetes and diabetic nephropathy a strong association has been reported between diabetic retinopathy and nephropathy. Of patients with Type I diabetes and diabetic nephropathy, 90–95% have evidence of diabetic retinopathy. A recent prospective biopsy series in patients with Type II diabetes have found that only 60–65% of those with Type II diabetes and diabetic nephropathy have diabetic retinopathy [32]. Thus, in patients with Type II diabetes, the absence of diabetic retinopathy is not as strong a predictor of the presence of an alternate form of renal disease accounting for proteinuria as it is in those with Type I diabetes. When indicated, tests including serum protein electrophoresis and serologies may help to identify other forms of renal pathology. In addition a patient with gross or persistent microscopic hematuria may require a renal biopsy.

Once a patient with Type II diabetes develops proteinuria, a decline in renal function appears to be inevitable. In these patients the presence of hypertension, poor blood sugar control, dyslipidemia and cigarette smoking all lead to a more rapid decline in renal function. The median duration from onset of proteinuria to the development of chronic renal failure is seven years with a rate of decline of GFR of 4 to 12 mL/min/year [26, 51–52]. Studies among Pima Indians found a cumulative incidence of ESRD of 40% at 10 years and 61% at 15 years after the onset of proteinuria [53]. Interestingly, this population, unlike Caucasian patients with Type II diabetes, do not show a dramatic increase in the incidence of cardiovascular disease. Therefore, attrition due to high cardiovascular mortality may account for some of the difference in cumulative incidences of ESRD reported in different studies.

ESRD

Once ESRD develops in patients with Type II diabetes, overall survival with any mode of renal replacement therapy is much shorter than for age-matched, non-diabetic patients. In one study of 78 patients with Type II diabetes and ESRD, 58% were alive at one year and only 14% at five years, irrespective of the mode of renal replacement therapy [54]. Most of these patients die of atherosclerotic cardiovascular disease. In patients with a history of cardiovascular disease, renal transplantation does not offer a survival advantage over dialysis. However, survival of patients without a history of vascular complications has been shown to vary with the mode of treatment among patients without prior atherosclerotic cardiovascular disease e.g. renal transplantation is associated with a much higher survival rate than hemodialysis [54].

Strategies for Preventing Progressive Nephropathy in Type II Diabetes

Fewer studies have examined therapeutic interventions to slow or halt the progression of nephropathy in patients with Type II diabetes than in those with Type I diabetes, in part because this heterogeneous, older population has a high incidence of cardiovascular mortality and presents many challenges to the conduct of clinical trials. Therapeutic interventions supported by some evidence of beneficial effect include glycemic control, control of hypertension, the use of specific antihypertensive agents, low protein diets, and the treatment of dyslipidemia.

Glycemic Control

The Diabetes Control and Complications Trial (DCCT) has shown that tighter glycemic control prevents the development of microalbuminuria in patients with Type I diabetes [55]. The United Kingdom Prospective Diabetes Study (UKPDS) randomized 3867 newly diagnosed patients with Type II diabetes to conventional diet therapy with a goal of a fasting blood glucose of less than 15.0 mmol/L, or to intensive treatment with sulphonylureas, metformin or insulin and a goal of a fasting plasma glucose less than 6.0 mmol/L [21]. Of the 1138 patients randomized to conventional diet treatment, ultimately, 702 received therapy with either sulphonylureas or insulin or metformin. Patients in the intensive treatment group were randomized to receive insulin or sulphonylureas initially with the subsequent addition of metformin in a subset of these patients. This study had a complex design and many changes were made in the protocol over the 14 years during which patients were recruited to it and during the median follow-up of 11 years. However, over the first 10 years of follow-up the authors demonstrated an 11% reduction in median HbAlc in the patients in the intensive group, compared to those in the conventional therapy group [21]. The intensive treatment group had a 25% reduction in the risk of microvascular endpoints. Most of this risk reduction was due to fewer patients requiring retinal photocoagulation. The study did not demonstrate that intensive blood glucose control reduced any diabetes-related cause of death or reduced all cause mortality. Similarly, it did not demonstrate any beneficial effect of intensive blood glucose control on individual macro-vascular endpoints, such as myocardial infarction (these endpoints included renal outcomes). Intensive blood sugar control led to a 34% reduction in albuminuria [21]. It is of interest that a subset of patients in this trial, who initially were randomized to intensive blood glucose control with metformin alone, achieved a statistically significant risk reduction of 32% for any diabetes related endpoint, 42% for diabetes-related deaths, and 36% reduction for all cause mortality. However, among the intensive treatment, metformin, and conventional groups, no significant difference was seen between the proportion of patients with urine albumin above 50 mg/L. Only overweight patients with Type II diabetes were randomized to initial intensive glucose control with metformin; these patients had not only a statistically significant decreased risk of diabetes-related end points compared to the conventional group but also had less weight gain and fewer hypoglycemic attacks than patients receiving insulin or sulphonylureas [56]. However, 537 non-overweight patients, who were already on maximal doses of sulphonylurea but still had high fasting plasma glucose levels, were allocated to receive either continued sulphonylurea therapy alone or the addition of metformin. The patients receiving both suplhonylureas and metformin had a statistically significantly higher risk of death than those who continued on sulphonylurea alone. This finding was unexplained [56].

Thus this complex trial (UKPDS), which did not report renal outcomes in any detail yet, at least suggests that intensive blood glucose control might slow the progression of diabetic nephropathy.

Control of Hypertension and the Use of Specific Anti-Hypertensive Agents

Many studies in patients with Type I diabetes have conclusively demonstrated that blood pressure control slows the rate of progression of renal disease [57–59]. However, a variety of small studies among patients with Type II diabetes have given conflicting results concerning the benefit of blood pressure control [60]. Embedded within the UKPDS study was a smaller study to determine whether tight blood pressure control reduced morbidity and mortality in hypertensive patients with Type II diabetes [61]. The authors allocated 758 patients to tight blood pressure control with a goal of less than 150/85 mmHg, and 390 patients to less tight control of blood pressure aimed initially at a target of less than 200/105 mm Hg (in the course of the study, this was modified to less than 180/105 mmHg). During the study, the mean difference in systolic and diastolic blood pressures between the two groups was 10 and 5 mmHg, respectively. In the group assigned to tight control of blood pressure the reductions in risk were 24% in diabetes related-end points, 32% in deaths related to diabetes, 44% in strokes and 37% in microvascular end points [61]. After six years of follow-up, a smaller proportion of those under tight control had a urinary albumin concentration of greater than 50 mg/L, a 29% reduction in risk, and a non-significant (39%) reduction in risk for proteinuria (greater than 300 mg/L) [61]. At nine years follow-up there was no significant reduction in risk for both a urinary albumin concentration of greater than 50 mg/L and proteinuria. There was no significant difference between the two groups, in plasma creatinine concentration or in the proportion of patients, who had a two-fold increase in creatinine concentration.

Of particular interest is to see whether specific anti-hypertensive agents might also protect the kidneys of patients with Type II diabetes. Australian investigators randomized 24 patients with Type II diabetes to either the angiotensin converting enzyme inhibitor (ACE) – perindopril, or the calcium channel blocker – nifedipine [62]. In hypertensive patients, 12 months of treatment with either agent significantly reduced urinary albumin excretion and preserved renal function, suggesting blood pressure control using either ACE inhibitors or calcium channel blockers exercised a beneficial effect. The UKPDS study randomized the group on tight blood pressure control to receive either atenolol – a beta blocker, or captopril – an ACE inhibitor [63]. In this study, reduction of blood pressure with either captopril or atenolol had a similar effect in reducing the incidence of diabetic complications [63].

In contrast to the above data, a multicentered study by Ravid and coworkers randomized 94 patients with Type II diabetes and microalbuminuria to either the ACE inhibitor – enalapril 10 mg/day or placebo, they followed them for five years [64]. More patients in the placebo group received long-acting nifedipine as required for blood pressure control. Compared to placebo, the ACE inhibitor decreased the number of patients, who progressed from microalbuminuria to proteinuria. Renal function as measured by reciprocal creatinine level was also better preserved in patients receiving enalapril.

Clearly ACE inhibitors have a beneficial effect in patients with nephropathy secondary to Type I diabetes. However, as outlined above, the beneficial effects of ACE inhibition have not been clearly established in patients with Type II diabetes mellitus. In such patients ACE inhibitors have some potential for untoward affects, such as hyperkalemia or acute renal failure due to pre-existing renal artery stenosis. Currently the Collaborative Study Group is conducting a multi-center clinical trial in 1600 patients with Type II diabetes randomized to receive either an angiotensin 2 receptor antagonist – irbesartan, a calcium channel blocker – amlodipine, or blood pressure control with conventional antihypertensive agents. Recruitment for this study is complete (as of January 1999) and the planned follow-up is 2 years. There is no outcome until the study ends and data is unblinded.

Low Protein Diets

Low protein diets may be beneficial in patients with renal impairment due to Type I diabetes [65–67]. However, to date, there is insufficient information to conclude that such diets slow the rate of decline in renal function in those with Type II diabetes. The Modification of Diet Renal Disease Study enrolled only 26 patients with Type II diabetes in its cohort of more than 800 and thus could not demonstrate a clear benefit of a low protein diet in slowing the rate of progression of renal disease in these patients [68]. Two studies in patients with Type II diabetes, one in Japan and the other in Canada, demonstrated a beneficial effect of a low-protein diet but less than 30 patients in each study received these diets [69–70].

The Treatment of Dyslipidemia

Dyslipidemia causes a rapid loss of renal function in animal models of renal disease. Similarly, in large epidemiologic studies in humans with Type II diabetes [71–72], dyslipidemia is a strong risk factor for the development of diabetic nephropathy and for a more rapid progression to ESRD. A small-randomized study in 34 patients with Type II diabetes demonstrated that the patients who received a cholesterol-lowering agent, had a slower rate of decline of renal function, compared to those receiving placebo [73]. Clearly, with the high risk of cardiovascular complications in those with Type II diabetes, cholesterol-lowering agents may have multiple beneficial effects.

References

1. U.S. renal data system, USRDS 1995 Annual Data Report. Bethesda, MD: National Institute of Health; 1995.
2. Humphrey LL, Ballard DJ, Forhnert PP, Chu C-P, O'Fallon M, Palumbo PJ. Chronic renal failure in non-insulin-dependent diabetes mellitus. Ann Intern Med 1989; 111: 788–796.
3. Raine AEF. Epidemiology, development and treatment of end-stage renal failure in type 2 (non-insulin-dependent) diabetic patients in Europe. Diabetologia 1993; 36: 1099–1104.
4. Michaelis D, Jutzi E. Epidemiologie des Diabetes mellitus in der Bevölkerung der ehemaligen DDR. Altersund geschlechtsspezifische Inzidenz- und Prävalenztrends im Zeitraum 1960–1987. Z Klin Med 1991; 46: 59–63.
5. Hasslacher C, Borgholte G, Panradl U, Wahl P. Verbesserte prognose von typ-I- und typ-II-diabetikern mit nephropathie. Med Klin 1990; 85: 643–646.
6. Lippert J, Ritz E, Schwarzbeck A, Schneider P. The rising tide of endstage renal failure from diabetic nephropathy type II – an epidemiological analysis. Nephrol Dial Transplant 1995; 10: 462–467.
7. Disney APS. Sixteenth report of the Australia and New Zealand Dialysis and Transplant Registry (ANZDATA). Woodville, Australia: The Queen Elizabeth Hospital; 1996.
8. Cowie CC, Port FK, Wolfe RA, Savage PJ, Moll PP, Hawthorne VM. Disparities in incidence of diabetic end-state renal disease according to race and type of diabetes. N Engl J Med 1989; 321: 1074–1079.
9. Pugh JA, Stern MP, Haffner SM, Eifler CW, Zapata M. Excess incidence of treatment of end-stage renal disease in Mexican Americans. Am J Epidemiol. 1988; 127: 135–144.
10. Newman JM, Marfin AA, Eggers PW, Helgerson SD. End-stage renal disease among native Americans, 1983-86. Am J Public Health 1990; 80: 318–319.
11. Nelson RG, Newman JM, Knowler WC, et al. Incidence of end-stage renal disease in type 2 (non-insulin-dependent) diabetes mellitus in Pima Indians. Diabetologia 1988; 31: 730–736.
12. Pettitt DJ, Saad MF, Bennett PH, Nelson RG, Knowler WC. Familial predisposition to renal disease in two generations of Pima Indians with type 2 (non-insulin-dependent) diabetes mellitus. Diabetologia 1990; 33: 438–443.
13. Kunzelman CL, Knowler WC, Pettitt DJ, Bennett PH. Incidence of proteinuria in type 2 diabetes mellitus in the Pima Indians. Kidney Int 1989; 35: 681–687.
14. Haneda M, Kikkawa R, Togawa M, et al. High blood pressure is a risk factor for the

development of microalbuminuria in Japanese subjects with non-insulin-dependent diabetes mellitus. J Diabet Complications 1992; 6: 181–185.
15. Ritz E. Hypertension and vascular disease as complications of diabetes. In: Laragh JH, Brenner BM, editors. Hypertension - Pathophysiology, Diagnosis and Management. New York, NY: Raven Press, 1990; 1705–1706.
16. Pinkney JH, Foyle WJ, Denver AE, Mohamed-Ali V, McKinlay S, Yudkin JS. The relationship of urinary albumin excretion rate to ambulatory blood pressure and erythrocyte sodium-lithium countertransport in NIDDM. Diabetologia 1995; 38(3): 356–362.
17. Rutherford PA, Thomas TH, Taylor R, Wilkinson R. Nephropathy and changes in sodium-lithium countertransport kinetics in type 2 (non-insulin-dependent) diabetes mellitus. Human Hypert 1994; 8(1): 29–35.
18. Gall MA, Rossing P, Jensen JS, Funder J, Parving HH. Red cell Na^+/Li^+ countertransport in non-insulin-dependent diabetics with diabetic nephropathy. Kidney International 1991; 39(1): 135–140.
19. Fujita, J, Tsuda K, Seno M, Obayashi H, Fukui I, Seino Y. Erythrocyte sodium-lithium countertransport activity as a marker of predisposition to hypertension and diabetic nephropathy in NIDDM. Diabetes Care 1991; 17(9): 977–982.
20. Ballard DJ, Humphrey LL, Melton LJ III, et al. Epidemiology of persistent proteinuria in type II diabetes mellitus: population-based study in Rochester, Minnesota. Diabetes. 1988; 37: 405–412.
21. UK Prospective Diabetes Study (UKPDS) Group. Intensive blood-glucose control with sulphonylureas or insulin compared with conventional treatment and risk of complications in patients with type 2 diabetes (UKPDS 33). Lancet 1998; 352: 837–853.
22. Sawicki PT, Didjurgeit U, Muhlhauser I, Bender R, Heinemann L, Berger M. Smoking is associated with progression of diabetic nephropathy. Diabetes Care 1994; 17: 126–131.
23. Paterson AM, Mancia G, Fitzgerald GA. Proceeding of the symposium on smoking: a risk factor for cardiovascular disease. Am Hear J 1988; 115 (suppl 2, part 2): S240–S294.
24. Deckert T, Feldt-Rasmussen B, Borch-Johnsen K, Jensen T, Kofoed-Enevoldsen A. Albuminuria reflects widespread vascular damage. The Steno hypothesis. Diabetologia 1989; 32(4): 219–226.
25. Nelson RG, Knowler WC, McCance DR, et al. Determinants of end-stage renal disease in Pima Indians with type 2 (non-insulin-dependent) diabetes mellitus and proteinuria. Diabetologia 1993; 36: 1087–1093.
26. Pugh JA, Medina R, Ramirez M. Comparison of the course to end-stage renal disease of type 1 (insulin-dependent) and type 2 (non-insulin-dependent) diabetic nephropathy. Diabetologia 1993; 36: 1094–1098.
27. Nowack R, Raum E, Blum W, Ritz E. Renal hemodynamics in recent-onset type II diabetes. Am J Kidney Dis 1992; 20: 342–347.
28. Myers BD, Nelson RG, Williams GW, et al. Glomerular function in Pima Indians with non-insulin-dependent diabetes mellitus of recent onset. J Clin Invest 1991; 88: 524–530.
29. Myers BD, Nelson RG, Williams GW, Bennett PH, Hardy SA, Berg RL, Loon N, Knowler WC, Mitch WE. Glomerular function in Pima Indians with noninsulin-dependent diabetes mellitus of recent onset. J Clin Invest 1991; 8(2): 524–530.
30. Schmidt K, Pesce C, Liu Q, Nelson RG, Bennett PH, Karnitschnig H, Striker LJ, Striker GE. Large glomerular size in Pima Indians: lack of change with diabetic nephropathy. JASN 1992; 3(2): 229–235.
31. Walker JD, Close CF, Jones SL, Rafftery M, Keen H, Viberti G, Osterby R. Glomerular structure in type-1 (insulin-dependent) diabetic patients with normo- and microalbuminuria. Kidney International 1992; 41(4): 741–748.
32. Schwartz MM, Lewis EJ, Leonard-Martin T, Lewis JB, Battle D, and The Collaborative Study Group. Renal pathology patterns in type II diabetes mellitus: relationship with retinopathy. Nephrol Dial Transplant 1998; 13: 2547–2552.
33. Gambara V, Mecca G, Remuzzi G, Bertani T. Heterogeneous nature of renal lesions in type II diabetes. J Am Soc Nephrol 1993; 3: 1458–1466.

34. Minetti EE, Cozzi MG, Granata S, Guidi E. Accuracy of the urinary albumin titrator stick 'Micral-Test' in kidney-disease patients. Nephrol Dial Transplant 1997; 12: 78–80.
35. Gall M-A, Rossing P, Skott P, et al. Prevalence of micro- and macroalbuminuria, arterial hypertension, retinopathy and large vessel disease in European type 2 (non-insulin-dependent) diabetic patients. Diabetologia 1991; 34: 655–661.
36. Savage S, Nagel NJ, Estacio RO, Lukken N, Schrier RW. Clinical factors associated with urinary albumin excretion in type II diabetes. Am J Kidney Dis 1995; 25: 836–844.
37. De F. Olivarius N, Andreasen AH, Keiding N, Mogensen CE. Epidemiology of renal involvement in newly-diagnosed middle-aged and elderly diabetic patients. Cross-sectional data from the population-based study 'Diabetes Care in General Practice', Denmark. Diabetologia 1993; 36: 1007–1016.
38. UK Prospective Diabetes Study Group. Study design, progress and performance. Diabetologia 1991; 34: 877–890.
39. Schrier RW, Savage S. Appropriate Blood Pressure Control in Diabetes (ABCD) trial: implications for complications. Am J Kidney Dis 1992; 20: 653–657.
40. Mogensen CE. Microalbuminuria predicts clinical proteinuria and early mortality in maturity-onset diabetes. N Engl J Med 1984; 310: 356–360.
41. Cooper ME, Frauman A, O'Brien RC, Seeman E, Murray RML, Jerums G. Progression of proteinuria in type 1 and type 2 diabetes. Diabet Med 1988; 5: 361–368.
42. John L, Sunder Rao PSS, Kanagasabapathy AS. Rate of progression of albuminuria in type II diabetes. Five-year prospective study from South India. Diabetes Care 1994; 17: 888–890.
43. Ravid M, Savin H, Lang R, Jutrin I, Shoshana L, Lishner M. Proteinuria, renal impairment, metabolic control, and blood pressure in type 2 diabetes mellitus. Arch Intern Med 1992; 152: 1225–1229.
44. Lebovitz HE, Wiegmann TB, Canaan A, et al. Renal protective effects of enalapril in hypertensive NIDDM: role of baseline albuminuria. Kidney Int 1994; 45 (suppl 45): S150–S155.
45. Schmitz A, Vaeth M. Microalbuminuria: a major risk factor in non-insulin-dependent diabetes. A 10-year follow-up study of 503 patients. Diabet Med 1988; 5: 126–134.
46. Mattock MB, Morrish NJ, Viberti GC, Keen H, Fitzgerald AP, Jackson G. Prospective study of microalbuminuria as predictor of mortality in NIDDM. Diabetes 1992; 41: 736–741.
47. Parving H-H, Gall M-A, Skott P, et al. Prevalence and causes of albuminuria in non-insulin-dependent diabetic patients. Kidney Int 1992; 41: 758–762.
48. Amoah E, Glickman JL, Malchoff CD, Sturgill BC, Kaiser DL, Bolton WK. Clinical identification of nondiabetic renal disease in diabetic patients with type I and type II diabetes presenting with renal dysfunction. Am J Nephrol 1988; 8: 204–211.
49. Fabre J, Balant LP, Dayer PG, Fox HM, Vernet AT. The kidney in maturity onset diabetes mellitus: a clinical study of 510 patients. Kidney Int 1982; 21: 7310–7318.
50. Suzuki Y, Ueno M, Hayashi H, et al. A light microscopic study of glomerulosclerosis in Japanese patients with non-insulin-dependent diabetes mellitus: the relationship between clinical and histological features. Clin Nephrol 1994; 42: 155–162.
51. Gall M-A, Nielsen FS, Smidt UM, Parving H-H. The Course of kidney function in type 2 (non-insulin-dependent) diabetic patients with diabetic nephropathy. Diabetologia. 1993; 36: 1071–1078.
52. Hasslacher C, Bostedt-Kiesel A, Kempe HP, Wahl P. Effect of metabolic factors and blood pressure on kidney function in proteinuric type 2(non-insulin-dependent) diabetic patients. Diabetologia 1993; 36: 1051–1056.
53. Nelson RG, Knowler WC, McCance DR, Sievers ML, Pettitt DJ, Charles MA, Hanson RL, Liu QZ, Bennett PH. Determinants of end-stage renal disease in Pima Indians with type 2 (non-insulin-dependent) diabetes mellitus and proteinuria. Diabetologia 1993; 36(10): 1087–1093.
54. Walker WG, Hermann J, Murphy R, Patz A. Elevated blood pressure and angiotensin II

are associated with accelerated loss of renal function in diabetic nephropathy. Trans Am Clin Climatol Assoc 1985; 97: 94–104.
55. Diabetes Control and Complications Trial Research Group. Effect of intensive therapy on the development and progression of diabetic nephropathy in the Diabetes Control and Complications Trial. Kidney Int 1995; 47: 1703–1720.
56. UK Prospective Diabetes Study (UKPDS) Group. Effect of intensive blood-glucose control with metformin on complications in overweight patients with type 2 diabetes (UKPDS 34). Lancet 1998; 352: 854–865.
57. Mogensen CE. Long-term antihypertensive treatment inhibiting progression of diabetic nephropathy. Br Med J 1982; 285: 685–688.
58. Parving H-H, Andersen AR, Smidt UM, Hommel E, Mathiesen ER, Svendsen PA. Effect of antihypertensive treatment on kidney function in diabetic nephropathy. Br Med J 1987; 294: 1443–1447.
59. Björck S, Nyberg G, Mulec H, Granerus G, Herlitz H, Aurell M. Beneficial effects of angiotensin converting enzyme inhibition on renal function in patients with diabetic nephropathy. Br Med J 1986; 293: 471–474.
60. Ritz E, Stefanski A. Diabetic nephropathy in type II diabetes. Am J Kidney Dis 1996; 27: 167–194.
61. UK Prospective Diabetes Study Group. Tight blood pressure control and risk of macrovascular and microvascular complications in type 2 diabetes: UKPDS 38. BMJ 1998; 517: 709–712.
62. Melbourne Diabetic Nephropathy Study Group. Comparison between perindopril and nifedipine in hypertensive and normotensive diabetic patients with microalbuminuria. Br Med J 1991; 302: 210–216.
63. UK Prospective Diabetes Study Group. Efficacy of atenolol and captopril in reducing risk of macrovascular and microvascular complications in type 2 diabetes: UKPDS 39. BMJ 1998; 317: 713–720.
64. Ravid M, Savin H, Jutrin I, Bental T, Katz B, Lishner M. Long-term stabilizing effect of angiotensin-converting enzyme inhibition on plasma creatinine and on proteinuria in normotensive type II diabetic patients. Ann Intern Med 1993; 118: 577–581.
65. Evanoff G, Thompson C, Brown J, Weinman E. Prolonged dietary protein restriction in diabetic nephropathy. Arch Intern Med 1989; 149: 1129–1133.
66. Evanoff GV, Thompson CS, Brown J, Weinman EJ. The effect of dietary protein restriction on the progression of diabetic nephropathy. A 12-month follow-up. Arch Intern Med. 1987; 147: 492–495.
67. Zeller KR, Jacobson H, Raskin P. The effect of dietary protein modification on renal function in diabetic nephropathy-preliminary report of an ongoing study. Kidney Int 1987; 31: 225.
68. Klahr S, Levey AS, Beck GJ, et al. The effects of dietary protein restriction and blood-pressure control on the progression of chronic renal disease. N Engl J Med 1994; 330: 877–884.
69. Pomerleau J, Verdy M, Garrel DR, Nadeau MH. Effect of protein intake on glycaemic control and renal function in type 2 (non-insulin-dependent) diabetes mellitus. Diabetologia 1993; 36: 829–834.
70. Shichiri M, Nishio Y, Ogura M, Marumo F. Effect of protein, very-low-phosphorus diet on diabetic renal insufficiency with proteinuria. Am J Kidney Dis 1991; 18: 26–32.
71. Nelson RG, Knowler WC, Pettitt DJ, Hanson RL, Bennett PH. Incidence and determinants of elevated urinary albumin excretion in Pima Indians with NIDDM. Diabetes Care 1995; 18: 182–187.
72. UK Prospective Diabetes Study Group. Urinary albumin excretion over 3 years in diet-treated type 2 (non-insulin-dependent) diabetic patients, and association with hypertension, hyperglycaemia and hypertriglyceridaemia. Diabetologia 1993; 36: 1021–1029.
73. Lam KSL, Cheng IKP, Janus ED, Pang RWC. Cholesterol-lowering therapy may retard the progression of diabetic nephropathy. Diabetologia 1995; 38: 604–609.

Acute Renal Failure in the Elderly

NORBERT LAMEIRE, ANKE NELDE, HEIDI HOEBEN and RAYMOND VANHOLDER
Renal Division, Department of Internal Medicine, University Hospital, 185, De Pintelaan, 9000 Gent, Belgium

Despite advances in the management of critically ill patients and technological advances in renal replacement therapy (RRT), acute renal failure (ARF) remains a dramatic syndrome with an ominous prognosis. Structural and functional changes in the aging kidney predispose elderly individuals to ARF. The greater incidence of concomitant systemic diseases including cardiac failure, diabetes mellitus and hypertension, and the presence of additional risk factors such as dehydration, investigations with contrast media and nephrotoxic medications, make the elderly very vulnerable. Obstructive uropathy is also more common in the elderly.

Demography and Incidence

The elderly are the fastest growing part of our population. In the United States, the portion of the population over age 65 years has grown from four per cent in 1900 to its current level of approximately 12.7%. It is predicted that by the year 2030 this proportion will reach 20%. In Europe the population above 60 years in 2025 is expected to be around 224 million people [1]. Most ARF in the elderly is associated with multiple system organ failure (MSOF) and occurs chiefly in patients admitted to intensive care units [2]. The true incidence of ARF in the elderly is difficult to estimate, because most published series use different diagnostic criteria of ARF. According to Groeneveld et al. [3], the age-related yearly incidence of ARF rose from 17 per million in adults under 50 years to 949 per million in the 80–89 age groups.

Structural and Functional Alterations in Aging Kidney

A detailed description of these changes, which is beyond the scope of this paper, can be found in Ref. [4]. Under normal conditions, these alterations in aging kidneys may have no major clinical impact because the renal functional reserve is sufficient to meet the excretory demands. However, the

Oreopoulos et al. (eds.), Nephrology and Geriatrics Integrated, 91–111.

adaptive capacity is limited and aging may adversely affect the course of a superimposed renal disease. The pre-existent reduction in functional reserve in the aging kidney may magnify an excretory defect caused by any new insult like volume changes or toxic drugs. Lameire et al. [5] have pointed out that in combination with dehydration a disturbance in the autoregulatory defence adaptations of renal blood flow and glomerular filtration rate leading to reductions in renal perfusion pressure, may rapidly provoke ischemic damage in aged kidneys [5]. Another mediator, nitric oxide (NO), may play a role in the propensity of the elderly for more frequent ARF. Studies have shown that NO synthesis blockade decreases renal blood flow, GFR, and glomerular capillary permeability (Kf) more in aging than in young rats; this suggests that NO may play a greater role in controlling renal function in advancing age than in the young [6].

Studies in a rat model of gentamicin-induced renal failure show that an increased glomerular NO production seems to protect renal function by counteracting the vasoconstrictor substances released during ARF [7].

When old and young animals are treated with equivalent doses of gentamicin, older animals show a more severe renal failure, reflected in a greater increase in serum creatinine and a more pronounced decrease in creatinine clearance. In basal conditions, aging rats showed a lower glomerular NO production, and a markedly blunted stimulation of NO synthesis by gentamicin [8].

Thus it can be deduced that a partial mechanism for the increased severity of gentamicin-induced ARF in older animals is the decreased production of glomerular NO. Aging tubular cells may be more vulnerable to ischemic damage because cellular antioxidant defences decline with age and oxidant injury may be a critical determinant of ischemic ARF. Miura et al. [9] suggest that, in addition to the changes in RBF and GFR, alterations in the metabolism and biochemistry of aging tubular cells may mediate age-related enhancement of ischemic renal cell injury.

Causes of Acute Renal Failure in the Elderly

In the elderly ARF is frequently multifactorial, as it is in other age groups. Elderly patients show the same spectrum of causes of ARF as young patients but, within that spectrum, there are significant differences [10]. Some forms of ARF have a particularly high incidence in the aged.

Prerenal ARF

The main cause of acute prerenal failure is a decreased perfusion of the kidney. Most of these hypoperfusion episodes are reversible with adequate fluid replacement but others go on to postischemic ATN. This evolution to ATN is more frequent in the elderly than in younger patients (23% versus 15%) [11]. In our series [12], 19% of ATN was due to hypovolemia. Decreased perfusion of the kidney can develop in many clinical settings, e.g. from a decrease in cardiac output or hypovolemia caused by gastrointestinal losses due to vomiting and/or diarrhea, bleeding, renal losses due to glycosuria and use of diuretics.

Frequently hypovolemia is due to dehydration, which affects approximately one per cent of all community hospital admissions in elderly individuals [13]. Up to 25% of non-ambulatory geriatric patients are mildly dehydrated [14]. In elderly nursing home residents particular risk factors for dehydration include acute febrile illnesses, multipharmacy intake – especially diuretics and laxatives, age over 85 years, and being bedridden [15]. In such persons urinary and lower respiratory tract infections are the most common diagnoses associated with fever. Hypernatremia, an indicator of dehydration, is seen in 25% of all febrile patients [15]. Untreated, the mortality, associated with dehydration, exceeds 50% [16].

In the elderly it is difficult to make the diagnosis of hypovolemic acute prerenal failure because the clinical signs and symptoms of dehydration often are unreliable. Furthermore, the traditional urinary parameters for differentiating prerenal from renal failure must be interpreted with caution, because they may merely reflect age-related disturbances in tubular handling of sodium and water. First, in view of the chronic reduction in urinary concentrating ability, urinary sodium and osmolality may not achieve 'prerenal' values during acute renal insults. Second, an elevated urinary sodium or urinary fractional excretion of sodium (FE Na) in an elderly patient may suggest an established parenchymal injury, but prerenal hypoperfusion may still be present and should be corrected. It has been known for some time that the FE Na is unreliable in sodium-retaining states such as chronic heart failure, decompensated cirrhosis, after diuretic therapy, after administration of contrast agents, in pigment-induced nephropathy, and in sepsis [17, 18].

The Renal Causes of ARF

1. *Renovascular Diseases*

Acute obstruction of the renal vasculature by thrombosis of the renal artery or its intrarenal branches or by emboli are more common in the elderly than was previously thought.

Cholesterol Embolization

Embolization from an ulcerating atheromatous aorta may occur spontaneously or as a consequence of surgical manipulation or bypass of vessels, angioplasty, or arteriography. Renal microembolization is responsible for one-third of ARF that develops after emergency operation for abdominal aortic aneurysm;

this may explain why, in this setting, patients may develop ARF without hypotension.

When ARF occurs after an angiographic procedure, the syndrome of renal cholesterol embolism usually appears after two to four weeks, in contrast with radiocontrast ARF, which develops a few days after the procedure. One may expect recovery of renal function in only 30–40% of these cases [19, 20]. However, even fully occluded arteries can be safely and effectively recanalized [21].

The most common presenting symptoms are flank pain with or without low-grade fever, and leukocytosis. Macroscopic or microscopic hematuria is not always present. The syndrome is characterised by accelerated hypertension, acute or chronic renal failure, acute deterioration of known or unknown pre-existing ischemic nephropathy, neurologic symptoms, visual disturbances, gastrointestinal hemorrhage, or pancreatitis. Ischemic changes of the feet or legs, which are common, present as purpura, livedo reticularis, gangrene, and non-healing vascular ulcerations. Common laboratory features are blood eosinophilia, an acute phase response and a low serum complement [22]. The diagnosis of cholesterol embolization can be established by kidney biopsy in 31%, muscle biopsy in 21%, skin biopsy in 17%, postmortem in 22% and clinically in only 9% of the cases.

Some believe that anticoagulant treatment, including streptokinase and tissue-type plasminogen activator predisposes to the development of cholesterol crystal embolization because it interferes with platelet-fibrin thrombus interaction and with the stabilisation of cholesterol crystals embedded within atheromatous plaques [23]. In contrast, total occlusion of both renal arteries, which usually is manifested by anuria, minimal output of urine may be seen in cholesterol emboli and hence the differential diagnosis from other forms of ARF may become difficult. Total or partial recovery of renal function has been observed with temporary RRT. Thus, in view of the contraindication to anticoagulant therapy, one should prefer peritoneal dialysis [24, 25].

Acute Renal Artery Thrombosis

ARF due to complete renal artery thrombosis occurs when the occlusion is bilateral or, with unilateral acute thrombosis in the presence of a nonfunctioning, contralateral kidney. Typically, in complete occlusion leading to total or segmental renal infarction, the patient complains of an acute onset of nausea, vomiting, flank pain, and fever. Approximately one-third of these patients have gross or microscopic hematuria. The most useful laboratory test is a markedly elevated plasma lactate dehydrogenase (LDH) level, with little or no elevation in plasma transaminases. In patients with acute renal-artery occlusion, the urinary concentrations of sodium, urea, creatinine, and osmolality may be similar to those found in the serum. The calculated FE Na is close to 100% [26].

The diagnostic work-up should include DTPA renal scanning, which demonstrates markedly diminished or absent renal perfusion, followed by aortography with delayed views to define reconstitution of the distal renal artery and a nephrogram. TEE is useful to localize aortic atheromatosis and may help identify those who are at risk before intra-aortic catheterisation is undertaken [27].

The optimal treatment for renal infarction is uncertain, but generally medical therapy is preferred. Although surgery can restore vascular patency, it is associated with a higher mortality rate; renal functional recovery is no better than with anticoagulation or thrombolytic therapy alone [28–30].

Early surgery remains the treatment of choice in patients with traumatic renal artery thrombosis, particularly if it is performed within the first few hours [31]. Medical therapy will improve renal function only if the occlusion is incomplete or if effective thrombolysis is initiated within 90 to 180 minutes, which represents the tolerance of normal renal tissue to ischemia [30].

In most cases the standard anticoagulant regimen in this setting has been intravenous heparin followed by oral warfarin. Thrombolytic therapy – with streptokinase or tissue-type plasminogen activator can effectively lyse the occluding thrombus [30, 32]. However, one should consider this modality only with early diagnosis when the ischemic renal tissue is still viable [30].

The risk of systemic bleeding can be minimized by local intra-arterial infusion of the thrombolytic agent, rather by intravenous administration [30, 32]. In patients with severe renal failure in whom there is no functional recovery within 4–6 weeks one can consider surgical revascularization. Late embolectomy has improved renal function in selected patients, indicating that the ischemic atrophy still can be reversed [33].

2. *Hemodynamically-Mediated ARF*

Direct interference with the protective autoregulatory mechanisms of RBF and GFR, either by disease or after pharmacological interventions may precipitate acute renal insufficiency. Drugs commonly prescribed to the elderly and known to impair renal autoregulation or to interfere with the vasodilatory capacity include prostaglandin-synthesis inhibitors, like aspirin and non-steroidal anti-inflammatory drugs (NSAIDs), and angiotensin-converting enzyme (ACE) inhibitors, or angiotensin receptor antagonists, and loop diuretics. If it is essential to treat with these drugs, the patient's renal function should be monitored closely and frequently.

a. *Non Steroidal Anti-Inflammatory Drugs (NSAID)*

Inhibition of the production of vasodilatory prostaglandins by NSAIDs can potentiate the renal vasoconstrictive effects of renal nerves, the alpha-adrenergic system, angiotensin II and vasopressin [34]. In the presence of reduced RBF, as in the 'normal' aged kidney, this prostaglandin inhibition may lead to ARF [35], particularly in elderly hypertensive patients, who have a significant reduction in urinary prostaglandin E2 secretion [36]. Well-known risk factors for NSAID-induced nephrotoxicity include age above 60 with atherosclerotic cardiovascular disease, pre-existing chronic renal insufficiency (serum creatinine > 180 mmol/L), and renal hypoperfusion states such as sodium depletion, diuretic use, hypotension, and sodium-avid states such as decompensated hepatic cirrhosis, nephrotic syndrome, and congestive heart failure [37]. There is, however, little evidence that NSAIDs impair renal function in otherwise healthy elderly individuals. In this cause of ARF, the hyperkalaemia sometimes is out of proportion to the degree of renal impairment, especially when these patients also receive potassium-sparing diuretics or ACE-inhibitors.

A large multicenter French study, covering one year, calculated that NSAIDs represented only 15.3% of all instances of drug-induced ARF but these drugs were incriminated in more than 25% of those over 60 years of age [38].

In a large epidemiological study in a general internal medicine practice only 0.5% of 1908 patients treated with iboprufen [39] suffered serious renal dysfunction. Although iboprufen was not causally related to the renal functional impairment, the drug is considered to be a risk factor in patients older than 65 years and in those suffering from coronary artery disease.

b. *ACE Inhibitors or Angiotensin Receptor Anatagonists*

Although we have relatively little experience with the recently marketed angiotensin receptor anatgonists, their intrarenal effects should be similar to the ACE inhibitors, and lead to the same spectrum of renal complications.

The syndrome of hemodynamic ARF caused by this class of drugs develops either in patients with a stenosis of the renal artery in a solitary kidney, or with bilateral renal artery stenosis. However, those with severe chronic heart failure, polycystic kidney disease, or intrarenal nephrosclerosis without renal artery stenosis also are at risk. In the elderly the frequency of ARF induced by ACE inhibitors has been estimated to vary between six to 23% in patients with bilateral renal-artery stenosis and increases to 38% in those with unilateral stenosis in a single kidney [40–42]. It has been calculated that ACE inhibitors were the cause of ARF in only 0.4% of an unselected population [38]. Elderly patients suffering from 'ischemic' kidney disease probably have a relatively high incidence of unsuspected bilateral renal artery stenosis. Frequently this overlooked disease is recognized after the acute deterioration of the chronically impaired renal function after starting therapy with ACE inhibitors.

3. *Acute Tubular Necrosis (ATN)*

The most frequent cause of ARF in both young and older patients is post-ischemic or postnephrotoxic ATN [10, 12]. The overall incidence of the non-oliguric form of ATN ranges between 25 and 87%. Characteristically the renal insults that cause this form of ATN include aminoglycoside nephrotoxicity, radiocontrast-induced ATN, rhabdomyolysis-induced ATN, and ATN complicating open heart surgery [43], but any insult that causes oliguric ATN can also result in the non-oliguric form of the disease. Although, for didactic reasons, we make the distinction between ischemic and toxic ATN, ATN in any age category frequently is the result of combined risk factors [12, 44]. Furthermore, the interaction between renal hypoperfusion and nephrotoxins is at least additive and probably synergistic. Particularly in older patients with ATN, several chronic premorbid conditions, i.e. congestive heart failure, hypertension, or diabetes mellitus predispose to the development of acute tubular necrosis.

a. *Post-Ischemic ATN*

In tertiary-care hospitals, this type of ATN accounts for approximately 50% of all ARF in the elderly [2, 10]. Complications of major surgery account for about 30% of all post-ischemic ATN. Another important factor in post-operative ATN is sepsis, particularly that arising in the abdomen.

Strong predictors of post-operative worsening of renal function are raised preoperative serum creatinine or blood urea levels [45]. Also advanced age and left ventricular dysfunction are associated with a greater risk of postoperative ATN. In contrast, advanced age alone is not predictive of postoperative renal failure. ATN is particularly frequent in aged people after elective or emergency operation for abdominal aortic aneurysm. The most common cause of transient renal ischemia during aortic aneurysm operation is peroperative hypotension due to hypovolemia. A major determinant of the post-operative ATN is the suprarenal aortic clamping time [46].

An important cause of renal failure after aortic clamping and unclamping is renal microembolization (see above), which is responsible for one-third of the postoperative ARF in this setting. Elective surgical repair of abdominal aortic aneurysm now is recommended in patients in their seventies and eighties (see for review Ref. [47]) but it has a mortality of 5%. However, following an operation for a ruptured aneurysm, ATN occurs in 30% of patients and carries a mortality of up to 74%.

Following coronary artery surgery, the three major risk factors were: old age, preoperative renal dysfunction, and postoperative hemodynamic instability, defined as the need of inotropic drugs. Although 16% of these patients developed ARF only 1.2% required dialysis. In the latter category, the mortality was 44% [48]. Of patients at risk for post-operative ATN an abnormally low urine output during cardiopulmonary bypass was one of the earliest peri-operative clinical markers [49].

b. *ATN Secondary to Sepsis*

Elderly individuals are more susceptible to infection and infection, particularly gram-negative septicemia, accounts for another 30% of cases of ARF. Although the absolute numbers of leukocytes in the elderly are similar to those in younger individuals, their function including that of the T-lymphocytes, declines with age [50]. Elderly patients with bacteremia may be afebrile and the main presenting manifestations of infection may be acute confusional states, general weakness or loss of appetite.

Also the elderly have a characteristic multisystem organ failure (MSOF) syndrome [51], which differs somewhat from that in young patients because of pre-existing multiple-organ chronic diseases. In the elderly this syndrome is most often precipitated in descending order of frequency by infection, metastatic carcinoma, cardiac arrhythmias, hemorrhagic shock, and acute myocardial infarction. In such patients the most common underlying chronic diseases are ischemic heart disease, chronic lung disease, hypertension, diabetes mellitus, carcinoma, cerebrovascular disease, chronic renal failure, and chronic liver disease, including cirrhosis. The mortality rate ranges from 46% when two organs have failed, to 67% for three, to 80% for four. In elderly patients with MSOF syndrome, ARF carries a greater than 80% mortality rate [52].

c. *Nephrotoxic ATN*

1. *Radio-Contrast-Induced ATN.* Especially in the elderly the routine use of iodinated contrast media in various radiological procedures is accompanied by severe side-effects, including nephrotoxicity. The development of radiocontrast-associated acute renal failure is influenced by the choice of low versus high osmolar contrast media, the baseline renal function, age, the presence of concurrent systemic disease, especially diabetes mellitus, and the state of hydration.

The use of low osmolar contrast material has been recommended in presence of diabetes mellitus and pre-existing renal failure. In patients with moderate pre-existing chronic renal failure, a hypotonic saline infusion before and after the procedure helps to prevent contrast-induced ARF [53]. Studies in elderly patients have yielded the same results [54].

2. *Antibiotics.* One of the most common causes of nephrotoxic ATN in the elderly are the aminoglycoside antibiotics. Erroneous estimate of GFR in such patients based on the serum creatinine concentration may lead to inappropriate dosing. Other risk factors for aminoglycoside nephrotoxicity are the duration of the treatment, volume depletion, and concurrent cephalothin use [55]. Also there is a significant association between concurrent use of loop diuretics and vancomycin nephrotoxicity in the elderly [56].

4. *Rhabdomyolysis*

Older people are particularly susceptible to rhabdomyolysis in clinical settings like acute immobilisation, trauma, infections, cerebrovascular accidents, and hypothermia. This complication is seen particularly during long surgical procedures, such as total hip arthroplasty, where there is prolonged muscle compression due to positioning, where there is vascular occlusion because of tourniquet use in orthopedic surgery or during vascular reconstructive procedures [57, 58]. Most of these patients develop mild ARF, most do not need dialysis, and most have an uneventful recovery. The frequency of this kind of ARF is usually underestimated.

5. *Acute Interstitial Nephritis (AIN)*

This syndrome, characterized by ARF and histological features of interstitial edema and inflammation is associated with a variety of agents, especially NSAIDs; clinically the latter is characterized by the combination of ARF and heavy proteinuria. Prompt recognition of this disease by renal biopsy may lead to early intervention with steroids and more rapid recovery of the renal function. Without treatment, renal failure may be prolonged and even permanent.

6. *Glomerulonephritis*

Acute glomerulonephritis is a common cause of ARF in the elderly and renal biopsies [59–61] show a high incidence of crescentic glomerulonephritis (39%), followed by other forms of glomerulonephritis (19%). Of the conditions associated with rapidly progressive glomerulonephritis, the idiopathic, and anti-GBM-associated glomerulonephritis are relatively common in older patients. Elderly women with the anti-GBM form appear to have a disease that is different from that seen in younger patients. Here, pulmonary hemorrhage is much less common and one rarely encounters circulating, antiglomerular-basement-membrane antibodies and linear deposition of IgG in the glomerular capillaries [62]. Any form of crescentic glomerulonephritis has a poor prognosis in the elderly.

The same principles apply to treatment of older adults with crescentic disease but one should exercise restraint in the use of powerful immunosuppressive agents such as corticosteroids, immunosuppressive drugs and plasmapheresis. The relative risk of death is 5.3 times higher in older (> 60 years) patients compared to younger patients [63] following agressive immunosuppression in rapidly progressive glomerulonephritis. Diffuse proliferative glomerulonephritis, which is common in association with infections, also causes ARF in the elderly. Clinical features of poststreptococcal glomerulonephritis in the elderly include hypertension in 82%, edema in 73%, dyspnea and pulmonary congestion in 41%, and oliguria in 75% [64]. Hence, it is easy to confuse postglomerular glomerulonephritis with congestive heart failure, and the combination of ARF, a nephritic urine sediment and pulmonary edema in an elderly patient must alert the clinician to this diagnosis. Poststreptococcal glomerulonephritis in the elderly seems to carry a favourable short-term prognosis [65].

Elderly patients suffering from ARF due to glomerulonephritis commonly have focal/segmental glomerulonephritis which, in the absence of ANCA testing, may include undiagnosed 'vasculitis' [66]. Compared with those patients younger than age 60, the elderly also have a higher incidence of vasculitis and Wegener's granulomatosis, but the incidence of systemic lupus erythematosus is significantly lower [59]. Because of the potential for reversing ARF in some forms of glomerulonephritis, one should not hesitate to perform a renal biopsy. This procedure does not carry a greater risk in the older patient than in the younger and one can obtain adequate renal tissue in 80–95%, with a complication rate of 2.2–9% [67]. After biopsy small capsular and retroperitoneal hematomas are common but are not of clinical significance. However, because of complex changes in the aged kidney or intercurrent diseases as arteriosclerosis or global sclerosis, the interpretation of the histological findings may be more difficult.

Postrenal ARF

An important cause of ARF in the elderly is urinary obstruction. In two major series, the incidence of postrenal obstructive ARF was 7.9 and 9% in patients over 65 and 70 years, respectively [10, 68]. ARF develops only with bilateral obstruction or obstruction in a solitary functioning kidney. The obstruction, which may be either intrinsic or extrinsic, can occur at any level of the urinary tract in the elderly.

Causes

Among the causes of lower-urinary-tract obstruction, the most common is prostatic enlargement due to benign prostatic hyperplasia or to prostatic adenocarcinoma.

The second most common cause of urethral obstruction in males is urethral stricture disease, which nowadays is frequent and often is secondary to iatrogenic causes and urethral trauma. Urethral obstructions are uncommon in females.

Benign prostatic hyperplasia affects 50% of men aged 50 and increases to 90% by the ninth decade of life [69]. A small fraction of these patients develop severe obstructive ARF that in some, progresses to irreversible renal failure. Some of them may present with symptoms of advanced renal failure, rather than with prostatism. Often the residual urine is infected, which may further impair tubular function and reduction in RBF and GFR. Prostatic carcinoma usually invades the ureterovesical junctions and causes bilateral hydroureteronephrosis with progressive renal insufficiency. The most efficient means of excluding a prostatic malignancy are rectal examination and the serum prostate-specific antigen (PSA) determination. In females the most common cause of postrenal failure is ureteral obstruction due to pelvic malignancy – in particular invasive carcinoma of the cervix. Such obstruction is especially common after radiation therapy.

One form of retroperitoneal fibrosis which may occur mainly in older patients may be due to leakage from atheromatous lesions in the aorta. The inflammation that attends such slow retroperitoneal leakage from aortic aneurysms may obstruct the ureters [70]. Those associated with abdominal aortic aneurysms represent 8.4% of all causes of retroperitoneal fibrosis [71]. Radiographically this 'inflammatory' abdominal aortic aneurysm causes medial displacement of the ureter similar to that seen in idiopathic retroperitoneal fibrosis. Even small inflammatory aneurysms may produce severe ureteral obstruction. Most of these patients are men who exhibit elevated erythrocyte sedimentation rates. Inflammatory aneurysms are of interest because several workers have reported successful corticosteroid treatment of the ureteral obstruction, when surgery was not an option [72]. Occasionally ureteral obstruction is encountered after arterial repair or replacement. Thus, at the time of aortoiliac aneurysm repair, it is important that the ureters are placed anterior to the laterally directed iliac grafts. If this is not done, ureteral obstruction may result.

One must exclude urinary tract obstruction in any patient who presents with ARF, because prompt intervention may bring improvement or complete recovery of renal function. Elderly men with unexplained ARF should undergo bladder catheterization.

An uncommon but classic manifestation of urinary tract obstruction is alternating anuria and polyuria; usually this is caused by fluctuating accumulation and release of urine behind a stone that changes its position. In rare cases, unilateral obstruction can lead to anuria and ARF; loss of function in the non-obstructed kidney may be due to vascular or ureteral spasm, mediated by autonomic activation [73].

Laboratory Findings

The urinary findings in obstructive ARF are similar to those in ATN. However, some patients may display high urinary osmolality and low urinary sodium concentrations, and so simulate prerenal failure. Often urinary microscopy is normal but it may reveal a few red or white blood cells. Depending on the cause of the obstruction, crystalluria and hematuria may point to post-obstructive ARF. Usually there is only mild proteinuria.

Postobstructive diuresis and hyperkalemic renal tubular acidosis are important clinical sequelae [72]. Postobstructive diuresis, as the name implies, is the profuse diuresis (> 4 L/day) that occurs after the release of the obstruction; it never occurs unless both kidneys, or a single functioning kidney, are completely obstructed. The period of total obstruction is usually short, often a few days to a maximum of one week. In most patients, after the obstruction is relieved, the urine output ranges from 4–20 litres per day but can reach 36–100 litres per day! In addition to the sometimes enormous losses of water and salt, patients may also become depleted of bicarbonate, calcium, magnesium and phosphate. At this stage one should avoid two particular therapeutic errors. The patient's volume and electrolyte status must be monitored carefully and adjusted appropriately during the diuretic phase. It is helpful to measure the total electrolyte losses in the urine. However, one can prolong the phase of post-obstructive polyuria by excessive administration of fluids. If the patient does not develop symptoms or signs of intravascular volume depletion, it is reasonable to infuse a daily volume somewhat less than the volume of urine passed in the preceeding 24 hours.

The development of hyperkalemic, hyperchloremic tubular acidosis reflects the patient's inability to lower the urinary pH below 5.5 during acid loading, or an inability to secrete renin during extracellular volume contraction (hyporeninemic hypoaldosteronism). Although usually this type of hyperkalemic tubular acidosis presents indolently, it tends to persist after correction of the obstruction. Patients who do not correct the hyperkalemia when the ARF is reversed by relieving the obstruction, should be investigated for the presence of tubular acidosis [72].

Diagnosis of Urinary-Tract Obstruction

Ultrasonography is safe, easily accessible initial investigation for the evaluation of patients with ARF. The diagnosis of obstruction is made on finding a dilated collecting system filled with urine. Ultrasonography has a high degree of sensitivity (90–98%) but a lower specificity (65–84%) in the detection of obstructive nephropathy [74]. Patients with highly distensible collecting systems or with pyelocaliectasis may be misdiagnosed as having hydronephrosis. False-negative studies are seen in patients with very early – less than 8 hours obstruction [75, 76]. In many of these, the patients were older and the obstructing process, usually prostatic carcinoma or retroperitoneal fibrosis, encased the retroperitoneal ureters and renal pelvis, preventing their dilatation [77]. In the elderly, volume depletion may obscure the presence of partial obstruction. When in such a patient there is strong suspicion of obstruction, repeat the ultrasonograhic examination after volume repletion.

Although intravenous pyelography and retrograde pyelography define the anatomical site and nature of the obstructive process much more accurately than does renal ultrasonography, these techniques no longer are recommended as the first step in the investigation of postobstructive ARF. Pyelography is of limited use because dye excretion is rarely sufficient to define the collecting system; and the contrast material has a higher nephrotoxic potential in the elderly patient. Retrograde pyelography is invasive, uncomfortable for the patient and, when the obstruction is severe, neither the catheters nor the dye may be able to pass the level of obstruction. However this examination may still be necessary in the preoperative evaluation because it can demonstrate the distal border of the ureteral obstruction, which may be important if one is considering an ureterolysis as in retroperitoneal fibrosis. Antegrade pyelography has several advantages in patients with obstructive ARF. First, if the renal pelvis is dilated on ultrasound, one can almost always introduce a fine needle into the renal pelvis under ultrasonographic guidance. Secondly, if the ureters are completely obstructed, the operator can proceed to a therapeutic nephrostomy. Third, this examination will demonstrate the proximal border of the ureteral obstruction; obstruction of the kidneys produces changes in the Doppler sonography waveform that produce an elevated resistive, or Pourcelot, index [78]. In pathologic hydronephrosis, arteriolar vasoconstriction (secondary to thromboxane production), increases the resistive index, thus distinguishing this disorder from kidneys that have dilated collecting systems but are not obstructed.

Computed tomography also can help in patients who have an unidentified cause of obstruction in whom ultrasound has been unsatisfactory. Although nuclear medicine imaging techniques are inferior to radiographic and ultrasonography studies demonstrating urinary-tract obstruction, they are useful in determining whether kidneys with severe anatomic hydronephrosis retain any significant degree of renal function.

Prevention and Amelioration of ARF in the Elderly

One should pay attention to those factors that would ensure an adequate cardiac output, normal perfusion pressure and adequate intraglomerular capillary pressure to ensure glomerular filtration and good oxygenation. Indeed correction of a disturbed circulation and/or volume depletion, or, where possible, even a moderate overexpansion of the extracellular volume, remains one of the most efficient measures to prevent clinical ATN. It should be stressed that this rehydration always should be done before one gives pressor agents or other 'prophylactic' drug treatments. Recent comprehensive reviews have been done on the use of mannitol, loop diuretics and other drugs in the prevention and/or attenuation of both experimental and clinical ATN [79, 80].

Regarding the use of these drugs one can reach the following conclusions:

1. A lack of controlled studies with mannitol and loop diuretics make controversial decisions about their efficiency in the prevention of ATN. However, in the absence of contraindications, and after adjustment of the hemodynamic status, their use should not be discouraged. It is more or less established that diuretics can convert an oliguric state to a non-oliguric state with adequate hydration. Whether this conversion carries a better prognosis has not been established, but it makes easier other aspects of treatment such as caloric supply. This, by itself, may improve the outcome more than the magnitude of the diuresis.
2. The role of low-dose dopamine is even more controversial. Its widespread use, especially in intensive care units all over the world, is more based on 'the mystique' that surrounds dopamine's effectiveness than on hard scientific data. Certainly, before 'renal dose' dopamine can be recommended for further application, we must conduct controlled trials.
3. Atrial Netriuretic Peptide (ANP) and its analogues have been used most

frequently in the field of renal transplantation. Up until now, the clinical results are disappointing, thus for the moment application of this drug can not be recommended. A recent update on clinical trials with atrial natriuretic peptide in non-transplant ATN was pessimistic about the beneficial effects of ANP therapy in this setting [81]. Preliminary encouraging results with dopamine, as inotropic agent, used with ANP should be confirmed. Also we should formulate more uniform recommendations on type of analogues, on doses to be used and on the route of administration.

4. Several studies have suggested that calcium-channel blockers prevent the development of ATN in cadaveric kidney transplantation and that they are able to reduce the risk of acute azotemia following the use of contrast media.

These encouraging results should be substantiated in further appropriate investigations.

Treatment of the Elderly with ARF

In general one treats ARF in the elderly the same as in other adults. Most elderly patients respond well to dialysis, whether it be peritoneal or hemodialysis. Although large prospective studies have not compared the different dialysis strategies with respect to outcome in patients with ARF, increasingly continuous extracorporeal therapies are recommended as an alternative to intermittent hemodialysis in the management of critically ill ARF patients in the ICU. These continuous techniques include continuous arteriovenous hemofiltration (CAVH), continous arteriovenous hemodiafiltration (CAVHD), continous venovenous hemofiltration (CVVH) and continuous venovenous hemodiafiltration (CVVHD).

The major advantages of these techniques are considerable: the slow continuous therapy and fluid removal, the purely convective solute transport, the high biocompatibility of the system, the high sieving capacity of the membranes, the isotonic ultrafiltration, the good clinical tolerance and hemodynamic response, the absence of rebound in solute concentrations, the stability of the desired body hydration, and the possibility of concomitant hyperalimentation. Recently Ash and Bever [82] pointed out that all patients have an ideal 'internal CAVHD system' that they can use without any penalty or royalty: the peritoneal dialysis system. However, especially in the critically ill ARF patient admitted to the ICU, the recently introduced techniques of continuous hemofiltration and hemodiafiltration have challenged the preeminence of peritoneal dialysis.

Currently for several reasons, peritoneal dialysis is less frequently used than hemodialysis in ARF:

1. There has been a change in the spectrum of patients who develop ARF: The underlying disease[s] are more serious than in the past; often they have

sepsis and hypercatabolism; the patients are older; and often ARF develops late in the course of a MOF syndrome. Compared to extra-corporeal dialysis, the lower efficiency of peritoneal dialysis in extracting solute and fluid limits its use in patients with ARF, who require significant volume and solute removal.

2. Often ARF is seen in patients who have had intra-abdominal surgery where the insertion of an intraperitoneal catheter may cause leakage and may be a source of infection.
3. By increasing the intra-abdominal pressure peritoneal dialysis may compromise lung function and therefore may not be suitable for patients with the acute respiratory distress syndrome [ARDS].
4. Continuous modes of renal replacement [CAVH, CAVHD, and CVVHD] have become increasingly popular for the treatment of ARF in the ICU because: it has greater ease and convenience of use; it provides a slow, continuous mode of volume control and blood purification, it is applicable in patients with low or unstable blood pressure, and it does not induce hemodynamic instability. Recently the principles of peritoneal dialysis, its application in ARF and the indications, contraindications and complications in the critically ill have been described in detail elsewhere [83, 84].

In one series of ARF in 246 elderly – total cumulative experience between 1960 and 1987, the survival was similar between the patients treated with peritoneal dialysis and those on hemodialysis [85].

In our experience the overall survival of patients with ARF who are treated in the ICU did not differ between those on peritoneal dialysis and those on all forms of hemodialysis including continuous as well as intermittent techniques [10].

Continuous equilibrium peritoneal dialysis has been performed in a variety of clinical settings from the ICU to the general medical ward, with a low incidence of catheter-related complications. However, some complications may develop during acute peritoneal dialysis.

In a series of 44 elderly patients with ARF, all treated by peritoneal dialysis, Sonnenblick et al. [86] observed peritonitis in 27%, sepsis in 13%, perforation of an organ in 8% and hemorrhage in 6%. In this series minor complications were observed such as hypotension, catheter obstruction, hypokalemia, hyperglycemia, dehydration, and hypothermia. Recently we summarized the place of intermittent hemodialysis in critically ill patients with ARF [87]. Continuous hemofiltration can be safe and effective in critically ill elderly patients. They have a greater than 40% in hospital survival [88]. As in the younger adult, prompt initiation of dialysis may alleviate the uremic symptoms and may prevent such complications as infection, gastrointestinal bleeding, and cardiac failure that are the major causes of death in the elderly with ARF [89]. The indications for dialysis in the elderly are the same as in the younger adult. One does not select a mode of dialysis, whether hemodialysis, hemofiltration, or peritoneal dialysis on the basis of the patient's age but on the basis of a number of patient and/or disease specific factors including the presence of hemodynamic instability, severe hypervolemia, hypercatabolism, compromised pulmonary function, bleeding potential, vascular access difficulties and others [90, 91].

Recovery of Renal Function and Prognosis of ARF in the Elderly

Usually one assesses the recovery of renal function in elderly patients surviving ARF on discharge from the hospital. The cumulative results in three series, comprising a total of 296 patients [5], indicated that 198 (67%) recovered renal function completely while only 8 (2.7%) did not recover sufficiently to remain free of dialysis. In one study [10] at least, the recovery of renal function of older and younger patients did not differ. In one study of long-term prognosis, 15 of 35 (43%) of elderly patients who survived ARF had a normal serum creatinine 39 months after discharge from the hospital [92].

Studies in mixed ARF populations indicate that some patients suffer a slow progressive deterioration of renal function, and that age is one determinant of long-term recovery [93–95]. A recent analysis of the long-term prognosis of elderly patients with ARF, who survived their stay in the ICU revealed that, 18 months after discharge from the hospital, only 10% were still alive. Preliminary data suggest that most of these patients died from a cause related to the disease responsible for the ARF [5]. Clearly there is no consensus on whether age is an independent predictive prognostic factor; however, recent studies have concluded that, in the elderly, that outcome has improved over the years [96, 97].

Because there is no uniformly accepted method for grading the severity of ARF, one cannot compare results from different units, compare new and conventional therapies, or predict the resources for ICU personnel and equipment and renal replacement therapy needed. More important, the nephrologist cannot confidently advise families about an individual patient's probability of survival and, therefore, cannot discuss with any confidence the troubling issue of whether or when to discontinue life-sustaining treatments.

Several risk models developed for critically ill patients have been applied to those with ARF, especially in the situation where ARF occurs as part of a multiple system organ failure (for review see Ref. [98]). Some individual renal units have developed their own prognostic equations that, like the Madrid scoring system, are simpler than the risk models and therefore can be applied more easily at the bedside [99]. A recent comparative validation of several scoring systems revealed that the Madrid scoring system was the most accurate in predicting the prognosis of ARF [100].

Until we have a validated method of assessing the severity of disease and predicting the outcome in the individual patient with ARF, one cannot conclude that, by itself, old age is an independent indicator of a poor prognosis [101].

However this certainly is not sufficient cause for the nephrologist to deny elderly patients the full range of therapeutic options.

References

1. Smith T. European health challenges. Brit Med J 1991; 303: 1395–1398.
2. Kumar R, Hill CM, McGeown MG. Acute renal failure in the elderly. The Lancet 1973; 1: 90–91.
3. Groeneveld ABJ,Tran DD, Van der Meulen J, Nauta, JJP, Thijs LG. Acute renal failure in the intensive care unit: predisposing, complicating factors affecting outcome. Nephron 1991; 59: 602–610.
4. Cameron JS, Macias-Nuñez JF. Renal function in the elderly. In: Davison AM, Cameron JS, Grünfeld JP, Kerr DNS, Ritz E, Winearls CG, editors. Oxford Textbook of Nephrology, 2nd edition. Oxford: Oxford University Press, 1998; 77–91.
5. Lameire N, Hoste E, Van Loo A, Dhondt A, Bernaert P, Vanholder R. Pathophysiology, causes, and prognosis of acute renal failure in the elderly. Renal Failure 1996; 18: 333–346.
6. Reckelhoff JF, Manning RD. Role of endothelium-derived nitric oxide in control of renal microvasculature in aging male rats. Am J Physiol 1993; 265 (suppl): R1123–R1165.
7. Rivas-Cabañero L, Rodriguez-Barbero A, Arevalo M, Lopez-Novoa JM. Effect of Ng-nitro-L-arginine methyl ester on gentamicin-induced nephrotoxicity in rats. Nephron 1995; 71: 203–207.
8. Valdivieso JM, Rivas-Cabañero L, Lopez-Novoa JM. Increased severity of gentamicin nephrotoxicity in aging rats is mediated by a reduced glomerular nitric oxide production. Eur J Pharmacol (in press).
9. Miura K, Goldstein RS, Morgan DG, Pasino DA, Hewitt WR, Hook JB. Age-related differences in susceptibility to renal ischemia in rats. Toxicol Apll Pharmacol 1987; 87: 284–296.
10. Lameire N, Matthys E, Vanholder R, De Keyser K, Pauwels W, Nachtergaele H, Lambrecht L, Ringoir S. Causes and prognosis of acute renal failure in the elderly. Nephrol Dial Transplant 1987; 2: 316–322.
11. Macias-Nuñez JF, Lopez-Novoa JM, Martinez-Maldonado M. Acute renal failure in the aged. Sem Nephrol 1996; 16: 330–338.
12. Lameire N, Verspeelt J, Vanholder R, Ringoir S. A review of the pathophysiology, causes and prognosis of acute renal failure in the elderly. Geriat Nephrol Urol 1991; 1: 77–91.
13. Snyder MA, Feigal DW, Arieff AI. Hypernatremia in elderly patients: a heterogenous, morbid and iatrogenic entity. Ann Int Med 1987; 107: 309–319.
14. Spangler PF, Risley, TR, Bilyew DD. The management of dehydration and incontinence in non-ambulatory geriatric patients. J Appl Behaviour Anal 1984; 17: 397–401.
15. Lavizzo-Mourey R, Johnson J, Stolley P. Risk factors for dehydration among elderly nursing home patients. J Am Geriatr Soc 1988; 36: 213–218.
16. Weinberg AD, Pals JK, Levesque PG, Beal LF, Cunningham TJ, Minaker KL. Dehydration and death during febrile episodes in the nursing home. J Am Geriatr Soc 1994; 42: 968–971.
17. Zarich S, Fang LST, Diamond JR. Fractional excretion of sodium: exceptions to its use. Arch Int Med 1985; 145, 108–112.
18. Vaz AJ. Low fractional excretion urine sodium in acute renal failure due to sepsis. Arch Int Med 1983; 143: 738–741.
19. Ouriel K, Andrus CH, Ricotta JJ, DeWeese JA, Green RM. Acute renal artery occlusion: when is revascularization justified? J Vasc Surgery 1987; 5: 348–355.
20. Salam TA, Lumsden AB, Martin LG. Local infusion of fibrinolytic agents for acute renal artery thromboembolism : report of ten cases. Ann Vascular Surg 1993; 7, 21–26.
21. O'Donovan RM, Gutierrez OH, Izzo JL Jr. Preservation of renal function by percuta-

neous renal angioplasty in high-risk elderly patients: short-term outcome. Nephron 1992; 60: 187–192.
22. Lye WC, Cheah JC, Sinniah R. Renal cholesterol embolic disease. Am J Nephrol 1993; 13: 489–493.
23. Bruns FJ, Segal DM, Adler S. Control of cholesterol embolization by discontinuation of anticoagulation therapy. Am J Med Sciences 1978; 275: 105–108.
24. McGowan JA, Greenberg A. Cholesterol atheroembolic disease. Report of three cases with emphasis on diagnosis by skin biopsy and extended survival. Am J Nephrol 1986; 6: 135–139.
25. Siemons L, van den Heuvel P, Parizel G, Buyssens N, De Broe ME, Cuykens JJ. Peritoneal dialysis in acute renal failure due to cholesterol embolization: two cases of recovery of renal function and extended survival. Clin Nephrol 1987; 28: 205–208.
26. Liano F, Gamez C, Pascual J, Teruel JL, Villafruela JJ, Orte L, Ortuno J. Use of urinary parameters in the diagnosis of total acute renal artery occlusion. Nephron 1994; 66: 170–175.
27. Coy KM, Maurer G, Goodman D, Siegel RJ. Transesophageal echocardiographic detection of aortic atheromatosis may provide clues to occult renal dysfunction. Am Heart J 1992; 123: 1684–1686.
28. Lessman RK, Johnson SR, Coburn JW, Kaufman JJ. Renal artery embolism: clinical features and long-term follow-up of 17 cases. Ann Intern Med 1978; 89: 477–482.
29. Moyer JD, Rao CN, Wildrich WC, Olson CA. Conservative management of renal artery embolus. J Urol 1973; 109: 138–143.
30. Blum U, Billman P, Krause T, Gabelmann A, Keller E, Moser E, Langer M. Effect of local low-dose thrombolysis on clinical outcome in patients with acute embolic renal artery occlusion. Radiology 1993; 189: 549–554.
31. Cosby RL, Miller PD, Schrier RW. Traumatic renal artery thrombosis. Am J Med 1986; 81: 890–894.
32. Steckel A, Johnston J, Fraley DS, Bruns FJ, Segel DP, Adler S. The use of streptokinase to treat renal artery thromboembolism. Am J Kidney Dis 1984; 4: 166–170.
33. Perkins RP, Jacobsen DS, Feder FP, Lipchik EO, Fine PH. Return of renal function after late embolectomy. N Engl J Med 1967; 276: 1194–1195.
34. Kafetz K. Nonsteroidal anti-inflammatory drugs and renal function in elderly people. Geriatr Nephrol Urol 1992; 1: 213–217.
35. Lamy PP. Renal effects of nonsteroidal antiinflammatory drugs. Heightened risk to the elderly? J Am Geriatric Soc 1986; 34: 361–367.
36. Mackenzie T, Zawada ET Jr, Johnson MD, Green S. The importance of age on prostaglandin E2 excretion in normal and hypertensive men. Nephron 1984; 38: 178–182.
37. Blackshear JL, Davidman M, Stillman MT. Identification of risk for renal insufficiency from non-steroidal antiinflammatory drugs. Arch Int Med 1983; 143: 1130–1134.
38. Kleinknecht D, Landais P, Goldfarb B. Pathophysiology and clinical aspects of drug-induced tubular necrosis in man. Contrib Nephrol 1987; 55: 145–158.
39. Murray MD, Brater DC, Tierney WM, Hui SL, McDonald CJ. Ibuprofen-associated renal impairment in a large general internal medicine practice. Am J Med Sciences 1990; 299: 222–229.
40. Hollenberg NK. Medical therapy of renovascular hypertension: efficacy and safety of captopril in 269 patients. Cardiovasc Rev Rep 1983; 4: 852–876.
41. Franklin SS, Smith RD. A comparison of enalapril plus hydrochlorothiazide with standard triple therapy in renovascular hypertension. Nephron 1986; 44 (suppl 1): 73–82.
42. Jackson B, McGrath BP, Matthews PG, Wong C, Johnston CI. Differential renal function during angiotensin converting enzyme inhibition in renovascular hypertension. Hypertension (Dallas) 1986; 8: 650–654.
43. Dixon BS, Anderson RJ. Nonoliguric acute renal failure. Am J Kidney 1985; Dis 6: 71–80.
44. Pascual J, Orofino L, Burgos J. Acute renal failure in the elderly. Geriatr Nephrol Urol 1992; 2: 51–61.

45. Novis BK, Roizen MF, Aronson S, Thisted RA. Association of preoperative risk factors with postoperative acute renal failure. Anaesth Analges 1994; 78: 143–149.
46. Myers BD, Moran SM. Hemodynamically mediated acute renal failure. N Engl J Med 1986; 314: 97–105.
47. Olsen PS. Renal failure after operation for abdominal aortic aneurysm in elderly patients. Geriatr Nephrol Urol 1993; 3: 87–91.
48. Andersson LG, Ekroth R, Bratteby LE, Hallhagen S, Wesslen O. Acute renal failure after coronary surgery. A study of incidence and risk factors in 2009 consecutive patients. Thor Cardiovasc Surg 1993; 41: 237–241.
49. Zanardo G, Michielon P, Paccagnella A, Rossi P, Calo M, Salandin V, Da Ros A, Michieletto F, Simini G. Acute renal failure in the patient undergoing cardiac operation. J Thor Cardiovascul Surg 1994; 107, 1489–1495.
50. Fillit H, Mayer L, Bona CA. Immunology of aging. In: Brocklehurst JC, Tallis RC, Fillit H, editors. Textbook of Geriatric Medicine and Gerontology. New York: Churchill Livingstone, 1992; 71–90.
51. Wang S, Fan L. Clinical features of multiple organ failure in the elderly. Chin Medical J 1990; 103: 763–767.
52. Wardle E N. Acute renal failure and multiple organ failure. Nephrol Dial Transplant 1994; 9 (suppl 4): 104–107.
53. Solomon R, Werner C, Mann D, D'Elia J, Silva P. Effects of saline, mannitol and furosemide on acute decreases in renal function by radiocontrast agents. N Engl J Med 1994; 331: 1414–1416.
54. Pfaffle AE, Moses JW, Chan R, Gleim GW, Zabetakis PM, Stugensky K, Michelis MF. Negative fluid balance and the occurrence of radiocontrast associated acute renal failure. Geriatr Nephrol Urol 1994; 4: 71–77.
55. Moore RD, Smith CR, Lipsky JJ, Mellits ED, Lietman PS. Risk factors for nephrotoxicity in patients treated with aminoglycosides. Ann Int Med 1984; 100: 352–357.
56. Vance-Bryan K, Rotschafer JC, Gilliland SS, Rodvold KA, Fitzgerald CM, Guay DRP. A comparative assessment of vancomycin-associated nephrotoxicity in the young versus the elderly hospitalized patient. J Antimicrobl Chemother 1994; 33: 811–821.
57. Lachiewicz PF, Latimer HA. Rhabdomyolysis following total hip arthroplasty. J Bone Joint Surg 1991; 73B: 576–579.
58. Biswas S, Gnanasekaran I, Ivatury RR, Simon R, Patel AN. Exaggerated lithotomy position-related rhabdomyolysis. Am Surgery 1997; 63: 361–365.
59. Moorthy AV, Zimmerman SW. Renal disease in the elderly: clinicopathological analysis of renal disease in 115 elderly patients. Clin Nephrol 1980; 14: 223–229.
60. Kingswood JC, Banks RA, Tribe CR, Owen-Jones J, Mackenzie JC. Renal biopsy in the elderly: clinicopathological correlations in 143 patients. Clin Nephrol 1984; 22: 183–187.
61. Preston RA, Stemmer CL, Materson BJ, Perez-Stable E, Pardo V. Renal biopsy in patients 65 years of age or older. An analysis of the results of 334 biopsies. J Am Geriatr Soc 1990; 38: 669–674.
62. Levi M, Schrier RW. Renal disease. In: Schrier RW, Saunders WS, editors. Geriatric Medicine. Philadelphia, 1990; 189–206.
63. Keller F, Michaelis C, Büttner P, Bennhold I, Schwarz A, Distler A. Risk factors for long-term survival and renal function in 64 patients with rapidly progressive glomerulonephritis (RPGN). Geriatr Nephrol Urol 1994; 4: 5–13.
64. Melby PC, Musick WD, Luger AM, Khanna R. Poststreptococcal glomerulonephritis in the elderly. Am J Nephrol 1987; 7: 235–240.
65. Washio M, Oh Y, Okuda S, Yanase T, Miishima C, Fujimi S, Ohchi N, Nanishi F, Onoyama K, Fujishima M. Clinicopathological study of poststreptococcal glomerulonephritris in the elderly. Clinical Nephrology 1994; 41, 265–270.
66. Davison AM, Johnston PA. Idiopathic glomerulonephritis in the elderly. Contrib Nephrol 1993; 105: 38–48.

67. Rakowski TA, Winchester JF. Renal biopsy in the elderly patient. In: Michelis MF, Preuss HG, editors. Geriatric Nephrology. New York: Field Rich, 1986; 37–39.
68. Pascual J, Orofino L, Liano F, Marcen R, Naya T, Orte L, Ortuño J. Incidence and prognosis of acute renal failure in older patients. J Am Geriatr Soc 1990; 38: 25–30.
69. Walsh PC. Benign prostatic hyperplasia. In: Walsh PC, Gittes RF, Perlmutter AD, Stamey TA, Saunders WB, editors. Campbell's Urology, 5th edition. Philadelphia, 1986; 1248–1265.
70. Serra RM, Engle JE, Jones RE, Schoolwerth AC. Perianeurysmal retroperitoneal fibrosis: an unusual cause of renal failure. Amer J Medicine 1980; 68: 149–153.
71. Wagneknecht LV, Hardy JC. Value of various treatments for retroperitoneal fibrosis. Europ Urol 1981; 7: 193–198.
72. Yarger WE. Obstructive urinary tract disease in the elderly. In: Martinez-Maldonado M, editor. Hypertension and Renal Disease in the Elderly. Boston: Blackwell Scientific Publications, 1992; 272–308.
73. Maletz R, Berman D, Peelle K, Bernard D. Reflex anuria and uremia from unilateral ureteral obstruction. Am J Kidney Dis 1993; 22: 870–873.
74. Stuck KJ, White GM, Granke DS, Ellis JH, Weissfeld JL. Urinary obstruction in azotemic patients: detection by sonography. Am J Radiol 1987; 141: 1191–1193.
75. Amis ES, Cronan JJ, Pfister RC, Yoder IC. Ultrasonic inaccuracies in diagnosing renal obstruction. Urology 1982; 19: 101–105.
76. Rascoff JH, Golden RA, Spinowitz BS, Charytan C. Non-dilated obstructive nephropathy. Archives of Internal Medicine 1983; 143: 696–698.
77. Lalli AF. Retroperitoneal fibrosis and inapparent obstructive uropathy. Radiology 1977; 122: 339–342.
78. Platt JF, Rubin JM, Ellis JH. Distinction between obstructive and nonobstructive pyelocaliectasis with duplex Doppler sonography. Am J Radiol 1989; 153: 997–1000.
79. Lameire N, Verbeke M, Vanholder R Prevention of clinical acute tubular necrosis with drug therapy. Nephrol Dial Transplant 1995; 10: 1992–2000.
80. Thadani R, Pascual M, Bonventre JV. Acute renal failure. N Engl J Med 1996; 34: 1448–1460.
81. Allgren RL. Update on clinical trials with atrial natriuretic peptide in acute tubular necrosis. Renal Failure 1998; 20: 691–695.
82. Ash SR, Bever SL. Peritoneal dialysis for acute renal failure: the safe, effective, and low-cost modality. Adv Renal Replacement Ther 1995; 2: 160–163.
83. Lameire N. Principles of peritoneal dialysis and its application in acute renal failure. In: Ronco C, Bellomo R, editors. Critical Nephrology. Dordrecht: Kluwer Academic Publishers, 1998; 1357–1371.
84. Goel S, Saran R, Nolph KD. Indications, contraindications and complications of peritoneal dialysis in the critically ill. In: Ronco C, Bellomo R, editors. Critical Nephrology. Dordrecht: Kluwer Academic Publishers, 1998; 1373–1381.
85. Rodgers H, Staniland JR, Lipkin GW, Turney JH. Acute renal failure: a study in elderly patients. Age Aging 1990; 19: 36–42.
86. Sonnenblick M, Slotki IN, Friedlander Y, Kramer MR. Acute renal failure in the elderly treated by one-time peritoneal dialysis. J Am Geriatr Soc 1988; 36: 1039–1044.
87. Lameire N, Van Biesen W, Vanholder R, Colardijn F. The place of intermittent hemodialysis in the treatment of acute renal failure in the ICU patient. Kidney Int 1998; 53 (suppl 66): S110–S119.
88. Bellomo R, Farmer M, Boyce N. The outcome of critically ill elderly patients with severe acute renal faiure treated by continuous hemofiltration. Artificial kidney and dialysis 1994; 17: 466–472.
89. Woodrow G, Turney JH. Cause of death in acute renal failure. Nephrol Dial Transplant 1992; 7: 230–234.
90. Owen WF Jr, Lazarus JM. Dialytic management of acute renal failure. In: Lazarus JM, Brenner BM, editors. Acute Renal Failure, 3rd edition. New York: Churchill Livingstone, 1993; 487–525.

91. Mehta RL. Therapeutic alternatives to renal replacement for critically ill patients in acute renal failure. Sem Nephrol 1994; 14: 64–82.
92. Gentric A, Cledes J. Immediatc and long-term prognosis in acute renal failure in the elderly. Nephrol Dial Transplant 1991; 6: 86–90.
93. Hall JW, Johnson WJ, Maher FT, Hunt JC. Immediate and long-term prognosis in acute renal failure. Ann Int Med 1970; 73: 515–521.
94. Kjellstrand CM, Ebben J, Davin T. Time of death, recovery of renal function, development of chronic renal failure and need for chronic hemodialysis in patients with acute tubular necrosis. Trans Am Soc Artif Internal Organs 1981; 27: 45–50.
95. Bonomini V, Stefoni S, Vangelista A. Long-term patient and renal prognosis in acute renal failure. Nephron 1984; 36: 169–172.
96. Turney JH, Marshall DH, Brownjohn AM, Ellis CM, Parsons FM. The evolution of acute renal failure 1956–1988. Quart J Med 1990; 74: 83–104.
97. Drüml W, Lax F, Grimm G, Schneeweiss B, Lenz K, Laggner AN. Acute renal failure in the elderly 1975–1990. Clin Nephrol 1994; 41: 342–349.
98. Halstenberg WK, Goormastic M, Paganini EP. Utility of risk models for renal failure and critically ill patients. Sem Nephrol 1994; 14: 23–32.
99. Liano F, Gallego A, Pascual J, Garcia-Martin F, Teruel JL, Marcen R, Orofino L, Orte L, Rivera M, Gallego N, Quereda DC, Ortuno J. Prognosis of acute tubular necrosis: an extended prospectively contrasted study. Nephron 1993; 63: 21–31.
100. Douma CE, Redekop WK, Van der Meulen JH, van Olden RW, Haeck J, Struijk DG, Krediet RT. Predicting mortality in intensive care patients with acute renal failure treated with dialysis. J Am Soc Nephrol 1997; 8: 111–117.
101. Pascual J, Liano F, Ortuno J. The elderly patient with acute renal failure. J Am Soc Nephrol 1995; 6: 144–153.

Hemodialysis in Elderly Patients

WENDY W. BROWN
St. Louis University School of Medicine, Director Clinical Nephrology, St. Louis VA Medical Center, St. Louis, Missouri, U.S.A.

As the general population in North America ages, those with end-stage renal disease age even more rapidly: the fasting growing segment of the dialysis population are those 65 years of age and older [1]. Table 1 shows the point prevalence and rates of end-stage renal disease (ESRD) by age group for the United States on Dec. 31, 1996: The incidence of ESRD per million people for the population as a whole was 1048; for those 65–74 years of age, it was 3518. Those 65 years of age and older represented 33.5% of the 283 932 patients with ESRD [1]. Table 2 shows the ESRD incidence data for the same period. Of new patients beginning renal replacement therapy, more than 46% were 65 years of age and older [1]. It is estimated that more than 60% of new patients will be 65 years of age and older by the year 2000 [2]. Geriatric patients are more likely to have diabetes and hypertension than younger patients, they are more likely to be members of a minority group, and frequently have limited social and financial resources [1, 3–7].

Whether we want to or not, as nephrologists, we are becoming geriatricians. It is critical that we educate ourselves about the special needs of the elderly dialysis patient. Table 3 lists some of the important issues in geriatric dialysis.

Table 1. ESRD point prevalence and rates by age group, Dec. 31, 1996*

Age	Count	% of Total		Incidence per Million
Total	283 932	100.0		1048
0–19 years	5 180	0.02		64
20–44 years	73 734	26.0		692
45–64 years	109 834	38.7		2280
65–74 years	58 549	20.6	} 33.5	3518
75+ years	36 635	12.9		2715

* Extrapolated from USRDS, 1998.

Oreopoulos et al. (eds.), Nephrology and Geriatrics Integrated, 113–126.

Table 2. Treated ESRD incidence counts and rates by age group, 1996*

Age	Count	% of Total		Incidence per Million
Total	73 091	100.0		270
0–19 years	1 129	0.02		13
20–44 years	12 622	17.3		117
45–64 years	25 417	34.8		542
65–74 years	19 456	26.6	} 46.4	1144
75+ years	14 467	19.8		1079

* Extrapolated from USRDS, 1998.

Table 3. Important issues in geriatric dialysis

- Demographics
- Indications for initiation of dialysis
- Co-morbidity
- Hemodialysis-associated morbidity
- Nutrition, immunity and infection
- Ethics

Indications for the Initiation of Dialysis

Older patients tend to become uremic at lower levels of serum creatinine than younger patients [6]. Population studies demonstrate that there is a 10% decrease in renal function per decade after the age 40 year, without a change in serum creatinine [8]. An eighty-year-old, therefore, with a serum creatinine of 1–1.5 mg/dl, has approximately one-half of the glomerular filtration of a 40-year-old. If the 80-year-old's serum creatinine doubles to 2 or 3 mg/dl, renal function may be only 25% of normal. In an octogenarian a serum creatinine of 4 or 5 mg/dl may represent a profound loss of renal function, which frequently is not recognized. Furthermore, uremia may present in a different manner in older patients: there may be unexplained dementia or change in personality or behavior, unexplained worsening of congestive heart failure or simply a change in the patient's sense of well-being. In addition, many of the manifestations of uremia may be attributed to the 'aging process' or to other diseases associated with aging [6]. A trial of dialysis may establish whether the patient's presentation is due to markedly diminished renal function or to a combination of disorders [6, 7].

Co-Morbidity in Elderly Dialysis Patients

Seventy-eight per cent of elderly people have at least one chronic illness; 30% have more than three [9]. Hemodialysis patients over 70 years of age have twice as many co-morbid conditions as younger patients: the older patient may have an average of five co-morbid diseases compared to 2.5 in younger patients [10]. Diabetes mellitus and hypertension account for 40–60% of end-stage renal disease in the elderly [1]. Other common co-morbid conditions in the geriatric patient include generalized atherosclerosis, heart disease, pulmonary disease, cancer, cerebrovascular disease, gastrointestinal disorders, arthritis and malnutrition. Co-morbid conditions that markedly shorten the survival of the elderly dialysis patient are pre-dialysis cardiac disease, hypertension, low serum albumin and diabetes mellitus.

Figure 1 shows adjusted, one-year death rates for dialysis patients by age and year of incidence of end-stage renal disease [1]. Patients 65–74 years of age had an annual mortality of approximately 30% in 1995, while those 75 years of age and older had an annual mortality of more than 45% [1]. This compares with the 1995 average annual mortality of 23.8% for the dialysis population as a whole [1]. Table 4 summarizes the one-year and five-year survival data for older dialysis patients from a number of different studies in various countries [1, 11–20]. The patients range in age from 60–89 years of age or older. One-year survival ranges from 54–92%, and five-year survival from 3.5–52%. The data are not adjusted for co-morbidity and are difficult to interpret; however, it is clear that a cohort of elderly dialysis patients do

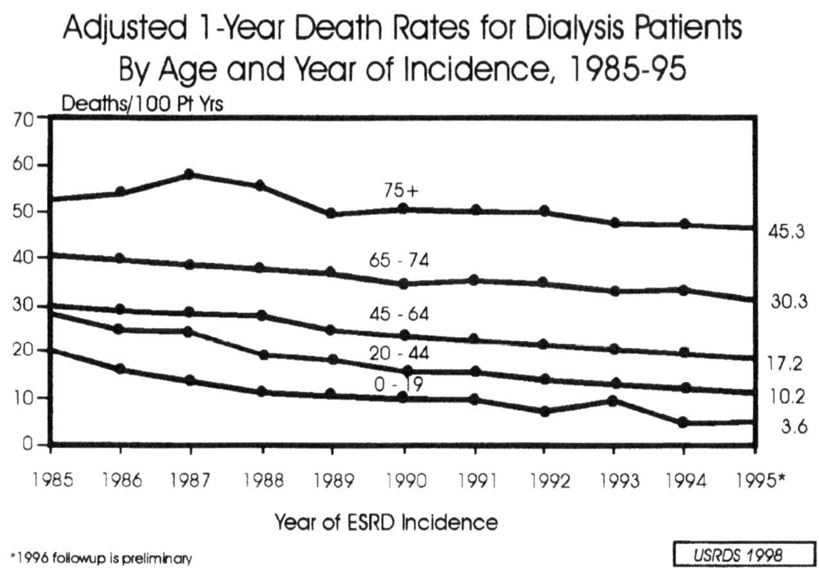

Figure 1.

Table 4. Survival of elderly hemodialysis patients

Source	Range (years)	1 year (%)	5 years (10%)
Westlie, 1984	70–87	78	22
Rotellar, 1985	65–85	70	15
Schaefer, 1985	68–78	90	50
	> 75	–	50
Panarello, 1989	60–78	92	52
EDTA, 1990*	75–84	75	20
EDTA, 1994*	75+	75	> 20
Japan, 1990*	75–89	54	18
Australia, 1990*	75–84	68	< 10
Canada, 1990*	65+	65	20
USRDS, 1991*	75–89	64.8	12
	80–84	59.8	9.3
	85+	53.6	3.5
USRDS, 1998*	65–74	69.7	–
	75+	54.7	–

* Registry.

relatively well on dialysis. One group of patients, ranging from 68 to more than 75 years of age, had a five-year survival of 50% [13].

Factors that have the greatest impact on survival include presence/absence of diabetes and cardiovascular disease, nutritional status, gender and race. Valderrabaño and colleagues reported the EDTA-ERA Registry five-year survival rates for patients aged 60 years or older at the start of treatment, stratified by age and primary renal disease. The data came from the years 1983 through 1992 (Fig. 2) [16]. Although survival decreased with increasing age for all patients, for those with 'standard primary renal disease', and for those with diabetes, at every age interval, survival was markedly worse among patients with diabetes. For example, the five-year survival for patients 60–64 years of age with 'standard primary renal disease' was more than 55%, but was less than 25% for those with diabetes. For patients 75 years of age and older with 'standard primary renal disease' the five-year survival was more than 25%, i.e. better than that in 60–64 year olds with diabetes. The 75-year-old patients with diabetes, however, had a five-year survival of approximately 12% [16].

Iseki and co-workers, who conducted a prospective four-year study of 1243 chronic hemodialysis patients [21], found a strong correlation between baseline serum albumin (serum albumin concentration obtained before the first dialysis session) and patient survival (Fig. 3). Patients, who began dialysis with serum albumin concentrations less than 3.5 gm/dl, had a five-year survival of less than 50%, compared to a more than 80% five-year survival for patients with baseline serum albumin concentration of 4.5 gm/dl or greater. It is striking that patient survival was decreased even for those with low 'normal' serum

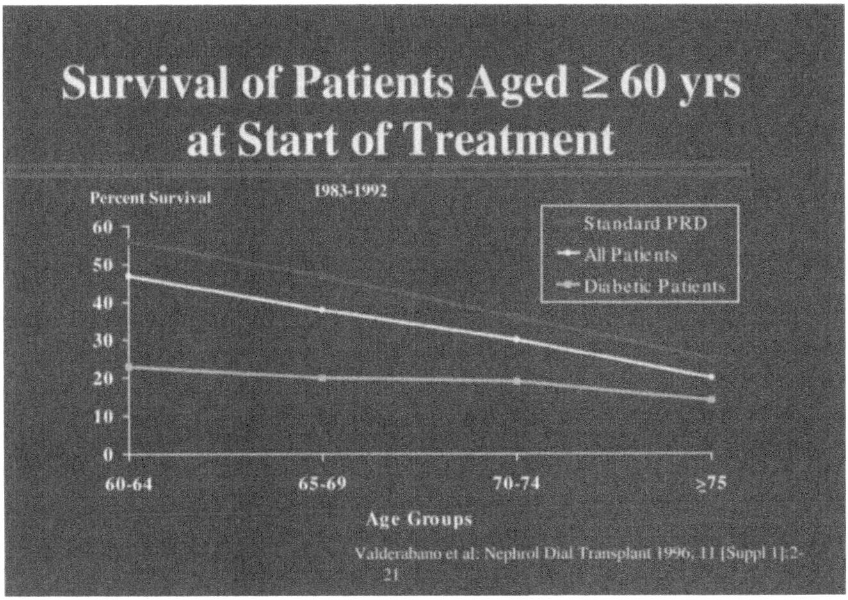

Figure 2.

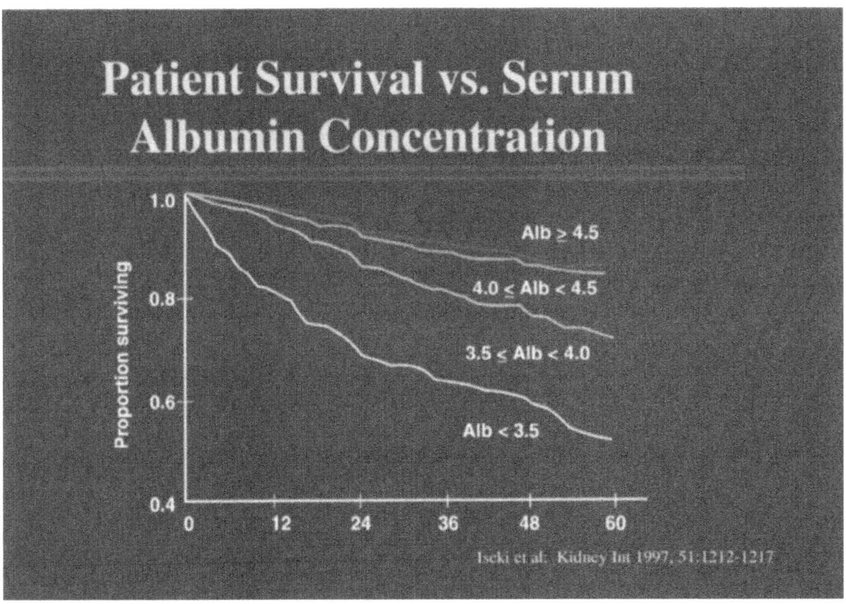

Figure 3.

albumin concentrations. Patients with baseline serum albumin concentration between 3.5 and 4 gm/dl had a five-year survival of approximately 70%.

Risk of Death in Dialysis Patients

There is a great deal of data regarding risk of death in hemodialysis patients, although we have not delineated the reasons for differences among various groups. Women dialysis patients have a lower mortality rate than men [1]. Young African-American patients have a higher mortality than young white patients [1]. After 50 years of age, African-American patients have a lower mortality than white patients [1]. Elderly white men with diabetes have the highest mortality [1, 22].

Interestingly, relative to the general population, the risk of death for dialysis patients decreases with increasing age. Dialysis patients 45 years of age have 20 times greater risk of death than age-matched non-dialysis patients. For those who are 75 years old, however, the risk of death is less than three times that of their age-matched cohort [23]. Presumably, these older patients have developed ESRD at a later age and are healthier than their younger cohorts! In the early days of dialysis, Chester and co-workers described nine patients older than 80 years of age, who had a two-year survival of 41% [10].

Cardiovascular Disease

Some of the factors that contribute to cardiovascular disease – the most common cause of death in the aged dialysis population [1, 24, 25] – are listed in Table 5. Two thirds of cardiovascular deaths are secondary to left ventricular hypertrophy with or without associated arrhythmias and one third are secondary to myocardial infarction [26]. The left ventricular hypertrophy and cardiac dilatation seen in these patients may be due to atherosclerosis or a non-atherosclerotic cause. After two years of treatment, peritoneal dialysis patients have a higher cardiac death rate than do hemodialysis patients. Foley and Parfrey speculated that this higher risk for peritoneal dialysis patients at two years may be secondary to increased 'uremia' associated with the loss

Table 5. Contributing factors to CV disease in dialysis patients

• Older age	• Pre-existing nephrotic syndrome
• Diet	• Diabetes
• Male gender	• Hypertension
• White race	• Hyperparathyroidism
• β blockers	• Anemia
• Smoking	• Hypoalbuminemia
• Hyperlipidemia?	

of residual renal function; in addition they noted that the excess cardiac death in these peritoneal dialysis patients appears to be related to hypoalbuminemia [27]. This increased risk of cardiac death may also be related to the increased lipid abnormalities seen in these patients [27]. The prevalence of cardiovascular-related deaths is highest in patients 65 years of age or older [24]. As a percentage of total deaths, however, cardiovascular deaths are approximately equivalent across all age groups (Fig. 4) [24].

Independent risk factors for left ventricular hypertrophy in dialysis patients over 65 years of age include increased systolic blood pressure, higher intradialytic weight gain [25], increasing age [1], lower hematocrit [25], and low systolic blood pressure [24]. A number of researchers are now studying the relationship between altered hemodynamics and physiology in patients with renal disease and the increased incidence of cardiovascular disease.

Using USRDS data, Becker and colleagues studied the relationship between systolic blood pressure and relative risk of death in ESRD patients. The data were adjusted for age, race, gender and diagnosis (diabetic vs. non-diabetic). Compared to the reference population with systolic blood pressure between 120 and 135 mmHg, the highest risk of death was for patients with a systolic blood pressure less than 120 mmHg. These patients had a relative risk of 1.7 (Fig. 5) [24]. In addition, they noted that the relative risk of death increased 1.43 times for each 10 mmHg decrease in mean arterial pressure [24]. Iseki and co-workers reached similar conclusions concerning diastolic blood pressure: the lower the diastolic blood pressure, the higher the death rate

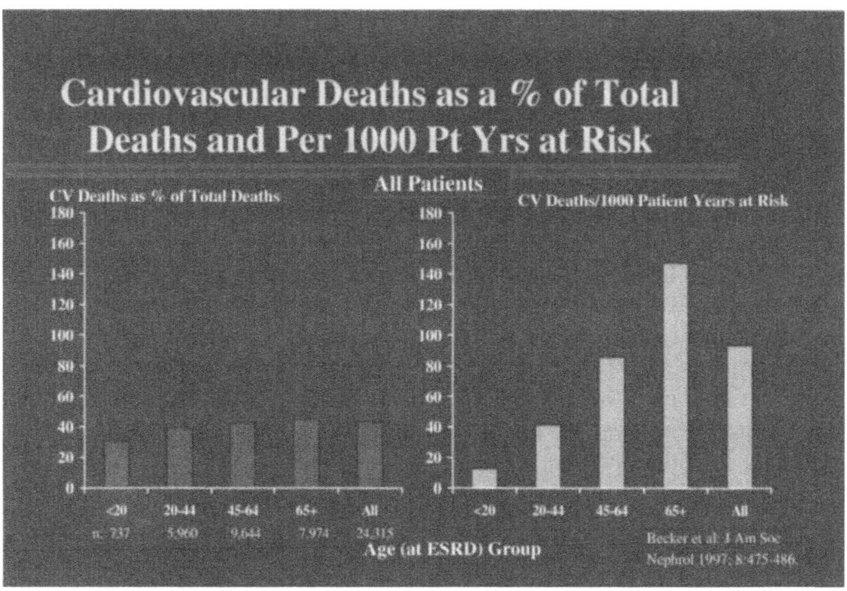

Figure 4.

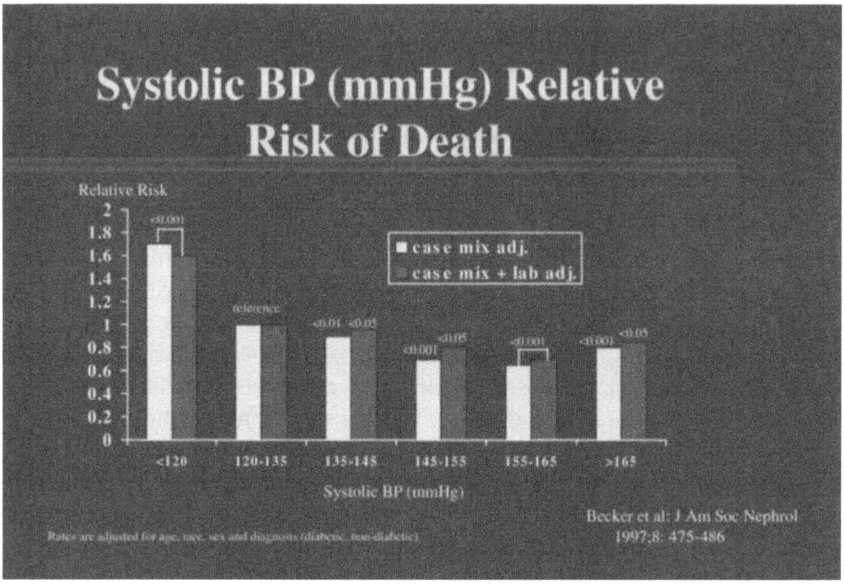

Figure 5.

[21]. They speculated that low diastolic blood pressure was a marker for malnutrition and/or cardiovascular disease in chronic hemodialysis patients [21].

Tucker studied the relationship between 24-hour ambulatory and clinic blood pressures and left ventricular mass index in patients with chronic renal failure. Although random clinic blood pressure measurements showed a positive relationship with left ventricular mass index, the strongest association was with 24-hour ambulatory blood pressure, particularly nocturnal blood pressure measurements [28]. Usually, blood pressure decreases at night in non-hypertensive patients and patients with essential hypertension. This nocturnal decrease is attenuated in patients with renal failure and in kidney transplant patients, and in some hypertensive patients without renal disease [29, 30]. In Tucker's study, the strongest predictor of increased left ventricular mass index in patients with chronic renal disease was this blunted nocturnal decrease in blood pressure [28]. Others have noted increased cardiovascular disease in those hypertensive patients without renal disease who also have a diminution in their nocturnal 'dipping' of blood pressure [31].

Vascular Access

Vascular access continues to be the Achille's heel of hemodialysis patients. In a study of vascular access survival in United States hemodialysis patients,

Woods and colleagues sought to identify factors that were associated with survival of permanent vascular access [32]. Interestingly, they found no difference in arteriovenous graft survival for patients younger or older than 65 years of age although, for both groups of patients, arteriovenous graft survival was significantly lower than fistula survival (Fig. 6) [32]. Arteriovenous fistula survival was better in patients less than 65 years of age. However, such survival was better than arteriovenous graft survival for both younger and older patients [32]. This finding is important because surgeons tend to construct arteriovenous fistulas less frequently in older patients, assuming that older blood vessels are too fragile or too atherosclerotic to permit adequate primary arteriovenous fistulae to develop. While there is some truth to this assumption, particularly because of the increased incidence of diabetes and atherosclerosis in the older patient [33], when primary arteriovenous fistulae are successful in these patients they have increased longevity compared to grafts. In the Woods study, arteriovenous fistulas in patients over the age of 65 years were 24% less likely to fail than arteriovenous grafts [32]. Recent years have seen a disturbing trend towards preferential placement of arteriovenous grafts, rather than fistulas, in patients of all age groups [32, 34, 35]. The data strongly suggest that this is inappropriate. Numerous papers have confirmed a decreased incidence of infection and thrombosis and other complications, and increased patency for primary arteriovenous fistulas compared to prosthetic grafts [3, 36–39]. Table 6 gives recommendations for vascular access in elderly patients. Access should be placed early, six months or more before the estimated need for dialysis. A primary arteriovenous fistula is the preferred dialysis access

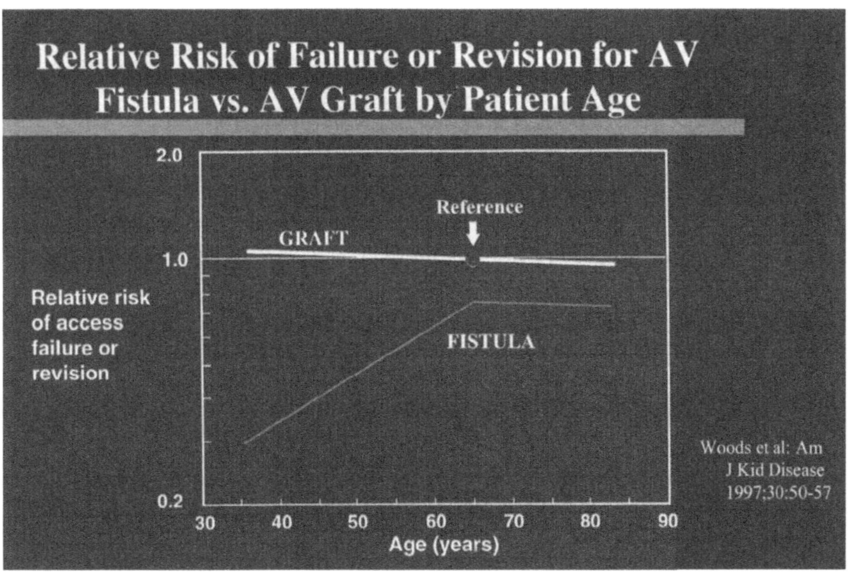

Figure 6.

Table 6. Recommendations for vascular access in elderly patients

- *Place access early*
- *Primary AV fistula preferred*
- Avoid hypotension and hypovolemia
- Replace blood loss promptly
- Liberalize dry weight
- *Ensure adequate nutrition*
- Titrate blood pressure
- Anti-platelet drugs

whenever surgically possible. Once hemodialysis is initiated, hypotension and hypovolemia must be avoided whenever possible [3, 40]. Elderly patients should be encouraged to drink enough fluid to gain the appropriate amount of weight between dialyses, particularly in the summer months and particularly for those living in hot and/or dry climates. Blood loss should be replaced promptly. Whenever possible, dry weight for elderly patients with access problems, particularly during the summer months, should be liberalized. Dietary intake should be reviewed regularly – many elderly patients are malnourished and have poor dietary habits. Malnutrition correlates with impaired healing, decreased immunity and susceptibility to infection. The Canadian Hemodialysis Morbidity Study found that hypoalbuminemia is the most significant predictor of vascular access thrombosis [41]. It has also been noted that malnourished geriatric patients without renal disease have antithrombin III and heparin co-factor II deficiencies [42]. In geriatric dialysis patients, correction of malnutrition may have the added benefit of decreasing the risk of vascular access thrombosis. Some patients with repeated thromboses may benefit from the administration of aspirin, other anti-platelet drugs [6, 43–46], or low doses of warfarin [36, 40].

Ethics and the Geriatric Dialysis Patient

The physician encounters many troublesome ethical issues in caring for the elderly patient with significant renal disease (Table 7). Access to ESRD treatment for geriatric patients has been an issue since the early days of dialysis

Table 7. Ethical issues in dialysis of the elderly

- Access to ESRD treatment
- Selection of ESRD modality
- Physician bias
- Quality of life/rehabilitation
- Initiation and termination of treatment
- Cardiopulmonary resuscitation

when treatment was offered primarily to young, employed, non-diabetic individuals without significant co-morbidity. Even as criteria for dialysis and transplantation have become more liberal, there has been tremendous variation between countries, among nephrologists and in different locations within the United States regarding the appropriateness of referring geriatric patients for renal replacement therapy [47–53]. In many instances, age has become a risk factor for denial of treatment [48–51, 54–60]. Chronologic age may be given preference over physiologic age, and frequently caregivers make assumptions about a patient's quality of life that reflect their personal biases. For the geriatric patient, decisions regarding renal replacement therapy should be individualized, as they are among younger patients. A number of studies have found that some older patients do surprisingly well on dialysis, and even enjoy increased socialization and life satisfaction after its initiation [10, 11].

'Quality of life' is very subjective. Physician bias and varying results among published studies may signal differences in patient, family and caregiver expectations and goals. Disney noted that 55% of dialysis patients 75–84 years of age were 'capable of normal activity', although 10% were considered disabled, 7–8% required frequent assistance and 2–3% required complete care [18]. Avram found no difference in Karnofsky score – a measure of functional capacity – between dialysis patients 70 years of age and older and younger dialysis patients [62]. In comparing older dialysis patients to age-, race-, and gender-matched patients without renal disease, Kutner and co-workers found greater functional disability and increased need for healthcare and social services among the dialysis patients, but noted improved functional status, independence and quality of life when anemia, physical rehabilitation and social services were addressed [63, 64]. Regarding rehabilitation, it is imperative to recognize that rehabilitation for an 80 year old on dialysis is not the same as for a younger patient. An 80-year-old has no expectation of returning to school or work; they may be satisfied with being able to care for themselves and play with their grandchildren.

As noted above, the most common cause of death among elderly patients with end-stage renal failure is cardiovascular disease. The second most common cause, at least in the United States, is withdrawal from dialysis [1]. Patients are most likely to stop dialysis if they are white, female, diabetic, more than 65 years of age [1], or a nursing home resident [65]. Nephrologists must apply the same ethical principles to older as they do to younger patients when assisting a patient and/or their family members in making decisions about initiating dialysis or terminating treatment. A number of publications now available can assist in this process [66–68]. Most patients who are competent want to participate in medical decision-making – geriatric dialysis patients are no different. For many older patients, age alone is not a consideration in deciding whether to withdraw from dialysis or to accept or decline ventilatory support or cardiopulmonary resuscitation. At least one study has noted that most older dialysis patients never considered termination of dialysis, and displayed similar attitudes toward cardiopulmonary resuscitation and respiratory support as did similarly aged patients who were not on dialysis [69]. Good communication and explanation of risk-benefit are critical when discussing end-of-life issues with any patient. Unless demented or otherwise incapacitated, the geriatric dialysis patient deserves the same consideration.

References

1. U.S. Renal Data System annual data report, Bethesda MD: National Institutes of Health, 1998.
2. Nissenson AR. Peritoneal dialysis in geriatric patients; an overview and introduction. Adv Perit Dial 1990; 6: 1.
3. Porush JG, Faubert RF. Chronic renal failure. In: Porush JG, Faubert RF, editors. Renal Disease in the Aged. Boston: Little Brown, 1991; 285–313
4. Glickman JF, Kaiser DL, Bolton WK. Aetiology and diagnosis of chronic renal insufficiency in the aged: the role of Renal Biopsy. In: Macias-Nuñez JF, Cameron JS, editors. Renal Function and Disease in the Elderly. London: Butterworths, 1987; 485–508.
5. Brown WW, Davis BB, Spry LA, et al. Aging and the kidney. Arch Intern Med 1986; 146: 1790–1796.
6. Brown WW. The Geriatric Dialysis Patient. Chapter 31. In: Henrich WL, editor. Principles and Practices of Dialysis, 2nd Edition. Baltimore: Williams and Wilkins, 1999; 460–476.
7. Winchester JF, Rakowski TA. End-stage renal disease and its management in older adults. In: Beck LH, editor. Genitourinary Problems. Clinics in Geriatric Medicine. Philadelphia: W.B. Saunders Company, 1998; 255–265.
8. Rowe JW, Andres R, Tobin JD. Age-adjusted normal standards for creatinine clearance in man. Ann Intern Med 1976; 84: 567–569.
9. Williams P, Ruch DR. Geriatric Polypharmacy. Hosp Prac 1986; 21: 104.
10. Chester AC, Rakowski TA. Argy WP, et al. Hemodialysis in the eighth and ninth decades of life. Arch Intern Med 1979; 139: 1001–1005.
11. Westlie L, Umen A, Nestrud S, Kjellstrand CM. Mortality, morbidity and life satisfaction in the very old dialysis patient. Trans Am Soc Artif Intern Organs 1984; 30: 21–30.
12. Rotellar E, Lubelzar RA, Rotellar C, Martinez-Camps E, Valls R. Must patients over 65 be haemodialyzed? Nephron 1985; 41: 152–156.
13. Schaefer K, Asmus G, Quellhorst E, Pauls A, Von Herath D. Optimum dialysis treatment for patients over 60 years with primary renal disease. Survival data and clinical results from 242 patients treated either by hemodialysis of hemofiltration. Proc Eur Dial Transplant Assoc Eur Renal Assoc 1985; 21: 510–523.
14. Panarello G, De Baz H, Cecchin E, Tesis F. Dialysis for the elderly: survival and risk factors. Adv Perit Dial 1989; 5: 49–51.
15. Brunner FP, Selwood NK. Results of renal replacement therapy in Europe, 1980–1987. Am J Kidney Dis 1990; 15: 384–396.
16. Valderrabaño F, Berthoux FC, Jones EHP, Mehls O. Report on management of renal failure in Europe, XXV, 1994 End Stage Renal Disease and dialysis report. Nephrol Dial Transplant 1996; 11 [Suppl 1]: 2–21.
17. Okada M. Mortality in chronic hemodialysis patients in Japan. Am J Kidney Dis 1990; 15: 410–413.
18. Disney APS. Dialysis treatment in Australia, 1982–1988. Am J Kidney Dis 1990; 15: 402–409.
19. Posen GA, Jeffrey JR, Fenton SSA, Arbus GS. Results from the Canadian Renal Failure Registry. Am J Kidney Dis 1990; 15: 397–401.

20. U.S. Renal Data System annual data report, Bethesda MD: National Institutes of Health, 1991.
21. Iseki K, Kiyoyuki M, Tokuyama K, et al. Low diastolic blood pressure, hypoalbuminemia, and risk of death in a cohort of chronic hemodialysis patients. Kidney Int 1997; 51: 1212–1217.
22. Furth S, Hermann JA, Powe NR. Cardiovascular risk factors, comorbidity, and survival outcomes in black and white dialysis patients. Sem Dial 1998; 11: 102–105.
23. Mignon F, Siohan P, Legallicier B, et al. The management of uraemia in the elderly: treatment choices. Nephrol Dial Transplant 1995; 10 [Suppl 6]: 55–59.
24. Becker BN, Himmelfarb J, Henrich WL, Hakim RM. Reassessing the cardiac risk profile in chronic hemodialysis patients: a hypothesis on the role of oxidant stress and other non-traditional cardiac risk factors. J Am Soc Nephrol 1997; 8: 475–486.
25. Neves PL, Silva AP, Bernardo I. Elderly patients in chronic hemodialysis: risk factors for Left Ventricular Hypertrophy. Am J Kidney Dis 1997; 30: 224–228.
26. Nally JV. Cardiac Disease in chronic uremia: investigation. Adv Renal Replacement Ther 1997; 4: 225–233, AM J Kidney Dis 1997; 30: 224–228.
27. Foley RN, Parfrey PS. Cardiac disease in uremia: clinical outcome and risk factors. Adv Renal Replacement Ther 1997; 4: 234–248.
28. Tucker B, Fabbian F, Giles M, et al. Left ventricular hypertrophy and ambulatory blood pressure monitoring in chronic renal failure. Nephrol Dial Transplant 1997; 12: 724–728.
29. Baumgart P, Walger P, Gemen S, et al. Blood pressure elevation during the night in chronic renal failure, hemodialysis and after renal transplantation. Nephron 1991; 57: 293–298.
30. Lipkin GW, Tucker B, Giles M, Raine AEG. Ambulatory blood pressure and left ventricular mass in cyclosporin and non-cyclosporin treated renal transplant recipients. J Hypertens 1993; 11: 439–442.
31. Verdecchia P, Porcellati C, Schillaci G, et al. Ambulatory blood pressure. An independent predictor of prognosis in essential hypertension. Hypertension 1994; 24: 793–801.
32. Woods JD, Turenne MN, Strawderman RL, et al. Vascular access survival among incident hemodialysis patients in the United States. Am J Kidney Dis 1997; 30: 50–57.
33. Schwab SJ. Opinion: what can be done to preserve vascular access for dialysis? Semin Dial 1991; 4: 142–153.
34. Woods JD, Bloembergen W, Young EW, et al. Predictors of permanent vascular access placement prior to ESRD in U.S. hemodialysis patients. (Abstr.) J Am Soc Nephrol 1996; 7: 1424.
35. Hirth RA, Turenne MN, Woods JD, et al. Predictors of type of vascular access in patients starting hemodialysis. JAMA 1996; 276: 1303–1308.
36. Besarab A, Dorrell S, Moritz M, et al. Opinion: what can be done to preserve vascular access for dialysis? Semin Dial 1991; 4: 160–162.
37. Glanz S. Opinion: what can be done to preserve vascular access for dialyis? Semin Dial 1991; 4: 157–158.
38. Palder SB, Kirkman RL, Whittemore AD, et al. Vascular access for hemodialysis. Ann Surg 1985; 202: 235–239.
39. National Kidney Foundation-Dialysis Outcomes Quality Initiative Clinical Practice Guideline for Vascular Access. Am J Kidney Dis 1997; 30 (Suppl 3): 150–191.
40. Waltzer WC. The surgical approach to dialysis access and transplantation in the elderly. In: Michelis MF, Davis BB, Preuss HG, editors. Geriatric Nephrology. New York: Field, Rich and Associates, 1986; 23–128.
41. Churchill DN, Taylor DW, Cook RJ, et al. Canadian hemodialysis morbidity study. Am J Kidney Dis 1992; 19: 214–234.
42. Kario K, Matsuo T, Kobayashahi H. Heparin cofactor II deficiency in the elderly: comparison with antithrombin III. Thromb Res 1992; 66: 489–498.
43. Fan P-Y, Schwab SJ. Vascular access: concepts for the 1990s. Editorial review. J Am Soc Nephrol 1992; 3: 1–11.

44. Kaufman JL. Opinion: what can be done to preserve vascular access for dialysis? Semin Dial 1991; 4: 160–162.
45. Harter HR, Burch JW, Majerus PW, et al. Prevention of thrombosis in patients on hemodialysis by low-dose aspirin. N Engl J Med 1979; 301: 577–579.
46. Domoto DT, Bauman JE, Joist JH. Combined aspirin and sulfinpyrazone in the prevention of recurrent hemodialysis vascular access thrombosis. Thromb Res 1991; 62: 737–743.
47. Fox RC, Swazey JP, Cameron EM. Social and ethical problems in the treatment of end-stage renal disease patients. In: Narins RG, editor. Controversies in Nephrology and Hypertension. New York: Churchill Livingstone, 1984; 45–70.
48. Rothenberg LS. Withholding and withdrawing dialysis from elderly ESRD patients: Part I. A historical review of the clinical experience. Geriatr Nephrol Urol 1992; 2: 109–117.
49. Berlyne GM. Over 50 and uremic. Nephron 1982; 31: 189–190.
50. Kjellstrand CM, Tyden G. Inequalities in chronic dialysis and transplantation in Sweden. Acta Med Scand 1988; 224: 149–156.
51. Kjellstrand CN, Logan GM. Racial, sexual and age inequalities in chronic dialysis. Nephron 1987; 45: 257–263.
52. Rozansky SJ, Jackson K. Rate of change of end-stage renal disease treatment incidence, 1978–1987. Has there been selection? J Am Soc Nephrol 1992; 3: 1502–1506.
53. Moulton LH, Port FK, Wolfe RA, et al. Patterns of low incidence of treated end-stage renal disease among the elderly. Am J Kidney Dis 1992; 20: 50–62.
54. Wetle T. Age as a Risk Factor for inadequate treatment. JAMA 1987; 258: 516.
55. Klahr S. Rationing of health care and the end-stage renal disease program. Am J Kidney Dis 1990; 16: 393–395.
56. Cassel CK. Issues of age and chronic care: another argument for health care reform. J Am Geriatr Soc 1992; 40: 404–409.
57. Pawlson LG, Glover JJ, Murphy DJ. An overview of allocation and rationing: implications for geriatrics. J Am Geriatr Soc 1992; 40: 628–634.
58. Cummings NB. Ethical issues in geriatric nephrology: overview. Am J Kidney Dis 1990; 16: 367–371.
59. Lamm RD. High technology health care. Am J Kidney Dis 1990; 16: 378–383.
60. Brodeur D. Ethical issues in geriatric nephrology. Am J Kidney Dis 1990; 16: 372–373.
61. Westlie L, Umen A, Nestrud S, Kjellstrand CM. Mortality, morbidity and life satisfaction in the very old dialysis patient. Trans Am Soc Artif Intern Organs 1984; 30: 21–30.
62. Avram MR, Pena C, Burrell D, et al. Hemodialysis and the elderly patient: potential advantages as to quality of life, urea generation, serum creatinine and less interdialytic weight gain. Am J Kidney Dis 1990; 16: 342–345.
63. Kutner NG, Brogan DJ. Assisted survival, aging, and rehabilitation needs: Comparison of older dialysis patients and age-matched peers. Arch Phys Med Rehabil 1992; 73: 309–315.
64. Kutner NG, Cardenas DD, Bower JD. Rehabilitation, aging and chronic renal disease. Am J Phys Med Rehabil 1992; 71: 97–101.
65. Husebye DG, Kjellstrand CM. Old patients and uremia: rates of acceptance to and withdrawal from dialysis. Int J Artif Organs 1987; 10: 166–172.
66. Initiation and Withdrawal of Dialysis in End-Stage Renal Disease: Guidelines for Physicians and the Care Team. New York: National Kidney Foundation, 1996.
67. The Kidney Foundation of Canada. Living with Kidney Disease. Montreal, Quebec: The National Office of the Kidney Foundation of Canada, 1995.
68. Moss AH. To use dialysis appropriately: the emerging consensus on patient selection guidelines. Adv Renal Replacement Ther 1995; 2: 175–183.
69. Holley J, Finucane TE, Moss AH. Dialysis patients' attitudes about cardiopulmonary resuscitation and stopping dialysis. Am J Nephrol 1989; 9: 245–251.

Peritoneal Dialysis in Older Individuals

JAMES F. WINCHESTER
Division of Nephrology and Hypertension, Department of Medicine, Georgetown University Medical Center, PHC 6003, 3800 Reservoir Road, Washington DC 20007, U.S.A.

Introduction

The number of healthy older individuals over the age of 65 years is increasing throughout the modern world, as are elderly patients with manageable morbid degenerative diseases. The older patient with renal disease presents the nephrologist with a long problem list, but a satisfying outcome when managed with expertise [1]. This paper will focus on peritoneal dialysis as the primary form of renal replacement therapy, and discuss its outcomes and complications, methods to improve the process, its effect on quality of life, and when such treatment becomes burdensome, or never should be started.

End-stage renal disease (ESRD) is defined as a loss of renal function to the point that renal replacement is necessary to prevent the syndrome of uremia. By the year 2040, 21% of the U.S. population will be over the age of 65, and by 2050, 5% will be over 85 [2]. Diabetes mellitus and hypertension account for 40–65% of ESRD in the elderly [3, 4], tubulointerstitial disease, obstructive uropathy, glomerulonephritides, and adult polycystic kidney disease for a further 37%, and the remainder has undiagnosed renal disorders. Currently, in the U.S., 47% of dialysis patients are over 65, and this fraction is expected to rise to over 60% by the end of the century [5]. There has been a substantial increase in elderly dialysis patients: In Europe from 11% in 1980 to 30% in 1987 [6]; and in Canada, dialysis patients over 65 increased from 25% in 1981 to 35% in 1989 [7]. Hemodialysis is the most frequent renal replacement therapy, followed by peritoneal dialysis (continuous ambulatory peritoneal dialysis (CAPD), machine-delivered, continuous, cyclic peritoneal dialysis (CCPD) or nocturnal intermittent peritoneal dialysis (NIPD)) that combined are used in 13.3% of the entire dialysis population [8]. CCPD and NIPD are examples of automated peritoneal dialysis (APD), the former employs a day-time dwell of peritoneal dialysate, whereas the latter has no daytime dwell. The elderly throughout the world use CAPD/APD and hemodialysis in almost equal proportions. According to the USRDS, there is a reciprocal relationship between age and the use of peritoneal dialysis; 46% of patients in the age group 0–19 use PD – a proportion that falls progressively

Oreopoulos et al. (eds.), Nephrology and Geriatrics Integrated, 127–135.

to about 12% by age 65 and over [8]. Only 5% of those over 65, use transplantation except in Norway where 55% of those over 65 have transplants [9]. Co-morbid conditions are common in elderly ESRD patients; 78% of such individuals have one chronic illness, 30% have three or more, and the management of these conditions requires polypharmacy [10, 11]. Moreover, some concurrent medical conditions may be undertreated – a fact that raises challenges for the nephrologist who seeks to optimize treatment [12].

Recently, the National Kidney Foundation in the U.S., has suggested that dialysis be introduced at an earlier stage – 15 ml/min for all patients, rather than previous standards of creatinine clearance of about 8–10 ml/min in non-diabetics, or 10–12 ml/min in diabetics. This recommendation was made in response to the high mortality of dialysis patients in the U.S. compared to other countries [13]. As U.S. specialists adopt these guidelines it is likely that the number of patients entering dialysis, currently 300 per million of the population [8], with incident rates exceeding 1000 per million of the population in those over 65 will increase.

As in the younger subject, one should pursue identification and treatment of reversible renal disorders, in a thorough manner. Similarly, predialysis management includes dietary control of protein and calories, diabetes, hypertension, etc., and, when indicated, hormone replacement with 1,25-dihydroxycholecalciferol, and erythropoietin. As has been shown, a multidisciplinary team approach and avoidance of urgent or emergency dialysis for acute uremic symptoms is associated with a decreased morbidity in the subsequent regular dialysis phase [14, 15].

Factors in the Selection of Peritoneal Dialysis Treatment

Indications for and contraindications to peritoneal dialysis are given in Table 1. The most important contraindications are dementia/depression (unless there is a competent partner to perform the dialysis), severe arthritis leading to technique failure, abdominal ostomies, peripheral vascular disease and aortic aneurysms. Impaired vision, impaired hearing, comprehension and level of education may complicate training of elderly patients, however, with skillful nursing and patient instruction; a successful outcome often is achieved [16, 17]. Ostomies constitute a relative contraindication to PD, especially if a 'presternal catheter' to gain access to the abdominal cavity has been used [18].

Complications of, and Clinical Experience with, Peritoneal Dialysis in Older Individuals

Elderly patients continued on erythropoietin benefit from improved quality of life [19], accompanying an increased hematocrit. Complications of dialysis are more common in the elderly on HD than on PD (Table 2). Specifically,

Table 1. Indications for and contraindications to peritoneal dialysis

Indications for PD	Contraindications to PD
Life-style choice	(Ostomy)
Cardiovascular instability	Peritoneal membrane inadequacy
No vascular access	Dementia
Difficult blood pressure control	Depression
	Inability to perform self-dialysis
	(Severe arthritis)
	Severe peripheral vascular disease
	Abdominal aortic aneurysm
	Active diverticular disease
	Blindness
	Poor skin healing, e.g. steroids
	Large blood mass

Table 2. Complications of peritoneal dialysis and hemodialysis that are more frequent in the elderly than in the young

Peritoneal Dialysis	Hemodialysis
Transfer to hemodialysis (low psycho-social rating) [47]	Vertricular arrhythmias [48]
Increased hospitalization [49]	Infections (vascular access related] [50]
Malnutrition [51]	Gastrointestinal bleed (including angiodysplasia) [52, 53]
Shorter technique survival [53]	

ventricular arrhythmias, vascular-access-related infections (artificial grafts or temporary access devices), and gastrointestinal bleeding (including angiodysplasia) are more common in the hemodialysis elderly compared to the young. On the other hand, the older peritoneal dialysis patient more frequently suffer from poor nutrition, more frequent transfer to hemodialysis, shorter technique survival, and more frequent hospitalization, than does the younger patient (Table 2).

Since dialysis adequacy (measured as Kt/V, relating time (t), urea distribution volume (V) and the amount of dialytic removal of urea (K)) directly correlate with outcome (morbidity and mortality) [20], one should carry out three day collections of dialysis fluid [21] and calculate the expected-to-predicted creatinine clearance [22].

In PD peritoneal access is achieved with a Tenckhoff catheter or a variation on this. The elderly are not more susceptible than the young to complications of peritoneal dialysis – peritonitis, catheter-related problems, hernias and hyperlipidemia [23]. Tunnel infections and catheter removal for infection may be less frequent in the elderly than in the young [24, 25].

Outcomes of Peritoneal Dialysis in Older Individuals

Outcome correlates directly with nutrition (as measured by serum albumin). Maintenance of a high serum albumin (> 3.5 g/dl) with dietary intervention is associated with higher survival [26]. Co-morbid conditions also influence outcome: e.g. in the 65+ age group, deaths/100 patient years is 7.0 for diabetics, and 6.6 for non-diabetics [20].

Survival statistics in elderly subjects for hemodialysis and CAPD are given in Table 3. Survival on peritoneal dialysis is quite variable depending on the center, country and registry, but does indicate that elderly patients can be maintained for prolonged periods of time. This survival is comparable to hemodialysis. However, CAPD survival may differ between Canada and the U.S., with a higher relative risk of death in the U.S. (As a result of the CANUSA study the adequacy of peritoneal dialysis (*Kt*/*V*) has been reappraised and a weekly *Kt*/*V* of 2.1 has been accepted as optimal.) [27]

The urea extracted during peritoneal dialysis, consists of that removed by peritoneal dialysis and that removed through residual renal function; in this respect, peritoneal dialysis alone may be insufficient because residual renal

Table 3. Survival of elderly dialysis patients (selected reports)

Reference	Age Range (years)	Percent Survival – One Year	Percent Survival – Two Year	Percent Survival – Five Year
USRDS 1997 [54]	45–64	81.6	–	–
(hemodialysis)	65–74	68.7	–	–
	75+	54.5	–	–
USRDS 1991 [20]	65–69	73.4	54.9	22.4
(hemodialysis)	70–74	68.2	47.4	16.9
	75–79	64.8	40.6	12
	80–84	59.8	34.1	9.3
	85+	53.6	27.6	3.5
Chester et al. [54] (hemodialysis)	70–85	–	42	–
Port et al. [55] (hemodialysis)	60–95	65	46	20
Rotellar et al. [56] (hemodialysis)	65–85	70	50	15
Disney [57]	65–74	77	65	34
(hemodialysis)	75–85	68	55	< 10
Canadian Registry [58] (peritoneal dialysis)				15
Nissenson [59] (peritoneal dialysis)				32
Segoloni [60] (peritoneal dialysis)				16

function declines with time. On the other hand, peritoneal dialysis slows the reduction in residual renal function compared to hemodialysis [28], perhaps because of less frequent episodes of hypotension, and less cytokine induced renal arterial vasoconstriction as a result of exposure of blood to dialysis membranes, or an induced state of overhydration. The Dialysis Outcome Quality Initiatives (DOQI) of the National Kidney Foundation contain guidelines for prescription of PD, and for the assessment of peritoneal membrane function and residual renal function in order to maintain the adequacy of peritoneal dialysis [29]. No studies of *Kt/V* in older patients have been published, but we can assume that the elderly patient is as likely to require optimal dose peritoneal dialysis as his/her younger counterpart.

Concurrent Diseases

There is some evidence that patients on peritoneal dialysis have fewer comorbid illnesses than their hemodialysis counterparts [30]. In either dialysis treatment method, the effect of age is likely to increase the number and severity of comorbid conditions, as outlined above. In this regard, the treating nephrologist needs to be vigilant about treating comorbid conditions. Recently, Redelmeier and associates have shown that, in patients with chronic illnesses, the treatment of unrelated medical conditions often is overshadowed by the primary illness, and consequently undertreated [31].

Peritoneal Dialysis in Nursing Homes and Daycare Centers

Compared to the availability of hemodialysis in nursing homes, peritoneal dialysis is available only to 10% of those on renal replacement therapy [32]. Because of the frequency of comorbid conditions in nursing-home residents [33], it is not surprising that the mortality rate of such patients is higher than the general older peritoneal dialysis patient (six and 12-month survivals of 53% and 29% respectively) [34]. A recent review of 10 years experience with PD in nursing homes has emphasized that survival expectations are limited in the very old and severely functionally impaired nursing-home resident [35].

Quality of Life

Quality of life (QoL) is important for all dialysis patients [36], including the elderly. The physician must weigh the need for dialysis (in discussion with the competent patient, or with family members of the non-competent patient) in relation to life expectancy, and complications of the primary disease or co-morbid conditions. It is especially important that the patient be given a free choice in selecting the mode of dialysis; in one study 'forcing' patients into CAPD was associated with a fall in QoL scores compared to those given free choice [37]. Although many studies on QoL and patient satisfaction are limited in scope, they do indicate that the elderly are more tolerant of, are less stressed by, and less depressed during, dialysis than their younger counterparts [38].

Stopping, or Never Starting, Therapy

The refusal to start dialysis therapy often may be the initial response of the patient, who views dialysis as 'high technology', burdensome, and expensive. This may be a valid decision, which must be honored in the competent non-depressed patient. Often one can suggest and undertake a 'trial' of dialysis with a clear end-point in mind, such as time to feel well, treatment of heart failure, meeting certain goals in ending one's life (e.g. need to be kept alive for a family wedding, graduation, etc.). Plans for end-of-life decisions should be discussed [39]. A more difficult problem to resolve is the ESRD patient who is not competent, or cognitive of his/her surroundings. Here it is important to work with families in a non-confrontational way to explain the likely outcome of the primary disease, and the benefits and complications to be expected from dialysis. Once viewed as a difficult and contentious subject, it is no longer taboo to stop long-term dialysis; indeed this is now one of the most common reasons for death in the elderly dialysis patient in the U.S. When the patient or family decides to withdraw from dialysis, the average time to death is 8.1 days [40], to 10 days [41]. Black patients [43] are 50–66% less likely to stop dialysis than white patients; this underlies the complex racial, cultural and religious differences, around treatment options, between patient groups. All dialysis patients should be encouraged to complete advanced directives regardless of age and these should be kept with the dialysis records. It is important to review the cognitive abilities, comprehension and possibility of depression in the patient contemplating discontinuation of dialysis. In the elderly cognition exhibits a heavy genetic influence [42]. Also the moral and ethical issues are complex for physician, patient and family; these must be dealt with squarely and in a logical manner [43]. In any case, withdrawal of dialysis should be viewed as a valid therapeutic option for the autonomous patient.

Conclusions

In the older individual treatment of end-stage renal disease is only one facet in the continuum of management of several diseases at one time. Renal replacement for the elderly patient with end-stage renal disease, should be viewed in much the same light as in the young, with the proviso that disease processes other than kidney disease may be present. Recently it has been shown that older patients rely on a partner more often than do the younger to help with peritoneal dialysis [44]. Co-morbid conditions should be treated aggressively, humanely and with thought for the patient's quality of life [45, 46]. The older peritoneal dialysis patient with complex medical problems, clearly requires the co-operation of physician, nurse, dialysis technician, social worker, dietician, physical medicine specialist, and a host of other sub-specialists and disciplines. The outcomes, however, often are highly satisfactory to both patient and health-care team.

Initiatives/Recommendations

Since the primary care physician is most often the nephrologist, it is important to provide dialysis patients with vaccination regimens, cancer screening, etc., as in the non-dialysis elderly. Maintenance of an intact peritoneal membrane is crucial to long-term peritoneal dialysis efficiency; in this regard, the elderly are no different from the young. The key to survival of the peritoneal membrane is avoidance of peritonitis. Thus all training programs must include in their curricula treatment of the elderly renal failure patient.

References

1. Winchester JF, Rakowski TA. End-stage renal disease and its management in the elderly. Clin Geriatric Med 1998; 14: 255.
2. Mignon F, Michel C, Mentre F, Viron B. Worldwide demographics and future trends of the management of renal failure in the elderly. Kidney Int 1993; 43: 18.
3. Porush JG, Faubert PF. Chronic renal failure. In: Porush JG, editor. Renal Disease in the Aged. Boston: Little Brown Co, 1991; 285.
4. Blagg CR. Chronic renal failure in the elderly. In: Oreopoulos DG, editor. Geriatric Nephrology. Boston: Martinus Nijhoff, 1986; 117.
5. Nissenson AR. Peritoneal dialysis in geriatric patients; an overview and introduction. Adv Perit Dial 1990; 6 (suppl): 1.
6. Geerlings W, Tufveson G, Brunner FP, et al. Combined report on regular dialysis and transplantation in Europe XXI 1990. Nephrol Dial Transplant 1990; 6 (suppl 2): 82.
7. Ismail N, Hakim RM, Patrikara A, Oreopoulos DG. Renal replacement therapies in the elderly. Am J Kidney Dis 1993; 22: 7591.
8. United States Renal Data System, USRDS 1998 Annual Data Report, Bethesda, MD, The National Institutes of Health, National Institute of Diabetes and Digestive and Kidney Diseases, 1998.
9. Mignon F, Siohba P, Legallicier B, et al. The management of uremia in the elderly: treatment Choices. Nephrol Dial Transplant 1995; 10: 551.
10. Williams P, Ruch DR. Geriatric polypharmacy. Hosp Prac 1986; 21: 104.
11. St Peter WL, Clark JL, Levos OM. Drug therapy in haemodialysis patients. Special considerations in the elderly. Drugs Aging 1998; 6: 441.
12. Redelmeier DA, Tan SH, Booth GL. The treatment of unrelated medical disorders in patients with chronic unrelated medical diseases. N Engl J Med 1998; 338: 1516.
13. Zarbock SF. Quality of care for dialysis patients: national initiative focuses on improved treatment. Home Care Provid 1997; 2: 62.
14. Levin A, Lewis M, Mortiboy P, et al. Multidisciplinary predialysis programs: quantification and limitations of their impact on patient outcomes in two Canadian settings. Am J Kidney Dis 1997; 29: 533.

15. Obrador GT, Pereira BJ. Early referral to the nephrologist and timely initiation of renal replacement therapy: a paradigm shift in the management of patients with chronic renal failure. Am J Kidney Dis 1998; 31: 398.
16. Callaghan L, Chu M, Cumings A, et al. You can't teach an old dog new tricks. In: Oreopoulos DG, Michelis MF, Hershorn S, editors. Nephrology and Urology in the Aged Patient. Dordrecht and Boston: Kluwer Academic Publishers, 1993; 317.
17. Kelman B. Challenges in the training of elderly CAPD patients. In: Oreopoulos DG, Michelis MF, Hershorn S, editors. Nephrology and Urology in the Aged Patient. Dordrecht and Boston: Kluwer Academic Publishers, 1993; 323.
18. Twardowski ZJ, Prowant BF, Pickett B, et al. Four-year experience with swan neck presternal peritoneal dialysis catheter. Am J Kidney Dis 1996; 27: 99.
19. Beusterien KM, Nissenson AR, Port FK, et al. The effects of recombinant human erythropoietin on functional health and well-being in chronic dialysis patients. J Am Soc Nephrol 1996; 7: 763.
20. United States Renal Data System, USRDS 1991 Annual Data Report, Bethesda, MD, The National Institutes of Health, National Institute of Diabetes and Digestive and Kidney Diseases, 1991.
21. Fischer A, Bock A, Brunner FP. Three consecutive day collection of dialysate and urine to identify non-compliance in CAPD patients. Nephrol Dial Transplant 1997; 12: 570.
22. Tzamaloukas AH, Braun M, Malhotra D, Murata GH. Estimated versus predicted creatinine generation as an indicator of compliance with the prescribed dose of continuous peritoneal dialysis. Int J Artif Organs 1996; 19: 151.
23. Nolph KD, Lindblad AS, Novak JW, Steinberg SM. Experiences with the elderly in the National CAPD Registry. Adv Perit Dial 1996; 6 (suppl): 33.
24. Holley JL, Bernardini J, Perlmutter JA, Piraino B. A comparison of infection rates among older and younger patients on continuous ambulatory peritoneal dialysis. Perit Dial Int 1994; 14: 77.
25. Nissenson AR, Gentile DE, Soderblom R. CAPD in the elderly: Southern California/Southern Nevada experience. Adv Perit Dial 1990; 6 (suppl): 51.
26. Lowrie EG, Lew NL. Death risk in hemodialysis patients: the predictive value of commonly measured variables and an evaluation of death rate differences between facilities. Am J Kidney Dis 1990; 15: 458.
27. Churchill DN, Thorpe KE, Vonesh EF, Keshaviah PR. Lower probability of patient survival with continuous peritoneal dialysis in the United States compared with Canada. Canada-U.S.A. (CANUSA) Peritoneal Dialysis Study Group. J Am Soc Nephrol 1997; 8: 965.
28. Lysaght MJ, Vonesh EF, Gotch F, et al. The influence of dialysis treatment modality on the decline of remaining renal function. Trans Am Soc Artif Intern Organs 1991; 37: 598.
29. NKF-DOQI clinical practice guidelines for peritoneal dialysis adequacy. Am J Kidney Dis 1997; 30 (3 Suppl 2): S67.
30. Port FK, Bloembergen WE, Erickson R, Held PJ. PD patients have fewer comorbid conditions and better quality of life at baseline. Peritoneal Dialysis Today 1998; 4: 7 (on line journal http//:www.multi-med.com/pdtoday/art0698-7.html).
31. Redelmeier DA, Tan SH, Booth GL. The treatment of unrelated disorders in patients with chronic medical diseases. N Engl J Med 1998; 338: 1516.
32. Schleifer CR. Nursing home dialysis: can we meet the challenge? Perit Dial Int 1997; 17: 234.
33. Anderson JE, Kraus J, Sturgeon D. Incidence, prevalence, and outcomes of end-stage renal disease patients placed in nursing homes. Am J Kidney Dis 1993; 21: 619.
34. Anderson JE, Sturgeon D, Lindsay J, Schiller A. Use of continuous ambulatory peritoneal dialysis in a nursing home; patient characteristics, technique success, and survival predictors. Am J Kidney Dis 1990; 16: 137.
35. Anderson JE. Ten year's experience with CAPD in a nursing home setting. Perit Dial Int 1997; 17: 255.

36. Rettig RA, Sadler JH, Meyer KB, et al. Assessing health and quality of life outcomes in dialysis: a report to the Institute of Medicine workshop. Am J Kidney Dis 1997; 30: 140.
37. Szabo E, Moody H, Hamilton T, et al. Choice of treatment improves quality of life. A study on patients undergoing dialysis. Arch Intern Med 1997; 157: 1352.
38. Burton HJ, Kline SA, Lindsay RM, Heidenheim AP. The relationship of depression to survival in chronic renal failure. Psychosom Med 1986; 48: 261.
39. Hofmann JC, Wenger NS, Davis RB, et al. Patient preferences for communication with physicians about end-of-life decisions. Ann Intern Med 1997; 127: 1.
40. Neu S, Kjellstrand CM. Stopping long-term dialysis. An empirical study of withdrawal of life-supporting treatment. N Engl J Med 1986; 314: 14.
41. Port FK, Wolfe RA, Hawthorne VM, et al. Discontinuation of dialysis therapy as a cause of death. Am J Nephrol 1989; 9: 145.
42. McClearn GE, Johansson B, Berg S, et al. Substantial genetic influence on cognitive abilities in twins 80 or more years old. Science 1997; 276: 1560.
43. Kjellstrand CM, Cranford R, Kaye M. Stopping Dialysis. Practice and cultural religious and legal aspects. In: Jacobs C, Kjellstrand CM, Koch KM, Winchester JF, editors. Replacement of Renal Function by Dialysis. Dordrecht and Boston: Kluwer Academc Publishers, 1996; 1480.
44. De Vecchi AF, Maccario M, Braga M, et al. Peritoneal dialysis in nondiabetic patients older than 70 years: comparison with patients aged 40 to 60 years. Am J Kidney Dis 1998; 3: 479.
45. Grapsa E, Oreopoulos DG. Dialysis in the elderly. In: Jacobs C, Kjellstrand CM, Koch KM, Winchester JF, editors. Replacement of Renal Function bv Dialysis. Dordrecht and Boston: Kluwer Academic Publishers, 1996; 896.
46. Oreopoulos DG. Dialyzing the elderly. Perit Dial Int 1997; 17 (Supp2): S7.
47. Carey H, Finkelstein S, Santacroce S, et al. The impact of psychosocial factors and age on CAPD dropout. Adv Perit Dial 1990; 6 (suppl): 26.
48. Capuano A, Sepe V, Cinafrone P, et al. Cardiovascular impairment , dialysis strategy and tolerance in elderly and young patients on maintenance haemodialysis. Nephrol Dial Transplant 1990; 5: 1023.
49. Gokal R. CAPD in the elderly – European and U.K. experience. Adv Perit Dial 1990; 6 (suppl): 38.
50. Dobkin JF, Miller PJ, Hutchinson JT, et al. Hemodialysis vascular access morbidity in the United States. Kidney Int 1993; 43: 1091.
51. Segoloni GP, Salomone M, Piccoli GB. CAPD in the elderly: Italian multicenter experience. Adv Perit Dial 1990; 6 (suppl): 41.
52. Chester AC, Rakowski TA, Argy WP, et al. Hemodialysis in the eighth and ninth decades of life. Arch Intern Med 1979; 139: 1900.
53. Posen GA, Fenton SSA, Arbus GS, et al. The Canadian experience with peritoneal dialysis in the elderly. Adv Perit Dial 1990; 6 (suppl): 47.
54. United States Renal Data System, USRDS 1997 Annual Data Report, Bethesda, MD, The National Institutes of Health, National Institute of Diabetes and Digestive and Kidney Diseases, 1997.
55. Port FK, Novello AC, Wolfe RA. Outcome of treatment modalities for geriatric end-stage renal disease. In: Michelis MF, Davis BB, Preuss HG, editors. Geriatric Nephrology. New York: Field Rich and Associates, 1986; 149.
56. Rotellar E, Lubelza RA, Rotellar C, et al. Must patients over 65 be hemodialyzed. Nephron 1985; 41: 152.
57. Disney AP. Dialysis treatment in Australia, 1982–1988. Am J Kidney Dis 1990; 15: 384.
58 Canadian Organ Replacement Registry: Kidney Foundation of Canada Report, 1989.
59. Nissenson AR, Gentile DE, Soderblom R. CAPD in the elderly: Southern California/Southern Nevada experience. Adv Perit Dial 1990; 6 (suppl): 51.
60. Segoloni GP, Salomone M, Piccoli GB. CAPD in the elderly: Italian multicenter study experience. Adv Perit Dial 1990; 6 (suppl): 41.

New Insights into Aging and Renal Osteodystrophy

KEITH A. HRUSKA
Renal Division, Department of Medicine, Barnes-Jewish Hospital/Washington University, St. Louis, Missouri 63110, U.S.A.

The Relationship Between Renal Osteodystrophy and Aging

As the population of the United States, Europe and Pacific Rim Asia ages, the people with chronic renal failure needing end-stage renal disease (ESRD) replacement therapy also are aging. As a result, an increasing number of individuals with the skeletal disorders of the aged are developing chronic renal failure (CRF). Attendant to CRF, renal osteodystrophy (ROD) of varying degrees of severity is almost uniformly present. In the past we have not adequately considered the effects of superimposing ROD on the skeleton of patients with the osteoporosis of aging. This brief pathophysiologic discussion considers some surprising analogies that arise when the two bone disorders are considered together.

The first of these analogies is that both are associated with an adynamic bone disorder that produces osteopenia: This form of low turnover osteopenia sometimes is referred to as 'senile osteoporosis'. Other investigators prefer the term 'involutional osteoporosis' or Type II osteoporosis to indicate the process that affects men and women over the age of 70 and makes them vulnerable to fractures of the hip and vertebrae [32, 33]. Whatever term is used for this disease, its pathogenesis is unknown despite considerable knowledge about several risk factors related to aging. This form of osteoporosis may involve a deficiency in stem cells or an increase in adipogenic differentiation leading to a lack of osteoprogenitors in the osteoblast differentiation program [36]. As a result, bone formation is severely decreased due to diminished osteoblast activity.

The second analogy between aging and ROD is that both involve defects in the osteoblast differentiation program. Such a defect associated with chronic renal disease recently has been discovered as a result of studies of a form of renal osteodystrophy that is becoming increasingly prevalent, namely a low-bone-turnover state, the adynamic bone disorder [18]. New pathophysiologic data indicate that chronic renal failure produces a deficiency in the osteoblast differentiation program that results in a low-bone turnover similar to senile osteoporosis. For purposes of this discussion, since both senile

Oreopoulos et al. (eds.), Nephrology and Geriatrics Integrated, 137–147.

osteoporosis and renal osteodystrophy are disorders of bone remodeling, the following section, will review the basic principles of bone remodeling.

Principles of Bone Remodeling

The term 'bone remodeling' describes the homeostatic processes that go on in the human skeleton following closure of the growth plates in the epiphyses. It is a process of initiation, activation, resorption and formation. We do not know why certain microscopic sites in the skeleton have been selected (initiation) as sites for the remodeling process, one possibility is microdamage or injury. Once the site of remodeling has been selected, bone remodeling begins under the influence of such factors as parathyroid hormone (PTH), tumor necrosis factor α (TNFα), and interleukin – 1(IL-1) (Fig. 1). These substances activate the differentiation program of two types of bone-cell progenitors – osteoblastic and osteoclastic. The activating factors influence osteoclastogenesis by increasing the production by marrow stromal cells and monocytic hematopoietic cells of important cytokines that stimulate osteoclast precursor growth and differentiation. Macrophage colony stimulating factor, M-CSF or CSF-1, is required early in the differentiation of osteoclast precursors, while the osteoprotegerin ligand (OPGL) is a key factor in the latter stages of this differentiation [21, 40]. Recently discovered, OPGL has been referred to as 'coupling factor', and it may be the means by which PTH and calcitriol stimulate the late stages of osteoclast development and thereby bone resorption [37, 40]. OPGL on the surface of bone marrow osteoprogenitors or pre-osteoblasts binds to its cognate receptor, RANK, on the surface of osteoclast precursors and stimulates osteoclast differentiation [21, 39, 40].

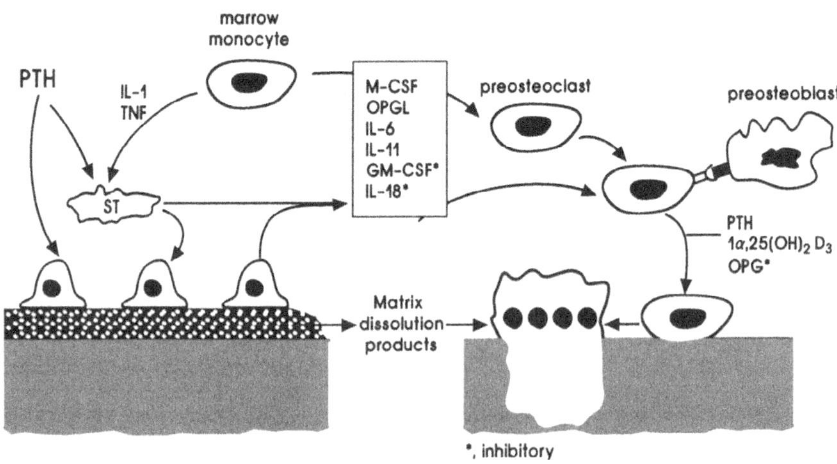

Figure 1. Activation of bone remodeling.

In addition, OPG, a soluble circulating receptor for OPGL, is an inhibitory regulator of the late stages of osteoclast differentiation [35].

The second cellular differentiation program that is stimulated at the time of remodeling activation is the osteoblast differentiation program. This program which is slower than osteoclastogenesis, produces preosteoblasts that move onto bone surfaces at the termination of bone resorption, when the osteoclasts depart from the resorption bay (Fig. 2). Osteoblast differentiation is initiated by mesenchymal stromal cells derived from stem cells. These cells exist as multipotential progenitors in the bone marrow; They are capable of switching into one of several differentiation programs including fibroblasts, osteoblasts, chondrocytes, myoblasts and adipocytes depending on the local stimulus. The senile form of osteoporosis seen with aging involves a deficiency in the pool of committed osteoprogenitors that participate in the osteoblast differentiation program.

The bone resorption phase of the remodeling cycle is characterized by movement of late-stage osteoclast precursors onto bone surfaces, and their transformation into polykaryons through cell fusion (Fig. 2). The multinucleated osteoclasts become highly polarized and form tight seals between the bone matrix and the plasma membrane in the area known as the clear zone. This seal is necessary for bone resorption because the major collagenolytic enzyme, cathepsin K, is activated at a low pH, and dissolution of bone mineral, hydroxyapatite, requires a low pH. The space under the osteoclast surrounded by the clear zone is acidified by insertion of vacuolar H-ATPases into a specialized area of the plasma membrane referred to as the ruffled border. In some respects, this border resembles the apical membrane of renal epithelial cells. The intercalated cells of the collecting duct are one of the few cells in the body (besides osteoclasts) capable of secreting protons using vacuolar H-ATPases.

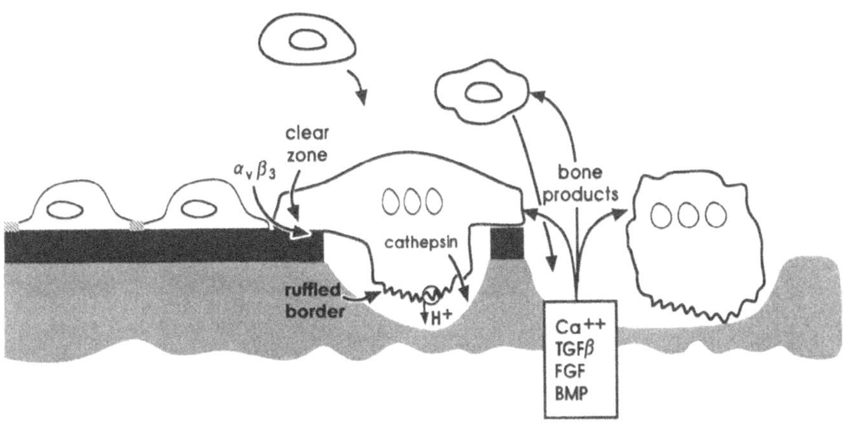

Figure 2. Bone resoption.

As bone resorption proceeds, accumulation in the resorption space of the products of resorption, such as Ca and TGF_{β}, signal the termination of resorption (Fig. 2). Some of the same factors released from bone matrix during resorption, such as TGF_{β} and FGF, serve as local growth factors for preosteoblasts moving into the resorption space left unoccupied by departing osteoclasts. After completion of the resorption cycles, many of the osteoclasts undergo apoptosis – a process that has not been carefully investigated in renal osteodystrophy or aging.

At the termination of resorption, cells from the osteoblast lineage, mostly newly differentiated preosteoblasts, move into the vacant resorption bay, become cuboidal osteoblasts, and begin to secrete new bone matrix (Fig. 3). This becomes mineralized in a highly organized regulated process, the order and molecular basis of which remains unknown. Bone formation during the remodeling process differs from that during development (endochondral bone formation) in that there is no cartilage intermediate step or stage. Bone formation is stimulated by osteoblast differentiation factors, which recently have been discovered through their role in endochondral bone formation. Their role in bone remodeling is less clear, but these factors, mainly members of the TGF_{β} superfamily (the bone morphogenetic proteins), FGF and the IGF's can render the bone anabolic in the appropriate setting. In the adult remodeling skeleton, bone formation proceeds until the quanta formed is just less than that resorbed. This underfilling of resorption lacunal in the remodeling process is the basis of the gradual decrease in bone mass with aging in the human after peak bone mass is achieved around the age of 25 years.

The osteoblast differentiation program that leads to cells competent to form bone (osteoblasts) has been progressively defined in recent years [1, 2]. We now know that marrow stromal cells, closely related to mesenchymal

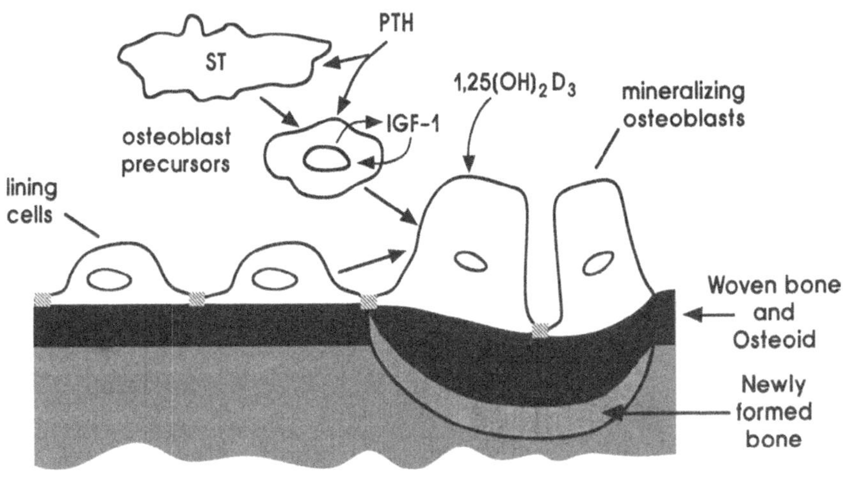

Figure 3. Bone formation.

stem cells, are capable of differentiating into osteoblasts. These stromal cells exist in two progenitor stages related to the osteoblast program: uncommitted and committed (referred to by Friedenstein as 'determined' or 'inducible') [13]. Osteoprogenitors do not express any of the markers of the osteoblast phenotype in significant quantity. Recent studies suggest that uncommitted osteoprogenitors express the antigens for the monoclonal antibodies SB10, SC26, and Stro-1 [29]. One of these antigens has been identified as the activated-leucocyte, cell-adhesion molecule, ALCAM, recognized by the SB10 antibody [4]. Preosteoblasts express some of the osteoblast phenotype markers such as alkaline phosphatase, but not those associated with mineralization of the extracellular matrix. The latter, such as osteocalcin and bone sialoprotein, which define the osteoblast, are expressly related to matrix maturation and mineralization (bone formation).

Bone tissue's vast capacity for regeneration and formation suggests that normally quiescent stem cells supply the initiating surge in cellular requirements for extensive new bone formation [36]. In the osteoporosis of aging, the deficiency in new bone formation appears to begin at the stem cell, which is unable to provide a steady supply of osteoprogenitors, thus resulting in a loss of the skeleton's self-renewal capacity [11–14, 19, 26, 30, 34]. A factor that might lead to a lack of osteoprogenitors from stem cells, is the aging skeleton's increased tendency for adipocyte differentiation in marrow space [3, 27]. At this time it is unclear whether this is due to increased expression of PPAR gamma or other unknown influences [7].

Several factors play a role in the growth and proliferation of osteogenic precursors. Leukemia inhibitory factor (LIF), which may be central to the persistence of stem cells, has osteogenic activities [6, 25, 31]. Also LIF inhibits the differentiation of preadipocytes, so it is one of the factors that should be considered in the osteoporosis of aging [28]. Both FGF-2 and TGF_{β}, which are potent mitogens for marrow stromal cells, are expressed and produced by stem cells and are stored in the bone extracellular matrix. Cell-surface proteoglycans (betaglycan), which are required for the presentation of FGF-2 to the receptors, act as reservoirs for TGF_{β}. FGF, a potent mitogen for stromal cells, is an osteogenic differentiation inhibitor [23], and thus may be an important factor in the osteoporosis of aging. However, many as-yet-unknown factors, which play roles similar to those discussed for LIF, FGF-2 and TGF_{β}, may turn out to be critical in the development of this bone disorder.

Renal Osteodystrophy

Osteitis Fibrosa

The several forms of renal osteodystrophy are distinguished by the pathology and pathogenesis of each type (Table 1). The main pathogenetic factor in ROD is secondary hyperparathyroidism that produces osteitis fibrosa cystica as its

Table 1. Histologic classification of renal osteodystrophy

Disorder	Description	Pathogenesis	Frequency (%)*
Osteitis fibrosa	Peritrabecular fibrosis, increased remodeling – resorption and formation	Secondary hyperparathyroidism, secondary role of cytokines and growth factors	50
Osteomalacia	Increased osteoid, defective	Aluminum deposition, plus unknown factors	7
Mixed disease	Features of both osteitis fibrosa and osteomalacia	Secondary hyperparathyroidism and aluminum deposition, plus unknown factors	13
Mild disease	Slightly increased remodeling	Early or treated secondary hyperparathyroidism	3
Adynamic renal bone disease	Hypocellular bone surfaces, no remodeling	Aluminum deposition, parathyroid hormone suppression, and other factors (deficiency of bone growth factors or increased suppressors of bone remodeling)	27

* The frequency at the start of therapy for end-stage renal disease is shown. Data are from Hutchison et al. [1]. Although the data are based on a small series, the distribution of disorders is similar to that generally seen in current clinical practice.

bone pathology (Table 1). Osteitis fibrosa consists of an accumulation of fibroblastic cells in the peritrabecular bone marrow space, which secrete a collagenous extracellular matrix that produces peritrabecular fibrosis. Secondly, rates of bone remodeling are increased due to a stimulation of activation frequency. This increased activity is characterized by both increased bone resorption and bone formation. The latter leads to a situation where production of bone matrix (osteoid) outstrips mineralization, and results in an accumulation of unmineralized osteoid. This accumulation is not as prominent in osteitis fibrosa as it is in osteomalacia, but it is present to some extent. While we believe that the basis of the increased rates of bone remodeling in CRD is direct action of PTH and other activators of remodeling such as TNF and IL-1, the pathogenesis of the 'fibrosa' is unknown.

We have developed the hypothesis that the accumulation of the fibroblastic cells in the bone marrow space of patients with the ROD of CRF represents early osteoprogenitors proliferating in response to PTH, but constrained from continuing through the osteoblast differentiation program by a diminishment of the program capacity induced by CRF. Recently we discovered the first component of the hypothesis – that PTH stimulates proliferation of a specific subset of osteoprogenitors in the broad class of uncommitted osteoprogenitors. This discovery is compatible with the second component of the hypothesis, that the 'fibrosa' component of osteitis fibrosa represents the synthetic and secretory activity of osteoprogenitors producing collagen in the marrow space in greater amounts than the differentiation program can accommodate.

ROD is caused by secondary hyperparathyroidism complicating CRF, but we propose that another factor, deficient in CRF, decreases the capacity of the osteoblast differentiation program. The pathology of the ROD disorder is characterized by a proliferation of fibroblastic cells (uncommitted osteoprogenitors) in the marrow space that secrete a type-I collagen ECM resulting in peritrabecular fibrosis. In addition, the high levels of PTH stimulate osteoclastogenesis and support osteoblast differentiation, thus resulting in increased bone remodeling. As a result, in this disorder, both bone resorption and bone formation are stimulated. In this context, we can consider that PTH is adapting to the otherwise diminished capacity of the osteoblast program.

Adynamic Bone Disorder

Accumulating clinical data regarding the adynamic bone disorder lend further support for the above concepts. One of the main causes of this disorder in the ESRD population is aggressive suppression of secondary hyperparathyroidism (Table 2) but other risk factors include age and glucocorticoid therapy. This form of renal osteodystrophy is characterized by major decreases in osteoblastic surfaces, mineral apposition rate and bone formation rate. Data regarding the adynamic bone disorder indicate that in the absence of excess parathyroid hormone, chronic renal failure is accompanied by a major decrease in osteoblastic activity while osteoclast activity is not diminished to the same degree. Over time this imbalance leads to osteopenia. Herein lie important parallels between the adynamic bone disorder of CRF and the senile form of osteoporosis; indeed, there are many histomorphometric and pathologic similarities between the two. However, current evidence suggests that senile osteoporosis may be related to a lack of sufficient stem cells to become osteoprogenitors, while our concept is that the adynamic bone disorder relates to lack of capacity in the differentiation program. Either defect results in an osteoblastic insufficiency and osteopenia.

There are several potential causes of a constraint in the osteoblast differentiation program in chronic renal failure, which include a deficiency in key bone-growth-factor levels responsible for osteoblast growth and differentia-

Table 2. Know causes of adynamic bone disorder

Suppression of PTH with calcitriol
Diabetes
Peritoneal dialysis
Age
Corticosteroids
Immobilization
Hypoparathyroidism

tion, or an increase in the activity of substances that inhibit osteoblast activity. Candidates exist for both class of pathogenetic substances. In the adult human, a significant component of the ambient bone morphogenetic protein-7 (BMP-7) levels may be endocrine and of renal origin. The BMP-7 knockout mouse has a renal phenotype (glomeruloagenesis), and the collecting duct is a major source of BMP-7 production. Thus, a parallel may exist between the erythropoietin deficiency in the anemia of chronic renal failure, and the adynamic bone disorder of chronic renal failure-that of a deficiency of an endocrine factor made in the kidney. Other bone growth factors that may be diminished in chronic renal failure include the fibroblast growth factors, sex hormones and the insulin-like growth factors (IGF's).

Senile Osteoporosis (Type II Osteoporosis)

We believe senile osteoporosis is a result of age-related changes in calcium homeostasis that affect both men and women [8]. Several studies have shown that plasma levels of 25-hydroxyvitamin D (25OHD) decrease with age [5, 16, 17, 20, 38]. The proposed basis for the decreased 25OHD levels are reduced vitamin intake, decreased sun exposure, and possibly decreased absorption. Plasma levels of $1,25(OH)_2D$ probably decrease with age, although this remains controversial [8]. Several studies suggest that calcium absorption is decreased by aging, but analysis of true calcium absorption [9, 10], and balance studies [15] minimize any reduction in net calcium absorption that occurs with aging although there is a decrease in the efficiency of absorption with aging. Possibly, the most important age-related change in calcium homeostasis is a progressive increase in PTH levels [24, 41]. Most likely the age-related increase in basal secretion and maximum secretory capacity [22] is related to parathyroid hyperplasia and chronic hypocalcemia, making it directly analogous to the secondary hyperparathyroidism of CRF.

The abnormalities in Ca homeostasis observed with aging do not provide a mechanism for the decrease in osteoprogenitors and the shift of mesenchymal stem cells towards adipogenesis. We do not know whether changes in $PPAR_\gamma$ levels or its cognate ligand, and, especially, changes in ligand concentration might account for the shift towards adipogenesis. One might consider adaptive the tendency towards hyperparathyroidism with aging; it may represent an attempt to compensate for underactivity in the osteoblast differentiation program (another situation analogous to chronic renal failure). Loss of a specific BMP influence with aging, such as might be produced through increased Noggin levels, could explain the decrease in osteoblast differentiation, and data from an animal model supports this concept. The superimposition of CRF on the osteoporosis of aging represents a further constraint on the osteoblast differentiation program (discussed above). Most likely the mechanisms of decreased osteoblast differentiation in aging and CRF differ, thus, the two entities likely are clinically additive in their impact on bone formation.

As a result, with improved survival of the aged with ESRD, fractures are likely to be a major complication.

Summary

Both aging and chronic renal failure, especially end-stage renal disease are characterized by a low bone turnover disorder. In aging, the senile form of osteoporosis may be related to a decrease in stem cells differentiating towards osteoprogenitors, while in CRF there is a decrease in the capacity of the osteoblast differentiation program in the absence of the influence of PTH. In both aging and CRF, secondary hyperparathyroidism is common. Thus, the effect of chronic renal failure on skeletal homeostasis in the elderly may be an additional factor that produces a deficiency of osteoprogenitors. Compensation through higher PTH levels produces an increase in resorptive activity. We do not know the long-term clinical result of superimposing CRF on senile osteoporosis because of the shortened survival of this population, but the risk of excess bone resorption becomes apparent as survival is increased.

This discussion of the pathogenesis of renal osteodystrophy and senile osteoporosis makes clear the need for improved and specific therapeutic approaches. At the present time, our treatments do not address the superimposition of chronic renal failure and renal osteodystrophy on the aging skeleton that may have osteoporosis.

References

1. Aubin JE, Kahn A. The osteoblast lineage-embryologic origins and the differentiation sequence. In: Favus MJ, editor. Primer on the Metabolic Bone Diseases and Disorders of Mineral Metabolism. Philadelphia, New York: Lippincott-Raven, 1996; 35–38.
2. Aubin JE, Liu F. The osteoblast lineage. In: Bilezikian JP, Raisz LG, Rodan GA, editors. Principles of Bone Biology. New York: Academic Press, 1996; 51–67.
3. Beresford JN, Bennett JH, Devlin C, Leboy PS, Owen ME. Evidence for an inverse relationship between the differentiation of adipocytic and osteogenic cells in rat marrow stromal cell cultures. J Cell Sci 1992; 102: 341–351.
4. Bruder SP, Ricalton NS, Boynton RE, Connolly TJ, Barry FP. Mesenchymal stem cell surface antigen SB-10 corresponds to activated leukocyte cell adhesion molecule and is involved in ostseogenic differentiation. J Bone Miner Res 1998; 13: 655–663.
5. Chapuy MC, Arlot ME, Duboeuf F, Brun J, Crouzet B, Arnaud S, Delmas PD, Meunier PJ. Vitamin D_3 and calcium to prevent hip fractures in elderly women. N Engl J Med 1992; 237: 1637–1642.
6. Cornish J, Callon K, King A, Edgar S, Reid IR. The effect of leukaemia inhibitory factor on bone in vivo. Endocrinology 1993; 132: 1359–1366.
7. Devchand PR, Keller H, Peters JM, Vazquez M, Gonzalez FJ, Wahli W. The PPARa-leukotriene B_4 pathway to inflammation control. Nature 1996; 384: 39–43.
8. Eastell R, Riggs BL. Vitamin D and Osteoporosis. In: Feldman D, Glorieux FH, Pike JW, editor. Vitamin D. San Diego: Academic Press, 1997; 695–711.

9. Eastell R, Yergey AL, Vieira NE, Cedel SL, Kumar R, Riggs BL. Interrelationship among vitamin D metabolism, true calcium absorption, parathyroid function, and age in women: evidence of an age-related intestinal resistance to 1,25-dihydroxyvitamin D action. J Bone Miner Res 1991; 6: 125–132.
10. Ebeling PR, Yergey AL, Vieira NE, Burritt MF, O'Fallon WM, Kumar R, Riggs BL. Influence of age on effects of endogenous 1,25-dihydroxyvitamin D on calcium absorption in normal women. Calcified Tissue Research 1994; 55: 330–334.
11. Egrise D, Martin D, Vience A, Neve P, Schoutens A. The number of fibroblastic colonies formed from bone marrow is decreased and the in vitro proliferation rate of trabecular bone cells increased in aged rats. Bone 1992; 13: 355–361.
12. Endo N, Nishida S, Ninto M, Tokunaga K, Kondo H, Ito A, Tanizawa T, Takahashi HE. CFU-F (Colony forming unit fibroblastic) assays as a parameter of bone forming activity in human: the comparison of ALP activity of CFU-F from bone marrow with histomorphometric indices of ilium. J Bone Min Res 1995; 10 (supplement 1): S469.
13. Friedenstein AJ. Determined and inducible osteogenic precursor cells. In: Anonymous, editor. Heart Tissue Growth, Repair and Remineralization. Amsterdam: Associated Scientific Publishers, 1973; 169–185.
14. Haynesworth SE, Goldberg VM, Caplan AI. Diminution of the number of mesenchymal stem cells as a cause of skeletal aging. In: Buckwalter JA, Goldberg VM, Wood SLY, editor. Musculoskeletal Soft-Tissue Aging: Impact on Mobility. Rosemont, 1994; 79–87.
15. Heaney RP, Recker RR, Stegman MR, Moy AJ. Calcium absorption in women: relationships to calcium intake, estrogen status, and age. J Bone Miner Res 1989; 4: 469–475.
16. Holick, M.F., L.Y. Matsuoka, and J. Wortsman. Age, vitamin D and solar ultraviolet. Lancet 1: 1104-1105, 1989.
17. Hollis B. Assessment of vitamin D nutritional and hormonal status: what to measure and how to do it. Calcif Tissue Int 1996; 58: 4–5.
18. Hruska KA. Growth factors and cytokines in renal osteodystrophy. In: Bushinsky DA, editor. Renal Osteodystrophy. Philadelphia: Lippincott-Raven, 1998; 221–261.
19. Kahn A, Gibbons R, Perkins S, Gazit D. Age-related bone loss: Aa hypothesis and initial assessment in mice. Clin Orthop Relat Res 1995; 313: 69–75.
20. Kochersberger G, Westlund R, Lyles KW. Calcium supplementation lowers serum parathyroid hormone levels in elderly subjects. J Gerontol 1990; 45: M159–M162.
21. Lacey DL, Timms E, Tan H-L, Kelley MJ, Dunstan CR, Burgess T, Elliott R, Colombero A, Elliott G, Scully S, Hsu H, Sullivan J, Hawkins N, Davy E, Capparelli C, Eli A, Qian Y-X, Kaufman S, Sarosi I, Shalhoub V, Senaldi G, Guo J, Delaney J, Boyle WJ. Osteoprotegerin ligand is a cytokine that regulates osteoclast differentiation and activation. Cell 1998; 93: 165–176.
22. Ledger GA, Burritt MF, Kao PC, O'Fallon WM, Riggs BL, Khosla S. Abnormalities of parathyroid hormone secretion in elderly women that are reversible by short-term therapy with 1,25-dihydroxyvitamin D_3. J Clin Endocrin Metab 1994; 79: 211–216.
23. Locklin RM, Williamson MC, Beresford JN, Triffitt JT, Owen M. In vitro effects of growth factors and dexamethasone on rat marrow stromal cells. Clin Orthop Relat Res 1995; 313: 27–35.
24. Marcus R, Madvig P, Young G. Age-related changes in parathyroid hormone and parathyroid hormone action in normal humans. J Clin Endocrin Metab 1984; 58: 223–230.
25. Metcalf D, Gearing DP. Fatal syndrome in mice engrafted with cells producing high levels of the leukaemia inhibitory factor. PNAS 1989; 86: 5948–5952.
26. Mets T, Verdonk G. Variations in the stromal cell population of human bone marrow during aging. Mech Ageing Dev 1981; 15: 41–49.
27. Meunier P, Aaron J, Edouard G, Vignon G. Osteoporosis and the replacement of cell populations of the marrow adipose tissue. Clin Orthop 1971; 80: 147–154.
28. Mori M, Yamaguchi K, Abe K. Purification of a lipoprotein lipase inhibiting protein produced by a melanoma cell line associated with cancer cachexia. Biochem Biophys Res Commun 1989; 160: 1083–1092.

29. Onishi T, Cheng S-L, Bruder S, Hruska K. Isolation and characterization of human bone marrow osteoprogenitor cells that proliferate in response to parathyroid hormone (PTH). J Bone Miner Res 1997; 12: S189 (Abstract).
30. Quarto R, Thomas D, Liang CT. Bone progenitor cell deficits and the age-associated decline in bone repair capacity. Calcif Tissue Int 1995; 56: 123–129.
31. Rathjen PD, Nichols J, Toth S, Edwards DR, Heath JK, Smith AG. Developmentally programmed induction of differentiation inhibiting activity and the control of stem cell populations. Genes and Development 1990; 4: 2308–2318.
32. Riggs BL, Khosla S, Melton LJI. A unitary model for involutional osteoporosis: estrogen deficiency causes both type I and type II osteoporosis in postmenopausal women and contributes to bone loss in aging men. J Bone Miner Res 1998; 13: 763–773.
33. Riggs BL, Melton LJI. Involutional osteoporosis. NEJM 1986; 314: 1676–1686.
34. Roholl PJM, Blauw E, Zurcher C, Dormans JAMA, Theurs HM. Evidence for a diminished maturation of preosteoblasts into osteoblasts during ageing in rats: an ultrastructural study. J Bone Miner Res 1994; 9: 355–366.
35. Simonet WS, Lacey DL, Dunstan CR, Kelley M, Chang MS, Luthy R, Nguyen HQ, Wooden S, Bennett L, Boone T, Shimamoto G, DeRose M, Elliott R, Colombero A, Tan HL, Trail G, Sullivan J, Davy E, Bucay N, Renshaw-Gregg L, Hughes TM, Hill D, Pattison W, Campbell P, Boyle WJ. Osteoprotegerin: a novel secreted protein involved in the regulation of bone density. Cell 1997; 89: 309–319.
36. Triffitt JT. The stem cell of the osteoblast. In: Bilezikian JP, Raisz LG, Rodan GA, editor. Principles of Bone Biology. San Diego: Academic Press, 1996; 39–50.
37. Tsukii K, Shima N, Mochizuki S, Yamaguchi K, Kinosaki M, Yano K, Shibata O, Udagawa N, Yasuda H, Suda T, Higashio K. Osteoclast differentiation factor mediates an essential signal for bone resorption induced by 1 alpha, 25-dihydroxyvitamin D3, prostglandin E2, or parathyroid hormone in the microenvironment of bone. Biochem Biophys Res Comm 1998; 246: 337–341.
38. Van Der Wielen RP, Lowik MRH, Van der Berg H, Degroot L, Haller J, Moreras O, Vanstaveren WA. Serum 25OHD concentrations among elderly people in Europe. Lancet 1995; 346: 207–210.
39. Yasuda H, Shima N, Nakagawa N, Mochizuki SI, Yanok K, Fujise N, Sato Y, Goto M, Yamaguchi K, Kuriyama M, Kanno T, Murakami A, Tsuda E, Morinaga T, Higashio K. Identity of osteoclastogenesis inhibitory factor (OCIF) and osteoprotegerin (OPG): a mechanism by which OPG/OCIF inhibits osteoclastogenesis in vitro. Endocrinology 1998; 139: 1329–1337.
40. Yasuda H, Shima N, Nakagawa N, Yamaguchi K, Kinosaki M, Mochizuki S-I, Tomoyasu A, Yano K, Goto M, Murakami A, Tsuda E, Morinaga T, Higashio K, Udagawa N, Takahashi N, Suda T. Osteoclast differentiation factor is a ligand for osteoprotegerin/osteoclastogenesis-inhibitory factor and is identical to TRANCE/RANKL. PNAS 1998; 95: 3597–3602.
41. Young G, Marcus R, Minkoff JR, Kim LY, Sergre GV. Age-related rise in parathyroid hormone in man – the use of intact and midmolecule antisera to distinguish hormone secretion from retention. Bone and Mineral 1987; 2: 367–374.

Older Transplant Recipients; Older Transplant Donors – What Are the Issues?

MARGARET J. BIA
Yale University School of Medicine, Renal Section, Department of Medicine, 333 Cedar St., New Haven, CT 06510, U.S.A.

The explosion in the incidence of ESRD in older individuals mandates a greater integration of geriatric knowledge into the practice of nephrology. Patients over 65 years old made up 40% of the ESRD population in 1989, a fraction that rose to 53% in 1993, and is expected to exceed 66–65% by the year 2000 [1]. This trend, along with the crisis in donor-organ supply, has had a major impact on renal transplantation and has affected our decisions concerning renal transplant recipients, and both cadaveric and living donors. I shall now address these three areas.

Renal Transplant Recipients

In the early years of renal transplantation, age was a major factor in determining the acceptability of a potential renal transplant recipient. Gone are the days when a candidate was rejected because she(he) is over 55 years old. Between 1988 and 1995, the number of recipients of cadaveric renal allografts over 50 years of age rose from 27% to 34% [2]. Similarly, in the same period the number of recipients of living donor kidneys, who were over 50 years old, doubled from 10 to 23% [2]. The greater representation of older patients in the renal transplant pool also is obvious when one observes the increasing number of patients over 50 and over 60 years of age who are waiting for a kidney. In 1997, 30% of all wait-listed patients were 50–64 years old and 7% were over 65. Most transplant centers reject a rigid age limit for renal transplantation but rather believe that it is the biologic, not the chronologic, age that is important in choosing a recipient.

As might be expected, patient survival following renal transplantation decreases with increasing age [3]. However the proper reference point for evaluating survival in older recipients should be the survival of age and morbidity-matched dialysis patients. Recently such comparisons have been made by examining data in all patients wait-listed for a kidney transplant and comparing the risk of mortality between those transplanted versus those remaining on dialysis during the period of observation [1, 4, 5]. Despite a higher initial

Oreopoulos et al. (eds.), Nephrology and Geriatrics Integrated, 149–154.

mortality in the early post transplant period, long-term mortality is significantly improved after a renal transplant (4). Wait- listed patients tend to be healthier than other dialysis patients and therefore have an improved survival (Fig. 1) [1]. However, even in these healthiest of dialysis patients, the relative risk of death is decreased significantly by a cadaveric renal transplant (Fig. 1). Recent data presented by Wolfe et al. at the annual meetings of the American Society of Nephrology demonstrated that this survival advantage of transplantation is apparent in all age groups, including patients over 60 years of age [5]. The Canadian transplant registry had similar results when it compared survival in 6400 patients over 60 years of age, matched for age, renal diagnosis and comorbid conditions between 1987–1993. Patients receiving a transplant had a mean five year survival rate of 81%, compared to 51% for those remaining on dialysis [6].

Thus renal transplantation not only is a viable option in older patients but may have a distinct survival advantage as well. This fact must be understood with the important caveat that comparisons between wait-listed dialysis patients and those receiving a transplant were generated in patients fit enough to qualify for transplantation which may exclude many older individuals on dialysis today. Therefore one must be cautious when applying these results to all older patients on dialysis. However these results confirm that transplantation is a viable option for older patients fit enough to qualify.

In our center, as well as others [7, 8], we often perform special tests in older patients, in addition to the routine recipient work-up (Table 1). Screening for potential vascular disease and gastrointestinal and genitourinary tract malignancy is evaluated more aggressively. A voiding cystourethragram, no longer routinely performed in most centers, may also be performed. One should make plans for postoperative support, mobility and rehabilitation to avoid a

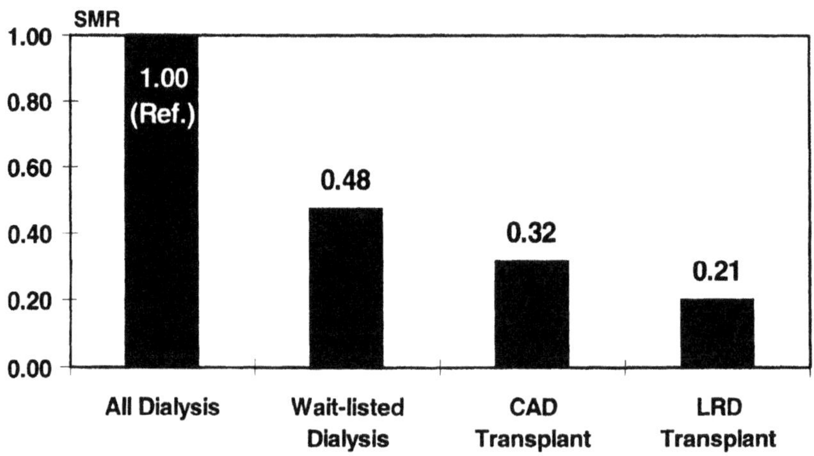

Figure 1. Adjusted mortality risk ratios by treatment modality for patients incident 1991–1996. Adjusted to age, sex and primary diagnosis (from Ref. [1]).

Table 1. Transplant work up: additional studies and needs in older recipients

Vascular	
	Cardiac – non invasive testing (echocardiogram; stress test)
	Peripheral – doppler studies
	Carotid – ultrasound (if bruits present)
GI	
	Endoscopy
	Barium enema
	Gallbladder ultrasound
	Prostatic surface antigen (PSA); voiding cystourethragram (VCUG)
Pre-Existing Bone Disease	
	Osteoporosis
	Renal osteodystrophy
Post-Operative Needs	
	Rehabilitation
	Eye care
	Support

prolonged hospitalization after transplant. Lastly, since the risk of renal allograft rejection is lower in older patients and the tendency for infection is higher, protocols for immunologic therapy should deliver less immunosuppression to older patients [8]. In older patients the major cause of renal allograft loss is not rejection but patient death due to cardiovascular disease and infection [1]. Hence, attention to details which prevent infection and cardiovascular disease are critical. Recent publications [8, 9] including that by the Clinical Practice Guidelines Committee of the American Society of Transplant Physicians [9], provides further details concerning the evaluation of individuals for transplant, including older patients.

Significant ethical issues here include the justification of using kidneys from the limited cadaveric donor pool for older patients who have a shortened life expectancy. In many centers, older patients are often encouraged to find a living donor. It has also been suggested that a 'Senior Citizen's Pool' be generated where kidneys from older donors be offered exclusively to older recipients awaiting transplant so that the shortened long-term graft survival of these older kidneys would be less relevant in patients with a shorter life expectancy [10]. Debate continues on this important and often emotionally charged topic.

Cadaveric Renal Donors

The increasing incidence of ESRD has created an enlarging list of patients awaiting transplant (38 000 in 1997). This number is expected to reach 60 000 by the year 2000. The increasing demand for cadaveric organs has 'pushed the envelope', leading us to consider the use of 'marginal' kidneys, including those from older donors. In 1995, one quarter of all cadaveric kidneys were from donors over 50 years old and the proportion continues to increase [2]. The down side of using kidneys from older donors is a decrease in long term graft survival [11, 12]. Although several single-center studies have found no difference in survival in these kidneys [11], UNOS (United Network for Organ Sharing) data demonstrate a significant decrease in survival with time [12].

Older kidneys are more susceptible to ischemic damage and subsequent rejection episodes. The shortened survival of kidneys from older donors may also come from a higher frequency of glomerulosclerosis in these kidneys. Many centers perform a kidney biopsy on all cadaveric donors over 55–60 years old. If glomerulosclerosis is present in more than 20% of glomeruli, a decision is then made to reject the kidney (putting it back into the pool) or, in some centers [7], two kidneys are placed into one recipient. Although the operation is longer, good results have been reported [7]. As mentioned above, use of a senior citizens' pool for older kidneys has been suggested to ensure a just use of these kidneys [10].

Kidneys from older donors may not survive as long as those from younger donors but still may offer the patient a survival advantage over dialysis. A recent study presented at the meetings of the American Society for Transplant Surgeons evaluated data from patients entered on the UNOS waiting list between 4/1/94 and 12/31/95. Patients were stratified for age, race, gender, sensitization and time since listing. Despite an increased risk of mortality in the initial post-transplant period, the risk of mortality at one year for candidates who received both older (> 55 years) and younger (< 55 years) donor kidneys was 38 to 96% less than for patients who remained on the waiting list an additional year (Table 2) [13]. This long-term-survival advantage of transplantation over dialysis, even in kidneys from older donors, was most apparent in diabetic recipients. Thus although older cadaveric kidneys do not last as long as younger kidneys, transplantation using these organs still may offer a survival advantage over remaining on dialysis.

Table 2. The impact of donor age on the mortality risk of transplantation (TX) vs. remaining on the waiting list (WL)[1]

Group	No. TX	Diabetes	Donor Age	Relative Risk of Mortality (TX versus WL)			
				1 Month	6 Month	1 Year	RR = 1 at Day
Kidney	110	Type 1	> 55	1.64	0.51	0.25*	82
	748		< 55	1.41	0.53*	0.25*	76
Kidney	815	None	> 55	2.94*	1.05	0.62	191
	5224		< 55	2.50*	0.68*	0.40*	119

* $p < 0.05$.

[1] Data from all adults on dialysis entered on the UNOS waiting list 4/1/98–12/31/95.

[2] Presented all the annual meeting of the American Society of Transplant Surgeons, May 1998.

Older Living Donors

The crisis in cadaveric organ shortage also is creating an increased demand for living donor organs. With national registry data that demonstrates excellent survival of kidneys from living unrelated donors [14], donors from spouses and friends are becoming commonplace and now constitute more of the living donor pool. When we (the Patient Care Committee of the American Society of Transplant Physicians) surveyed U.S. transplant centers in 1995 for their age cut-off for living donors, 27% had no age exclusion while 70% used > 70 years old [15]. The use of grandparents to serve as donors for children requiring a renal transplant is no longer an unusual event. This increasing acceptance of older living donors raises many questions about the longevity of the allograft and also about the risk to the donor.

Some short-term studies have reported good survival of kidneys from living donors over 55–65 years old while others have reported a compromised survival [11]. Clearly more long term data are needed in this area. Most centers follow a rigorous donor work-up protocol that would exclude donors with serious medical issues or depressed GFR (although the definition of depressed GFR varies among centers [15]). Also we must evaluate the long-term renal safety of uninephrectomy in donors over 60 years because earlier studies evaluating long term donor safety consisted mainly of individuals who donated at an earlier age. As the crisis in organ supply and demand continues and the the use of living donors expands, I suspect that, in the coming years, the question of 'who can be a renal donor' will be addressed to many nephrologists in and out of the transplant world. It will demand our best command of medical, ethical as well as legal knowledge to generate the answers to this question.

Summary

An increasing volume of data compels us to consider the issue of age in making decisions regarding both renal-transplant recipients and donors. We can summarize these geriatric issues in transplantation as follows:

(1) The explosion of a geriatric population of patients with ESRD, and data showing a survival advantage of transplantation over wait-listed dialysis patients calls us to become expert in transplanting patients over 60 years old.

(2) The critical shortage in cadaveric organ supply is creating a variety of solutions including expanding the donor pool with older kidneys in which long-term survival may be shorter than in kidneys from younger donors.

(3) The donor shortage and data that demonstrates improved survival of living related and unrelated donor transplants, has stimulated older (> 60 years old) individuals to donate to a relative, spouse or friend.

Future efforts should be directed toward continued research designed to evaluate the efficacy and safety of these trends. We also need to provide improved training in geriatrics for nephrologists so that we and transplant surgeons can deliver better medical care to an aging population of patients with ESRD.

References

1. U.S. Renal Data Systems. USRDS 1997. Annual Data Report. The National Institutes of Health, National Institutes of Diabetes and Digestive and Kidney Diseases. Bethesda, MD, 1997.
2. 1996 Annual Report of The U.S. Scientific Registry of Transplant Recipients and The Organ Procurement and Transplantation Network. Transplant Data 1988–1995. UNOS, Richmond, VA and the Division of Transplantation, Bureau of Health Resources Development, Health Resources and Services Administration, U.S. Department of Health and Human Services, Rockville, MD, 1996.
3. Terasaki PI, Cecka JM, Gjertson DW, Takemoto S, Cho YW, Yuge J. Risk and long-term kidney transplant survival. In: Cecka JM, Terasaki PI, editors. Clinical Transplants. CA: UCLA Tissue Typing Laboratory, 1996; 443–458.
4. Port FK, Wolfe RA, Mauger EA, Berling DP, Kaihong J. Comparison of survival probabilities for dialysis patients versus cadaveric renal transplant patients. J Am Med Assoc 1993; 270: 1339–1343.
5. Wolfe RA, Ashby VB, Milford EL, Ojo AO, Etttenger RE, Agodoa YC, Held PJ, Port FK. Patient survival for wait-listed (WL) dialysis versus cadaveric renal transplant (TX), patients in the U.S. (abstract). J Amer Soc Nephrol 1997; 8: 708A.
6. Schaubel D, Desmeules M, Mao Y, Jeffrey J, Fenton S. Survival experience among elderly end stage renal disease patients: a controlled comparison of transplantation and dialysis. Transplant 1995; 60: 1389–1394.
7. Scandling JD. Emerging options for renal transplantation in older patient. Nephrology Rounds 1998; 2(3).
8. Becker BN, Ismail N, Becker YT, MacDonnell RC, Helderman JH. Renal transplantation in the older end stage renal disease patient. Seminar in Nephrol 1996; 16: 353–362.
9. Kasiske BL, Ramos EL, Gaston RS, Bia MJ, Danovitch GM, Bowen RA, Lundin PA, Murphy KJ. The evaluation of renal transplant candidates: clinical practice guidelines. J Am Soc Nephrol 1995; 6: 1–34.
10. Gjertson DW, Terasaki PI, Cecka JM, Takemoto S, Cho YW. Senior Citizen pool for aged Kidneys. Trans Proc 1997; 29: 129.
11. Kauffman HM, Bennett LE, McBride MA, Ellison MD. The Expanded donor. Transplant Rev 1997; II: 165–190.
12. Terasaki PI, Gjertson DW, Cecka JM, Takemolo S, Cho YW. Significance of donor age effect on kidney transports. Clin Transplant 1997; II: 366–372.
13. Edwards E, Basadonna G. The impact of donor age on the mortality risk of transplantation vs remaining on the waiting list (WL) for kidney (K) and kidney/pancreas (KP) patients (abstract). Proc Am Soc Transplant Surg, May 1998: No. 165.
14. Terasaki PI, Cecka JM, Gjertson DW, Cho YW. Spousal and other living renal donor transplants. In: Cecka JM, Teresaki PI, editors, Clinical Transplants. CA: UCLA Tissue Typing Laboratory, 1997; 269–284.
15. Bia MJ, Ramos EL, Donovitch GM, Gaston RS, Harmonld E, Leichtman AB, Lundin PA, Neylon J, Kasiske BL. Evaluation of living donors: the current practice of U.S. transplanters. Transplant 1995; 60: 322–327.

Hydronephrosis and Renal Deterioration in the Elderly due to Abnormalities of the Lower Urinary Tract and Ureterovesical Junction

PERRY M. SUTARIA and DAVID R. STASKIN
Division of Urology, Beth Israel Deaconess Medical Center, Harvard Medical School, Boston, MA 02215, U.S.A.

The geriatric population presents a unique challenge to the health care provider. The incidence of common lower urinary tract disorders, such as benign prostatic hypertrophy (BPH), prostate cancer and incontinence increase dramatically with aging. In their more severe forms, these disorders may predispose to hydronephrosis and ultimately to renal deterioration. This review of lower urinary tract and ureterovesical junction (UVJ) physiology and pathophysiology, will focus on: (1) anatomic UVJ obstruction from prostate cancer, or severe bladder hypertrophy; (2) functional obstruction from compression or stretching of the UVJ during bladder distention from urinary retention; and (3) bladder decompensation in the female. We will present a diagnostic and treatment algorithm and discuss future trends in the geriatric population. Clearly, the geriatric health care provider always must consider the lower urinary tract when confronted with acute renal deterioration, because prompt diagnosis and treatment of significant, lower-urinary-tract disease can maximize recovery of renal function.

In the elderly a primary objective of urologic care of the lower urinary tract is to manage the storage and emptying functions of the bladder and bladder outlet. In these patients voiding dysfunction may present as bothersome irritative or obstructive lower urinary tract symptoms or incontinence. However, the more severe forms of lower urinary tract pathology may compromise renal function by causing ureteral obstruction, hydronephrosis and ultimately obstructive nephropathy and renal failure.

Lower urinary tract (bladder, prostate and urethra) and ureterovesical junction (UVJ) causes of ureteral obstruction include anatomic encroachment or functional compression of the UVJ. Anatomic obstruction may be due to extrinsic invasion by prostate cancer or to hypertrophy of the bladder musculature surrounding the ureteral tunnel. Functional compression of the UVJ occurs with bladder overdistention, which increases ureteral resistance through the ureteral tunnel. Benign prostatic hyperplasia (BPH) and carcinoma of the prostate are common in the elderly male. The incidence of both BPH and prostate cancer increases rapidly with age and both may contribute to urinary retention and bladder overdistention, as well as to direct invasion of the UVJ.

Oreopoulos et al. (eds.), Nephrology and Geriatrics Integrated, 155–165.

Although outlet obstruction in the elderly female is rare in comparison, urinary retention secondary to bladder decompensation is more common, and may impair upper tract emptying.

Lower Urinary Tract Function and Dysfunction

Normal lower urinary tract function is a complex interaction between physiology, pharmacology, neurology and anatomy. Of the many complex classifications that have been devised to characterize normal and abnormal voiding patterns, the clearest and most direct separates voiding into two distinct processes: (1) bladder filling and storage, and (2) bladder emptying [1].

Normal bladder filling and storage depends on two properties. The bladder must progressively fill with urine at low intravesical pressures, and the bladder outlet must remain closed. Bladder filling is under sympathetic (adrenergic) control. Sympathetic stimulation of beta-receptors in the bladder wall lead to smooth muscle relaxation, which allows the bladder to fill at low pressures. Sympathetic alpha-receptor stimulation in the area of the bladder outlet lead to smooth-muscle contraction and increased outlet resistance so there is no leakage during the filling and storage phase. The combined sympathetic beta and alpha effects allow the bladder to fill at low pressures without urinary leakage.

Normal bladder emptying, which is slightly more complex, also depends on two basic functions. The bladder outlet must relax and the bladder detrusor muscle must have an effective and coordinated contraction of adequate strength and duration. The relaxation of the outlet is both voluntary and autonomic (decreased sympathetic tone) and bladder contraction is under parasympathetic, autonomic control. The voiding mechanism first involves the voluntary relaxation of the striated muscle of the outlet via the pudendal nerve. The smooth muscle of the outlet also relaxes by a decrease in sympathetic alpha-receptor stimulation. Finally the bladder contracts in a co-ordinated manner via parasympathetic, cholinergic stimulation through the pelvic nerve.

Similarly lower urinary tract dysfunction can be divided into: (1) a failure to store urine, and (2) a failure to empty urine. Anatomically the lower urinary tract is separated into two functional areas: (1) the bladder, and (2) the bladder outlet. Virtually all pathologic voiding conditions can be characterized using these four categories.

Failure to store urine results from an increase in bladder pressure or a decrease in outlet resistance, alone or in combination. Failure to empty urine result from a decrease in bladder activity or an overactive bladder outlet, alone or in combination. Combinations of storage and emptying problems are also common in the elderly. The extreme form of failing to empty is overflow voiding, which may present as incontinence (failure to store). The geriatric patient also may present with detrusor hyper-reflexia with impaired contractility (DHIC); this condition is defined as uninhibited bladder contractions sufficient to cause incontinence but not to empty the bladder to completion (again this is a combination of storage and emptying disorders).

UVJ Function and Dysfunction

The ureterovesical junction (UVJ) is an anatomic structure with important physiologic functions. The UVJ allows unidirectional urine flow and the passage of urine boluses at low pressures into the bladder. Anatomically the UVJ begins when the ureter enters the bladder wall and pierces the detrusor muscle (ureteral hiatus). The ureter then runs underneath the bladder mucosa for 1.5–2 cm and terminates at the ureteral orifice. The intravesical portion of the ureter is surrounded by the trigonal musculature and fascia (Waldeyer's sheath) and runs just below the bladder mucosa. The intravesical ureter is quite pliant and is backed by a strong plate of bladder muscle (Fig. 1) [2]. This arrangement results in passive occlusion of the ureter with bladder filling, like a flap valve, and in unidirectional urine flow through the UVJ. Reflux is thought to occur when the portion of submucosal ureter is of inadequate length, thereby rendering the flap valve ineffective and allowing the retrograde passage of urine from the bladder to the upper tracts.

UVJ dysfunction is broadly categorized as congenital or acquired. Congenital anomalies lie outside the scope of this discussion and in general do not play a major role in renal deterioration in the elderly. The acquired lesions are either anatomic or functional (physiologic). Anatomic dysfunction is simply anatomic blockage or encroachment upon the UVJ with subsequent obstruction, hydronephrosis and renal deterioration. Examples of intrinsic anatomic UVJ obstruction include ureteral tumors and stones. Extrinsic UVJ compression can be from locally advanced prostate cancer, bladder cancer, other locally advanced pelvic and metastatic malignancies, inflammatory lesions such as retroperitoneal fibrosis and prior pelvic radiation. Functional UVJ obstruction is due to a failure to empty the bladder (retention) because of poor bladder contractility or increased outlet resistance. Functional obstruction can be categorized as either low-pressure urinary retention or high-pressure retention, depending on the compliance of the bladder wall and on the resistance of the bladder outlet to leakage. Animal models have examined these factors in detail [3]. Each of these types of retention have a unique physiology and pathophysiology regardless of the causes of the infravesical obstruction and likely play a significant role in the renal deterioration of the elderly.

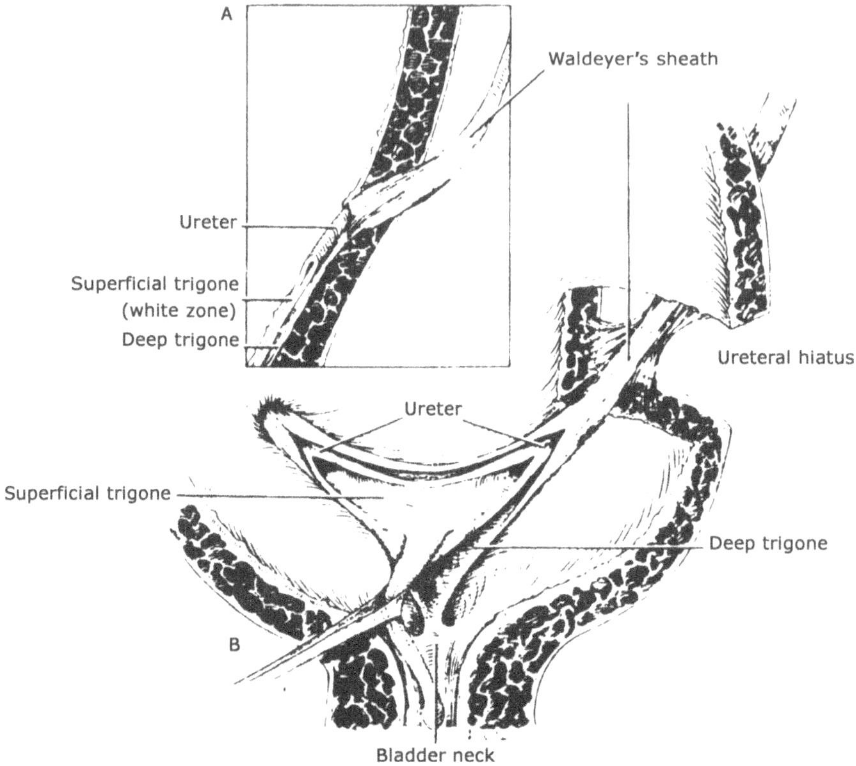

Figure 1. The normal ureterovesical junction and trigone. (A) section of the bladder wall perpendicular to the ureteral hiatus shows the oblique passage of the ureter through the detrusor and also shows the submucosal ureter with its detrusor backing. Waldeyer's sheath surrounds the prevesical ureter and extends inward to become the deep trigone. (B) Waldeyer's sheath continues in the bladder as the deep trigone, which is fixed at the bladder neck. (From Tanagho 1963.)

Common Lower Urinary Tract and UVJ Causes of Hydronephrosis and Renal Deterioration in the Elderly

The many causes of hydronephrosis and renal deterioration in the elderly are shown in Table 1. We will concentrate on lower urinary tract pathology where obstruction is the classic cause of upper tract damage. Obstruction may develop at any level along the distal ureter, UVJ, bladder, prostate or urethra and can be intrinsic e.g., ureteral carcinoma, ureteral stone or ureteral stricture or extrinsic e.g., retroperitoneal fibrosis or radiation therapy. We mention these processes chiefly to draw attention to their pathophysiologic mechanisms because they represent only a small percentage of elderly patients with sig-

Table 1. Causes of hydronephrosis and renal deterioration in the elderly

Upper Urinary Tract	
Extrinsic ureteral obstruction	
Inflammatory:	retroperitoneal fibrosis, abdominal aortic aneurysm, appendicitis, radiation therapy, inflammatory bowel disease
Anatomic:	crossing vessel
Neoplastic:	retroperitoneal tumor (lymphoma, sarcoma, metastatic)
Traumatic:	surgical ligation
Intrinsic ureteral obstruction	
Stone, stricture (stone, iatrogenic), ureteral cancer	
Physiologic/congenital	
Diuresis, UPJ obstruction, congenital megaureter,	
Lower Urinary Tract and Ureterovesical Junction	
Congenital:	reflux, UVJ obstruction, megaureter, ureterocele, duplex systems posterior urethral valves, ectopic ureter
UVJ Obstruction	
Anatomic obstruction	
Intrinsic:	ureteral Ca, stones
Extrinsic:	prostate Ca, bladder Ca, chronic obstruction with detrusor hypertrophy
Functional obstruction – Retention	
High pressure retention:	compression from "intravesical pressure"
Low pressure retention:	compression from "stretch and stress"
Bladder outlet obstruction:	bladder neck dysfunction, prostatic obstruction (BPH, prostate Ca)
Sphincteric dysfunction:	detrusor sphincter dyssynergy
Urethral disease:	stricture, cancer, stone

nificant hydronephrosis and renal deterioration. Discussion will focus on: (1) anatomic obstruction at the UVJ from malignant prostatic disease, or severe bladder hypertrophy; (2) functional obstruction resulting from compression or stretching the UVJ during bladder distention from urinary retention, most commonly associated with benign prostatic disease in the male; and (3) bladder decompensation in the female.

Anatomic UVJ Obstruction

Prostate cancer, which represents 36% of all new cancers, is the cause of 14% of all cancer deaths in men [4]. The median age at diagnosis is 72 years and the increase in incidence with aging is nearly exponential; specifically, the incidence of prostate cancer more than doubles between ages 65–75 [5]. Prostate cancer increases faster with age than any other major cancer, and the burden of prostate cancer will continue to grow.

Extension of prostatic carcinoma into the bladder (localized metastatic disease) can obstruct the ureters, regardless of bladder volume or detrusor activity. This type of silent hydronephrosis may present as uremia rather than renal colic because the disease progress is insidious. Fortunately, ureteral obstruction from prostatic carcinoma is rare; it is treated by stenting of the ureters and hormonal therapy (orchiectomy or antiandrogen). Also it is important to realize that many patients who are being followed for local or distant metastatic disease rarely present in uremia from ureteral obstruction; more often, they suffer from uremia secondary to urinary retention [6]. The differential diagnosis can be made by passing a Foley catheter.

Anatomic obstruction also can be secondary to severe detrusor hypertrophy associated with chronic obstruction. In the elderly, this usually is due to benign prostatic disease such as BPH. In this circumstance, the UVJ is obstructed by bladder muscle hypertrophy. Since outlet obstruction is not the sole cause of the renal deterioration, bypassing the infravesical obstruction with a Foley catheter will not totally relieve the upper tract obstruction and correct the uropathy. Often it is necessary to place ureteral stents or carry out percutaneous renal decompression to ensure recovery of renal function.

Functional UVJ Obstruction

Functional obstruction of the UVJ is strictly due to infravesical obstruction at the bladder neck, the prostate e.g., carcinoma or BPH or urethra e.g., stricture or malignancy. The end result is urinary retention. In the elderly male, the most common cause of urinary retention is benign prostatic hyperplasia (BPH). BPH is the most common benign neoplasm in the elderly. By 85 years of age, 90% of men will have identifiable BPH within their prostate gland [7] and, by age 75 up to 25% of men will require medical or surgical intervention for their symptoms [8]. In a significant number of these patients, the upper urinary tracts also are at risk. A combined analysis of 25 BPH studies showed that 7% of patients with clinical symptoms of BPH will have hydronephrosis and up to 33% of them will have associated renal insufficiency [9]. Also patients with BPH have a risk of urinary retention that increases about 1% per year [10], and as the male population ages, retention with associated renal insufficiency will become a more prominent feature of benign prostatic disease.

Acute and chronic urinary retention ultimately can produce renal insufficiency in some patients. It presents in two basic forms: (1) low intravesical pressure retention and (2) high intravesical pressure retention, each of which has a unique pathophysiology and each ultimately can lead to renal deterioration. In the 'healthy bladder' without outlet obstruction, the bladder stores fluid at low pressure, thus allowing the upper tracts to empty at low renal pelvic and ureteral pressures, thereby preserving upper tract function. In addition, normal emptying also occurs at low pressures, which prevents detrusor hypertrophy, loss of bladder-wall compliance and eventual detrusor decompensation.

In urinary retention, changes in the compliance and contractility of the bladder ultimately determine the degree of elevation of intravesical pressure. The resting resistance of the bladder outlet determines both the 'overflow' pressure – that required to allow urinary leakage during chronic retention, and the constant pressure that is maintained within the bladder. The frequency and duration of detrusor contractions also determine the chronic intravesicle pressure [11] and the resistance to ureteral urine flow [12, 13].

In the normal bladder, without overdistention, the urine, by peristalsis enters a low pressure reservoir (the bladder) through a tunnel of low resistance (the intravesicle ureter). Low pressure retention develops when the bladder volume increases without an increase in intravesicle pressure. This increase in volume even without an increase in pressure, can lead to UVJ obstruction, hydronephrosis and renal deterioration. Increased bladder volumes apply 'tension' and 'stretch' forces to the ureter as it courses through the bladder wall. Chronic low pressure retention stretches the intravesicle ureter and exposes this portion to increased detrusor-wall tension proportional to the radius (ie. the volume) of the bladder according to LaPlaces' law [14, 15]. Both effects contribute to UVJ obstruction. The normal intravesical ureter acts as a unidirectional 'flap valve' and any increase its length provides additional resistance to the flow of urine from the upper tracts. This increases the upper tract emptying pressures and produces functional (physiologic) UVJ obstruction. Similarly the increase in wall tension (when the bladder diameter increases) produces an increase in the compressive force that is applied to the intravesicle ureter and also may lead to hydronephrosis and renal deterioration.

Chronic obstruction also can lead to high pressure urinary retention, independent of the bladder volume. Patients who compensate for bladder outlet obstruction by increasing bladder activity and detrusor contractile strength may be subject to a higher risk of detrusor hypertrophy and functional ureteral obstruction [16]. In some patients the intrinsic properties of the bladder, such as its smooth muscle tone, its extracellular matrix composition and the resistance of the outlet predispose to a poorly compliant, high-pressure reservoir that in turn can lead to upper tract damage [17]. In this circumstance the mechanism of damage is more obvious; persistent high pressures within the bladder provide a direct resistance to the low-pressure emptying of the renal pelvis and ureter. In addition, the increased pressures directly compress and obstruct the UVJ. Ultimately this leads to hydronephrosis and, if left untreated by medication, surgery or Foley catheter, ends in renal deterioration.

The Female Patient

In the absence of spinal-cord disease, hydronephrosis and renal deterioration due to lower urinary tract or UVJ dysfunction is rare in the elderly female. Also, urinary retention from increased outlet resistance (obstruction) is unusual. However, certain conditions predispose to retention, e.g. iatrogenic obstruction from operations for incontinence, severe atrophic vaginitis with urethral stenosis, or other rare malignant or benign growths within the urethra. In the female, hydronephrosis also can be associated with obstruction at the UVJ or distal ureters from large cystoceles with or without uterine prolapse. Rarely obstruction may be due to a large retroflexed uterus [18] or larger uterine fibroids [19].

A more common cause of retention in the female patient is detrusor decompensation (poor bladder contractility). In general, females have low outlet resistance to leakage (detrusor 'leak point' pressure) so that the female, who is incontinent (overflow incontinence) at low bladder pressures, generally is protected from upper tract damage. In rare circumstances where bladder compliance is poor, upper tract damage can occur when residual urine is high and where outlet resistance is also high. In these cases, women suffer the same pathophysiology previously discussed in men. Therefore, females with acute renal deterioration and hydronephrosis also require lower urinary tract evaluation. While significant pathology is rare, a lower urinary tract abnormality, when found, is often easy to correct; thus prompt diagnosis and treatment can ensure maximum renal recovery.

Diagnosis and Treatment of Hydronephrosis and Renal Deterioration in the Elderly

In the elderly evaluation of the lower urinary tract for causes of hydronephrosis and renal deterioration follows an uncomplicated diagnostic and treatment algorithm (Fig. 2). An elderly patient with acute renal deterioration requires an initial imaging study to identify hydronephrosis; its absence is a good indication that the lesion likely is pre-renal or renal – rarely retroperitoneal fibrosis. If hydronephrosis is present, one must determine if the patient is in urinary retention, either with imaging studies, or by simply placing a Foley catheter.

If retention is present and the hydronephrosis resolves, the patient needs to be evaluated for either decreased bladder contractility – neurogenic, from chronic obstruction, or increased outlet resistance – BPH, prostate cancer, urethral stricture alone or in combination. This can be done with urodynamic studies to assess both the bladder and the outlet and with cystoscopy to search for anatomic obstruction. The treatment will be based on the cause of the retention.

If retention is present, but hydronephrosis persists after Foley drainage, one should suspect anatomic UVJ obstruction from detrusor hypertrophy secondary to chronic retention. Again the evaluation includes urodynamic studies and cystoscopy. The obstruction is relieved promptly with either a percutaneous nephrostomy tube or ureteral stent, while attention is directed to diagnosis and treatment of the cause of chronic retention. Once the retention is resolved, the UVJ obstruction usually dissipates, but the patient may need long-term, chronic decompression.

Hydronephrosis without retention requires a search for causes of ureteral or UVJ obstruction, or for unusual physiologic or congenital causes of per-

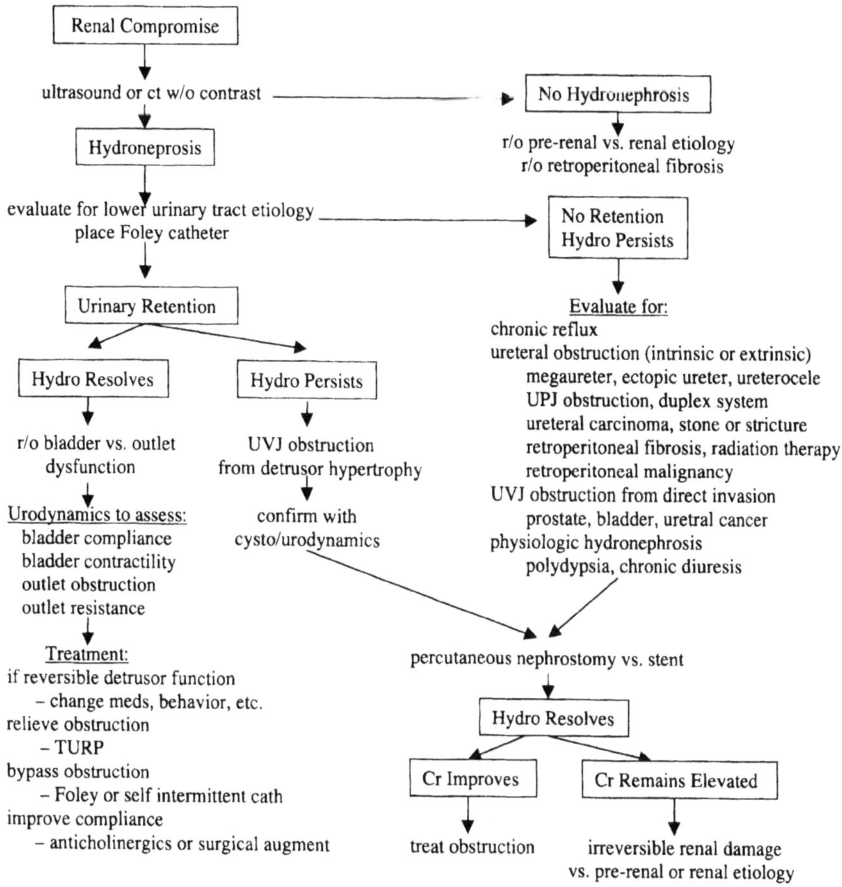

Figure 2. Diagnostic and treatment algorithm for renal compromise and hydronephrosis in the elderly.

sistent hydronephrosis. Again one needs to relieve the obstruction immediately with either a percutaneous nephrostomy tube or ureteral stents. Long-term treatment is directed to the relief of the obstructing process or, if no treatment is possible, to continue mechanical drainage. Ultimately the degree of renal recovery will direct further investigation. If renal function does not improve after decompression, one must entertain the possibility of irreversible renal damage from obstruction or coexisting pre-renal and/or renal dysfunction.

Conclusion

In the elderly, lower tract dysfunction may predispose to upper tract deterioration. Clearly the increasing incidence with aging of common lower-urinary-tract pathology – BPH, prostate cancer, incontinence, and subsequent voiding dysfunction, predisposes them to upper tract damage. In addition, there is an increasing trend towards 'conservative' (medical) therapy for obstructive voiding symptoms in men and urge incontinence in women. We know that BPH can predispose to 'silent' hydronephrosis and ultimately to renal deterioration. It remains to be seen whether the increased use of medical therapy (alpha blockers) to control symptoms will delay surgical intervention, allowing growth of the prostate to continue and, in turn, lead to a higher incidence of 'silent' hydronephrosis and renal damage in the conservatively treated man. Similarly, the increased use of anticholinergics for urge incontinence (or the side effects of these medications when used for other conditions) also may increase the incidence of urinary retention in the elderly. When one chooses to treat voiding complaints in the elderly with medical therapy post void residual urine must be monitored to avoid inadvertent urinary retention.

Prostate cancer in the elderly male also is of great concern. The incidence of prostate cancer rises with aging and the geriatric population is expanding rapidly; thus in the future we will diagnose more prostate cancer and these people will live longer with their cancers. Again we will see an increase in the incidence of local complications such as outlet obstruction with retention or direct ureteral invasion. Similarly, the increasing popularity of surgical treatment for stress incontinence will expose elderly women to iatrogenic bladder outlet obstruction, especially since intrinsic voiding function may deteriorate with aging. These patients need to be monitored carefully. Clearly, the geriatric health-care provider always must consider the lower urinary tract when he or she is confronted with acute renal deterioration or hydronephrosis. The prompt diagnosis and treatment of significant lower urinary-tract disease will assure each elderly patient maximum recovery of renal function.

References

1. Wein AJ, Barrett DM. Voiding Function and Dysfunction: A Logical and Practical Approach. Chicago: Year Book Medical Publishers, 1988.
2. Tanagho EA, Pugh RCB. The anatomy and function of the ureterovesical junction. Br J Urol 1963; 35: 151–165.
3. Blok C, Van Venrooij GEPM, Mokhless I, Coolsaet BLRA. Dynamics of the ureterovesical junction: Its resistance to upper urinary tract outflow in pigs. J of Urol 1986; 136: 1127–1131.
4. Wingo PA, Tong T, Bolden S. Cancer statistics, 1995. Cancer J Clin 1995; 45: 8–31.
5. Pienta KJ, Esper PS. Risk factors for prostate cancer. Ann Intern Med 1993; 118: 793–803.
6. Colombel M, Mallame W, Abbou CC. Influence of urological complication on the prognosis of prostate cancer. Eur Urol 1997; 31 (Suppl): 21–24.
7. Isaacs JT, Coffey DS. Etiology and disease process of benign prostatic hyperplasia. Prostate 1989; 2 (suppl): 33–50.
8. O'Brien WM. Benign prostatic hypertrophy. Am Fam Phys 1991; 44: 162–171.
9. McConnell JD, Barry MJ, Bruskewitz RC, et al. Benign prostatic hyperplasia: diagnosis and treatment. Clinical Practice Guidelines. No. 8, AHCPR Publication No. 94-0582.

Rockville, MD: Agency for Health Care Policy and Research, Public Health Service, U.S. Department of Health and Human Services, 1994.

10. McConnell JD. Epidemiology, etiology, pathophysiology and diagnosis of benign prostatic hyperplasia. In: Walsh PC, Retik AB, Vaughan ED Jr, Wein, AJ, editors. Campbell's Urology, Seventh Edition. Philadelphia: Saunders, 1998; 1429–1452.
11. Styles RA, Neal DE, Griffiths CJ, Ramsden PD. Long-term monitoring of bladder pressure in chronic retention of urine: the relationship between detrusor activity and upper tract dilation. J Urol 1988; 140: 330–334.
12. Blok C, van Venrooij GEPM, Coolsaet BLRA. Dynamics of the ureterovesical junction: Effectiveness of its ureteral peristalsis in high pressure pig bladders. J of Urol 1985; 134: 825–827.
13. Blok C, Coolsaet BLRA, Mansour M, Razzouk A. Dynamics of the ureterovesical junction: interaction between diuresis and detrusor instability at the ureterovesical junction in pigs. J of Urol 1986; 136: 1123–1126.
14. Steers WD. Physiology and pharmacology of the bladder and urethra. In: Walsh PC, Retik AB, Vaughan ED Jr, Wein, AJ, editors. Campbell's Urology, Seventh Edition. Philadelphia: Saunders, 1998; 870–915.
15. Staskin DR. Hydroureteronephrosis after spinal cord injury. Effects of lower urinary tract dysfunction on upper tract anatomy. Urol Clin North Am 1991; 18: 309–316.
16. Kerr LA, Bauer SB, Staskin DR. Abnormal detrusor function precipitating hydronephrosis identified by extended voiding cystometry. J of Urol 1994; 152: 89–92.
17. Styles RA, Ramsden PD, Neal DE. Chronic retention of urine. The relationship between upper tract dilation and bladder pressure. Br J Urol 1986; 58: 647–651.
18. Keating PJ, Walton SM, Maouris P. Incarceration of a bicornuate retroverted gravid uterus presenting with bilateral ureteric obstruction. Br J Gynaecol 1992; 99: 345–347.
19. Monga AK, Woodhouse CR, Stanton SL. Pregnancy and fibroids causing simultaneous urinary retention and ureteric obstruction. Br J Urol 1996; 77: 606–607.

The Geriatric Patient with Obstructive Uropathy

SAULO KLAHR
Simon Professor of Medicine, Department of Medicine, Washington University School of Medicine at Barnes-Jewish Hospital, St. Louis, MO 63110-1092, U.S.A.

Definitions

'Obstructive nephropathy' refers to the renal disease caused by impaired flow of urine or tubular fluid. 'Obstructive uropathy' refers to the structural or functional changes in the urinary tract that impede the normal flow of urine. 'Hydronephrosis' describes dilatation of the urinary tract [1].

Incidence and Prevalence

Obstructive uropathy is common and occurs at all ages. Hydronephrosis has been found at postmortem in 3.5–3.8% of patients with equal distribution between males and females. After the age of 60, obstructive uropathy is more frequent in males due to the increased incidence of benign prostatic hyperplasia and carcinoma of the prostate. In the U.S. in 1985 about 166 patients per 100 000 population were hospitalized with a presumptive diagnosis of obstructive uropathy. At discharge it was the fourth leading diagnosis among males with kidney and urological disorders with a rate of 242 per 100 000 discharges. In females, obstructive uropathy ranked sixth among the diagnoses at discharge in patients with kidney and urological disorders with a rate of 94 per 100 000 population. In 1985, in the U.S., 387 per 100 000 patient visits were ascribed to obstructive uropathy [2]. Some 450 000 surgical procedures are performed yearly for benign prostatic hyperplasia, making this the most common operation in males. In 1985, about 80% of these operations were done on men age 65 or older. In the United States from 1989 to 1993, a five-year span, 4869 patients with the diagnosis of obstructive nephropathy began treatment for end-stage renal disease (ESRD) [3]. During this period, obstructive nephropathy accounted for 2% of the patients being treated under Medicare regulations for ESRD. Among the 4869 patients with obstructive nephropathy treated for ESRD, 6.9% were younger than 20 years of age, 35.7% were between the ages of 20 and 64, and 57.4% were older

Oreopoulos et al. (eds.), Nephrology and Geriatrics Integrated, 167–177.

than 64 years. Males comprised 73.8% of those with obstructive nephropathy who were being treated for ESRD.

Clinical Considerations

Changes in renal function that occur with normal aging have an important impact on the routine clinical management of urinary tract obstruction in the geriatric patient. During the period of obstruction, older patients run a greater risk of volume overload, from continuous salt intake, and of hyperkalemia and acid-base disturbances. Also the salt-losing tendency and abnormalities of water conservation that follow the relief of obstruction may be more severe in the geriatric patient. Contrast material must be used cautiously in the diagnosis of obstructive nephropathy in elderly patients because of the increased susceptibility of the aging kidney to injury. Geriatric patients have a greater propensity to develop congestive heart failure or pulmonary edema during obstruction or during the dehydration that follows relief of obstruction. Since lower urinary tract obstruction is more common and instrumentation is needed more frequently in the elderly, infections of the urinary tract are common in this group [4].

The physician should consider all of these factors when managing geriatric patients with urinary-tract obstruction.

Causes of Urinary Tract Obstruction in the Elderly (Table 1)

Intrinsic Causes of Urinary Tract Obstruction

Intraluminal Causes

Intraluminal obstruction can be intrarenal or extrarenal. A common cause of *intrarenal obstruction*, the deposition of uric acid crystals in the tubular lumen (uric-acid nephropathy), is seen most commonly in hematological malignancies, particularly during treatment with alkylating agents. The severity of the obstruction bears a direct relationship to the levels of uric acid in the plasma.

The second most common cause of death in patients with multiple myeloma is renal failure. This may be due to deposition of Bence-Jones protein in the lumen of the renal tubules because histological studies of end-stage kidneys of patients with multiple myeloma show (in the tubules) a lamellar deposition of a protein that is immunologically similar to Bence-Jones protein. Also, it has been observed that the incidence of renal failure is higher in patients with multiple myeloma and Bence-Jones proteinuria. Further, the severity of the renal disease correlates well with the quantity of Bence-Jones protein excreted. Against this concept, however, most of these patients with early renal failure have striking alterations in renal tubule cell morphology, but no histological evidence of protein deposition. Thus, in these patients renal insufficiency may be related to the toxic rather than the obstructive effects of Bence-Jones protein. Further, in multiple myeloma large retroperitoneal myelomatous masses may produce extrinsic obstruction of the ureter.

Probably the most common *causes* of intraluminal obstruction are renal calculi and blood clots. Renal calculi – composed of magnesium ammonium sulphate (struvite) – develop in patients with persistently alkaline urine and frequent urinary tract infections – a clinical combination often observed in the elderly. The prevalence of this type of renal stones in the elderly is unknown, but 15% of all renal calculi are struvite stones. No one knows whether the primary event leading to stone formation is an abnormality in urinary acidification or infection with urea-splitting organisms, but the frequency of urinary-tract infections is significantly greater in all types of kidney stone diseases and struvite stones may occur in individuals on chronic alkali therapy alone. Regardless of the exact mechanism of stone formation, infection with urea-splitting organisms, most commonly *Proteus* and less frequently *Klebsiella* and *Pseudomonas*, leads to alkalinization of the urine and increased concentration of ammonia. This environment favors the precipitation of triple-phosphate crystals.

Intramural Causes

Such causes of urinary tract obstruction can be (1) *functional* or (2) *anatomical*. In the elderly the two major functional abnormalities – those related to dynamic abnormalities in the urinary tract are neurogenic bladder and bladder-neck dysfunction.

Neurogenic Bladder

Abnormalities of urine storage in the bladder are characterized by incontinence and not infrequently by sustained increases in intravesical pressure, which can impair ureteral and renal function [5]. Alterations in the elastic and other properties of the bladder wall may produce a non-compliance state in which the bladder resists filling at a higher than normal pressure. Pathological processes that damage the musculature and its elastic fibers alter the normal bladder's accommodation response. Prolonged catheterization, drainage via suprapubic tubes, chronic infection, interstitial cystitis and radiation can result in permanent transmural injury and fibrosis of the bladder. Usually increased vesical pressures – greater than 40–50 cm of water – are associated with ureteral dilatation and the development of vesicoureteral reflux. In addition, inflammation and ultimately fibrosis of the trigone that follows long-term chronic catheterization seems to lead to vesicoureteral reflux, even at moderate bladder pressures [5]. These complications develop particularly in elderly patients, when chronic catheterization is used to manage incontinence.

In addition to changes in the anatomic characteristics of the bladder wall, neurological abnormalities may impair the storage ability of the bladder [6].

Table 1. Causes of urinary tract obstruction in the elderly

I. Intrinsic Causes
- A. Intraluminal
  - 1. Intrarenal: uric acid; multiple myeloma
  - 2. Extrarenal: calculi; blood clots
- B. Intramural
  - 1. Functional
    - (a) Neurogenic bladder: diseases of the brain, spinal cord or of peripheral innervation
    - (b) Bladder neck dysfunction
  - 2. Anatomical
    - (a) Tumours (polyps, carcinoma)
    - (b) Infections
    - (c) Strictures (post-radiation)

II. Extrinsic Causes
- A. Reproductive system
  - 1. Males: prostatic enlargement either benign prostatic hyperplasia or adenocarcinoma
  - 2. Females: uterus prolapse, fibro-adenoma, carcinoma of the cervix
- B. Gastrointestinal tract
  - Malignancies
- C. Vascular system
  - Aneurysmal dilatation
- D. Retroperitoneal space
  - 1. Fibrosis
  - 2. Surgical complications
  - 3. Tumours: primary or metastatic
  - 4. Hemorrhage (hematomas)

Damage to the pelvic nerve, as may occur, for example, during a radical pelvic operation for carcinoma of the cervix, rectum or prostate, in time produces a subtle abnormality of storage function that appears to be due to injury of the preganglionic parasympathetic motor axon. The bladder becomes 'hypertonic' and resists filling with a greater-than-normal pressure. The pressure/volume relationship is determined by the strength of the urethral continence mechanism, which determines the intravesical pressure at which the urethra begins to release urine. As soon as the intravesical pressure equals the urethral pressure, urine is lost from the urethra. Therefore, the peak intravesical pressure is approximately equal to peak intraurethral pressure. After pelvic neural transection, there is no neural mechanism to allow sphincteric relaxation with an increase in intravesical pressure.

Bladder Neck Dysfunction

This abnormality, which has a peak incidence in the fourth to sixth decades of life [7], is an uncommon cause of obstructive nephropathy. Contracture of the vesical neck with difficulty in urination may complicate any form of prostatectomy, but is more common after transurethral resection.

Extrinsic Causes of Urinary Tract Obstruction

Prostatic Enlargement

Enlargement of the prostate to the point where it produces obstruction of the urethra is an almost universal finding in aging men [8]. Because of considerable progress in prostatic surgery, benign prostatic hyperplasia is no longer a leading cause of death in the elderly but it remains a major cause of morbidity. The prostate weighs approximately 1 g at birth, increases to about 4 g before puberty, and then grows to about 20 g by age 20. On average, there is no further change in prostatic weight for approximately 20–30 years. Then a second growth spurt begins and results in a mean weight of approximately 60 g by age 70. The frequency of symptomatic prostatic hyperplasia in American men above the age of 50 varies from 50–75% in most series [9]. In a small fraction of men, the gland atrophies with age, presumably because of atherosclerosis of the arteries that supply blood to the gland.

In white men symptoms of urethral obstruction are unusual before 55 years of age; however, the disorder appears to be more common and manifests itself approximately 10 years earlier in black men. Japanese men have a lower incidence of urethral obstruction than European and American men. There is no close relationship between the degree of enlargement and the development of symptoms, and there can be severe obstruction of the urethra as a result of regional changes within the prostate in the absence of generalized growth [10]. The discrepancy between the size of the gland and symptoms is due to the fact that benign prostatic hyperplasia begins in the periurethral area of the gland. The exact age at which this process commences is uncertain but it probably occurs after 40 years. As the tissue in the periurethral area enlarges, it compresses the urethra and may produce obstructive symptoms before enlargement beyond the prostatic capsule. Thus obstruction may develop before one can recognize an increase in prostatic weight [11].

Clinical Manifestations. Usually the symptoms of prostatic hypertrophy include disturbances in micturition – urgency, frequency, decreased urinary stream and the finding of an enlarged prostate on rectal examination. Rarely, prostatic enlargement may be accompanied by symptoms that are so mild that the patients are unaware of them or choose to ignore them. Usually mild disturbances in micturition are discovered only after careful and direct questioning. With progressive obstruction, the residual urine increases and eventually results in overflow incontinence. An enlarged prostate that causes obstruction may produce hypertrophy of the detrusor with eventual detrusor decompensation, trabeculate formation and bladder diverticuli. This hypertrophy of the detrusor also may cause obstruction of the intramural ureter and dilatation of the upper urinary tract with progressive renal damage. Reflux of urine into the ureters (found in up to 14% of such patients) also contributes to renal damage [12].

Clinical Consequences of Urinary Tract Obstruction

Obstructive uropathy is a common cause of renal failure. The symptoms and signs of obstructive uropathy often are nonspecific. The associated clinical abnormalities may be dominated by impaired renal function, by manifestations related to urinary tract infection, and sometimes by extrarenal manifestations of the underlying pathologic process responsible for the obstructive uropathy, such as tumors or metastases from distal tumors.

Renal Failure Associated with Obstructive Uropathy

Bilateral obstruction of the urinary tract can cause acute or chronic renal failure. Acute renal failure also may occur when a solitary kidney is obstructed. If acute renal failure presents with complete anuria or if periods of anuria alternate with periods of polyuria, one should entertain the possibility of obstructive uropathy. With partial or intermittent obstruction, polyuria may be a consequence of the concentrating defect that occurs in obstructed kidneys [13–15]. Under such conditions, thirst may be a prominent symptom. Patients presenting with the signs and symptoms of chronic uremia may have undetected, longstanding, urinary-tract obstruction. Such obstruction may appear in the setting of underlying parenchymal renal disease of another etiology and manifest itself by a change in the rate of progression of renal insufficiency. In some patients, however, obstruction may be the only cause of end-stage renal failure. Occasionally, in patients with retroperitoneal fibrosis in whom the obstruction develops in a slow and progressive manner, an initial presenting complaint may be far-advanced renal failure. One should consider urinary-tract obstruction in patients with uremia and no previous history of renal disease and a relatively benign urine sediment. Also it should be considered in those with known renal disease, who develop an abrupt and otherwise unexplained decrease in renal function.

Pain and Renal Enlargement

Sometimes pain may be the presenting complaint in patients with urinary-tract obstruction, usually those with acute or rapidly developing obstruction. Acute ureteral obstruction may be characterized by steady, crescendo pain radiating downward toward the groin, the testicles, or labia [16]; however, there may be no pain, especially in patients with chronic slowly progressive obstruction. Occasionally, such patients may complain of dull flank pain usually related to increased fluid intake or to the use of diuretics [17]. Flank pain during micturition is said to be pathognomic of ureterovesical reflux. Sometimes kidney size may increase notably in long-standing obstruction. These patients may have an increase in abdominal girth or a palpable flank mass.

Urinary-Tract Infection

There is a striking association between urinary tract infection and obstruction of the urinary tract [18]. Infection tends to be more common with obstruction of the lower urinary tract – located below the ureterovesical junction. Several factors may condition the development of infection in the setting of obstruction: (1) the increase of residual urine in the bladder, because urine is an excellent culture medium and (2) altered properties of the bladder that facilitate bacterial adhesion and growth [19]. The greater predisposition to infection in certain patients with urinary tract obstruction may be due to alterations in the glycoprotein composition of epithelial cells of the bladder. Obstruction of the upper urinary tract is not necessarily accompanied by infection. One should suspect obstruction associated with urinary tract infection when the infections are repetitive or recurrent, or when the organisms are resistant to usual therapeutic agents to which the cultured bacteria have demonstrated susceptibility.

Hypertension

Acute or chronic obstructive uropathy, either unilateral or bilateral, may be accompanied by a significant elevation in blood pressure [20–25]. The hypertension, which could be coincidental or related to the obstruction, may relate either to increased ECF volume, owing to decreased sodium excretion, or to an abnormal release of renin and increased generation of angiotensin II. In patients with bilateral obstruction, the demonstration of increased exchangeable sodium and the (usual) prompt reversal of the hypertension after catheter drainage and diuresis suggest that the hypertension is due to abnormal retention of salt and water subsequent to the obstruction. Thus, these patients would have a volume-dependent type of hypertension. In addition, in hypertensive patients with bilaterally hydronephrotic kidneys the concentrations of renin in renal venous blood and peripheral venous blood are normal. After corrective surgery, reversal of the hypertension brings an osmotic diuresis and a negative salt and water balance, further suggesting that this is a type of volume-dependent hypertension.

On the other hand, hypertension in patients with unilateral ureteral obstruction may be renin-dependent [20, 22, 24]. Elevated values for renal-vein renin have been found in patients with unilaterally hydronephrotic kidneys. After appropriate surgery, the hypertension abated and the renin values returned to normal [20]. Animal studies have demonstrated increased renin release following acute ureteral obstruction [26]. In dogs, acute unilateral ureteral obstruction is associated with an increase in blood pressure and a rise in ipsilateral, renal-vein renin in spite of a concurrent rise in renal blood flow. The causal relationship between renin release and the increase in blood pressure is suggested by the fact that pretreatment with desoxycorticosterone acetate (DOCA) and salt abolished the rise in renin and blood pressure. In contrast, chronic studies in animals have shown that the renin release is not sustained and that the peripheral renin is normal with prolonged unilateral ureteral occlusion. This suggests that chronic, established hypertension in the setting of unilateral obstruction may not be related to increased renin secretion [27]. Since corrective surgery may reduce the hypertension in some patients, other abnormalities not related to renin may be operating in obstruction. It has not been established whether these abnormalities relate to subtle changes in volume or to the lack of release of vasodepressive substances by the obstructed kidney.

Polycythemia

The polycytemia reported in a few instances of obstructive uropathy probably is related to increased production of erythropoietin by the obstructed kidney [28]. In experimental animals, unilateral obstruction results in elevated plasma levels of erythropoietin that precede the increase in hemoglobin levels.

Hyperkalemic Hyperchloremic Acidosis

Certain patients with obstruction may have hyperkalemic hyperchloremic acidosis (renal tubular acidosis type 4) as a clinical manifestation of partial obstruction of the urinary tract [29, 30]. The reasons for the decreased excretion of hydrogen and potassium in this circumstance have been described elsewhere [31, 32].

Gross Hematuria

Gross hematuria may be associated with obstruction, particularly when it is due to stones. Long-standing obstructive uropathy may lead to increased kidney size with readily palpable kidneys.

Diagnostic Approach to the Patient with Obstructive Uropathy

The approach to the patient with obstructive uropathy varies with the clinical setting and presenting symptoms, the spectrum of which extends from those presenting with acute pain to those with acute renal failure and anuria. Thus, the diagnostic approach and the urgency with which the diagnosis must be made are highly variable. When one suspects urinary-tract obstruction, certain preliminary information is essential; e.g. a history of similar symptoms, the presence or absence of urinary-tract infection, and the kinds of drugs ingested. Questions directed toward eliciting lower urinary tract symptoms are clearly important. Review of hospital records may reveal abrupt changes in urine output. Physical examination with particular reference to the flank and abdomen is important. Tenderness may or may not be present in the costovertebral angle. Muscle rigidity over the kidney and rebound tenderness may be elicited, particularly if the patient has acute infection. Analysis of the urine may provide important information. The presence of hematuria alone may suggest that the obstructive lesion is a calculus, a sloughed papilla, or a tumor. The urine sediment should be examined carefully for the presence of crystals. Sulfonamide, cysteine, or uric-acid crystals may indicate the type of stone causing the ureteral obstruction that has resulted in acute renal failure. In the laboratory, one should determine renal function by such measures as levels of creatinine or blood urea nitrogen.

Upper Urinary Tract Obstruction

Usually the diagnosis of upper urinary-tract obstruction is relatively easy but occasionally, it may be difficult. When evaluating a patient with hydronephrosis, one should keep in mind that not all dilated collecting systems are caused by obstruction. Several radiological techniques can be used to demonstrate upper urinary tract obstruction (Table 2).

Table 2. Techniques used to diagnose upper urinary tract obstruction

Plain films of the abdomen (KUB)
Sonography (ultrasound)
Excretory or intravenous pyelography (IVP)
Retrograde pyelography
Isotopic renography
Computed tomography
Magnetic resonance imaging
Pressure flow studies (Whitaker test)

Lower Urinary-Tract Obstruction

This refers to obstruction below the ureterovesical junction. Such obstruction may be evaluated by cystoscopy, radiologic tests and urodynamic tests.

References

1. Klahr S. Urinary tract obstruction. In: Schrier RW, Gottschalk CW, editors. Diseases of the Kidney, 6th edition. Boston: Little Brown, 1997; 709–738.
2. National Kidney and Urologic Diseases Advisory Board: The scope and impact of kidney

and urologic diseases in Long Range Plan, Chapter 1, Washington DC, National Institutes of Health, NIH Publication 90-583, 1990; 7–35.
3. United States Renal Data System 1996 Annual Data Report II. Incidence and prevalence of ESRD. Am J Kidney Dis 1996; 18 (Suppl 2): S34–S47.
4. Mukamel E, Nissenkorn I, Boner G, Servadio C. Occult progressive renal damage in the elderly male due to benign prostatic hypertrophy. J Am Geriatr Soc 1979; 24: 403–406.
5. McGuire EJ. Physiology of the lower urinary tract. Am J Kidney Dis 1983; 2, 402–408.
6. Bradley WE. Neurologic disorders affecting the urinary bladder. In: Karane RJ, Siroky MB, editors. Clinical Neuro-Urology. Boston: Little, Brown, 1979; 245–255.
7. Gillenwater JY. Pathophysiology of obstructive uropathy. In: Coggins CH, Cummings NB, editors. Prevention of Kidney and Urinary Tract Disease, DHEW (NIH 78-855), Vol. 5. Washington DC: U.S. Department of Health, Education and Welfare, 1978; 169–187.
8. Walsh PC. Begnign prostatic hyperplasia. In: Harrison JH, et al., editors. Campbell's Urology 4th edition, Vol. 2. Philadelphia: Saunders, 1979; 949–966.
9. Rotkin ID. Epidemiology of benign prostatic hypertrophy: review and speculations. In: Grayhack JT, Wilson JD, Sherbenske MJ, editors. Benign Prostatic Hyperplasia, DHEW (NIH 76-1113). Washington, DC: U.S. Department of Health, Education and Welfare, 1975; 105–117.
10. Chapman I, Lapi N, Fethiere W. Prostatic enlargement and low urinary tract obstruction. Geriatrics 1964; 19: 231–239.
11. Semple JE. Surgical capsule of benign enlargement of prostate: its development and action British Medical Journal 1963; 1: 1640–1643.
12. Kogan SJ, Freed SZ. Post-operative course of vesicoureteral reflux associated with benign obstructing prostatic disease. Journal of Urology 1974; 112: 322–325.
13. Earley LF. Extreme polyuria in obstructive uropathy. Report of a case of 'water losing nephritis.' in an infant, with a discussion of polyuria. N Engl J Med 1956; 225: 600-603.
14. Knowlan D, Corrado M, Schreiner GD, Baker R. Periureteral fibrosis, with a diabetes insipidus-like syndrome occurring with progressive partial obstruction of a ureter unilaterally. Am J Med 1960; 28: 22–31.
15. Mees EJD. Reversible water losing state, caused by incomplete ureteric obstruction. Acta Med Scand 1960; 168: 193–202.
16. Rishola L. Studies on renal colic and its treatment of posterior splanchnic block. Acta Chir Scand Suppl 1954; 184: 1–9.
17. Covington T Jr, Reeser E. Hydronephrosis associated with overhydration. J Urol 1950; 63: 438.
18. Santoro J, Kaye D. Recurrent urinary tract infections. Pathogenesis and management. Med Clin North Am 1978; 62: 1005–1020.
19. Korhonen TK, Väisänen V, Kallio P, Nurmiaho-Lassila EL, Ranta H, Siitonen A, Elo J, Svenson SB, Svanborg-Edén C. The role of pili in the adhesion of *Escherichia coli* to human urinary tract epithelial cells. Scand J Infect Dis Suppl 1982; 33: 26–31.
20. Belman AB, Kropp KA, Simon NM. Renal-pressor hypertension secondary to unilateral hydronephrosis. N Engl J Med 1968; 278: 1133–1139.
21. Garrett J, Polse SL, Morrow JW. Ureteral obstruction and hypertension. Am J Med 1970: 49: 271–273.
22. Nemoy NJ, Fichman MP, Sellers A. Unilateral ureteral obstruction. A cause of reversible high renin content hypertension. JAMA 1973; 225: 512–513.
23. Palmer JM, Zweiman FG, Assaykeen TA. Renal hypertension due to hydronephrosis with normal plasma renin activity. N Engl J Med 1970; 283: 1032–1033.
24. Squitieri AP, Ceccarelli FE, Wurster JC. Hypertension with elevated renal vein renins secondary to ureteropelvic junction obstructio. J Urol 1974; 111: 284–287.
25. Weidmann P, Beretta-Piccoli C, Hirsch D, Reubi FC, Massry SG. Curable hypertension with unilateral hydronephrosis. Studies on the role of circulating renin. Ann Intern Med 1977; 87: 437–440.

26. Kaloyanides GJ, Bastron RD, DiBona G. Effect of ureteral clamping and increased renal arterial pressure on renin release. Am J Physiol 1973; 225: 95–102.
27. Vaughan ED Jr, Bühler FR, Laragh JH. Normal renin secretion in hypertensive patients with primarily unilateral chronic hydronephrosis. J Urol 1974; 112: 153–156.
28. Jaworski, ZF, Wolan CT. Hydronephrosis and polycythemia. A case of erythrocytosis relieved by decompression of unilateral hydronephrosis and cured by nephrectory. Am J Med 1963; 34: 523–528.
29. Batlle DC, Arruda JA, Kurtzman NA. Hyperkalemic distal renal tubular acidosis associated with obstructive uropathy. N Engl J Med 1981; 1: 304–373.
30. Pelleya R, Oster JR, Perez GO. Hyporeninemic hypoaldosteronism, sodium wasting and mineralocorticoid-resistant hyperkalemia in two patients with obstructive uropathy. Am J Nephrol 1983; 3: 223–227.
31. Purcell H, Bastani B, Harris KP, Hemken P, Klahr S, Gluck S. Cellular distribution of H(+)-ATPase following acute unilateral ureteral obstruction in rats. Am J Physiol 1991; 261: F365–376.
32. Klahr S. Pathophysiology of obstructive nephropathy: a 1991 update. Semin Nephrol 1991; 11: 156–168.

Urinary Incontinence in the Elderly

LARRY T. SIRLS[1] and THOMAS RASHID[2]
[1] *Urodynamics Laboratory, William Beaumont Hospital, Royal Oak, Michigan, U.S.A.;*
[2] *William Beaumont Hospital, Royal Oak, Michigan, U.S.A.*

Urinary incontinence, a common and troublesome manifestation of voiding dysfunction in the elderly, must be viewed as a single symptom within the spectrum of bladder dysfunction. Other symptoms of such dysfunction include urgency, increased urinary frequency, nocturia, slow stream, hesitancy, feeling of incomplete bladder emptying, etc. Abnormalities in the voiding cycle may range from those that simply annoy patients to the severe and disabling.

Urinary incontinence is treatable and curable, but the approach to it in the elderly differs significantly from that in younger patients. This chapter will outline the epidemiology and the pathophysiology of urinary incontinence in the elderly population. It will present a detailed clinical assessment, that emphasizes the history and physical exam and discuss guidelines for additional testing, the objectives of the tests and their influence on treatment decisions. Behavioral and medical therapies will be emphasized, with a brief discussion of alternative therapies and surgical interventions.

Epidemiology

The most dramatic population change in the twentieth century has been in the age composition. Since the century began, the percentage of Americans 65 and older has tripled. In the 1980s the increase in the number of Americans over 65 years of age was more than twice that of the total population – 2.1% compared to 1% [2, 3]. In 1990, the population in the United States was 249 million and those 65 years and older accounted for nearly 25% [1]. This trend is projected to continue well into the twenty-first century.

The increase in life expectancy is accompanied by a rising pandemic of chronic disease, mental disorders and associated disabilities [4]. One of the most common of these disabilities encountered is urinary incontinence, which is described as a 'social cancer,' bringing with it risk of embarrassment, isolation and depression. Urinary incontinence predisposes to perineal rashes, pressure ulcers, urinary tract infections, urosepsis, falls, and fractures. In community-dwelling older persons, the prevalence of urinary incontinence is

Oreopoulos et al. (eds.), Nephrology and Geriatrics Integrated, 179–198.

15–30%; in acute care settings, approximately 33%; and among institutionalized older persons about 50% [5, 6]. The cost of managing urinary incontinence in the U.S. was more than $10 billion in 1987 – a sum that exceeded the amount devoted to dialysis and coronary artery bypass surgery combined [7]. Clearly, because future demographic shifts project great increases in elderly, we can expect a substantial increase in the absolute numbers of incontinent older persons.

Urinary incontinence is abnormal at any age and it will continue to increase as disease and functional impairment becomes more common with aging [8]. Physicians caring for the elderly should realize that incontinence is treatable, but that it requires a special evaluation and approach to treatment.

Survey of Voiding Function

Voiding can be thought of as two relatively distinct phases, one of bladder filling and storage, and one of bladder emptying. Bladder filling and storage require three components; (1) storage of increasing volumes of urine at low pressure, (2) a urethral sphincter mechanism that is closed at rest and during increases in intra-abdominal pressure, and (3) absence of involuntary bladder contractions or bladder overactivity. Bladder emptying requires; (1) an adequate, sustained bladder-muscle contraction, (2) relaxation of the urethral sphincter mechanism and (3) absence of anatomic obstruction. When one applies these simple rules to voiding dysfunction, any type of voiding dysfunction can be logically described, and treatment options rationally follow.

Aging and Continence

The lower urinary tract undergoes significant changes with aging. At the cellular level, changes in the detrusor smooth muscle cause decreased bladder contractility. Then an incomplete dysfunctional pattern develops that leads to a higher prevalence of involuntary detrusor contractions [9, 10]. In addition, bladder capacity decreases and the post-void residual volume (PVR) increases usually by 50–100 ml. In the aging man, prostatic enlargement produces bladder outlet obstruction in 50% [10]. In the aging woman, there is a decline in maximal urethral closure pressure and length [11]. Finally, the elderly excrete most of their fluids at night and an increase in sleep disorders is accompanied by 1–2 episodes of nocturia.

Urinary continence requires not only an intact lower urinary tract but an adequate mentation and mobility, which may be uncertain in the elderly. Although these age-related changes do not cause urinary incontinence directly, they may predispose the individual to urine loss.

Transient Urinary Incontinence

Transient urinary incontinence accounts for approximately 50% of incontinence observed in the elderly. Often appropriate early management can cure this reversible form of incontinence and prevent it from becoming established. The causes of transient incontinence can be recalled by using the mnemonic 'DIAPPERS' (misspelled with an extra 'p' (Table 1) [12]. Delirium may cause incontinence that abates after treatment of the underlying cause.

Symptomatic urinary tract infection (UTI) may cause frequency, urgency and dysuria – all of which may lead to incontinence. However, assymptomatic UTI, present in 10–30% of the elderly, usually does not cause incontinence [13, 14]. Up to 80% of elderly women attending incontinence clinics have atrophic vaginitis [15]. Commonly, these patients present with urgency and dysuria, and the vaginal mucosa is pale, thin and friable on physical examination. This entity is readily treated with low-dose estrogen (orally or vaginally). Frequently pharmaceuticals cause transient urinary incontinence in the elderly, precipitating urine loss by a variety of mechanisms [16]. Psychological disturbances such as depression or neurosis also may cause transient incontinence.

Excessive urine output due to diuretics, metabolic abnormalities and large fluid intake will cause frequency, nocturia, and incontinence. Restricted mobility, common in the elderly, frequently contributes to incontinence. Finally stool impaction, by stimulating correct receptors, may produce an overflow type of incontinence in up to 10% of patients [17]. In every patient, a transient cause of urinary incontinence should be sought and, if identified, continence may be restored in the majority.

Functional Incontinence

Some consider functional incontinence to be a disorder specific to the elderly and secondary to alterations in mental status or mobility. However, this generalization is of doubtful validity. This diagnosis implies a normal lower urinary tract which the elderly patient may not have. Therefore in accepting the

Table 1. Transient causes of urinary incontinence based on the mnemonic, DIAPPERS. (Pannil et al., J Amer Geriatr Soc 1988; 36: 902–910.)

D	Delirium/confusional state
I	Infection-Urinary (symptomatic)
A	Atrophic urethritis/vaginitis
P	Pharmaceuticals
P	Psychological, especially depression
E	Endocrine (hypercalcemia, hyperglycemia)
R	Restricted mobility
S	Stool impaction

diagnosis of functional incontinence one may fail to appropriately investigate the patient's complaint and thus risk misdiagnosis. In addition, many patients with impaired cognitive function or immobility are not incontinent. However, measures that improve a patient's motivation, environmental demands such as bedside commode, medical status, and mobility may relieve the voiding dysfunction [8].

Established Incontinence

If incontinence persists after attention to transient and functional causes one shall examine the lower urinary tract. A simple classification describes voiding dysfunction as primarily one of the filling/storage phase or the emptying phase of micturition. Generally failure in either category is not absolute, but often is relative.

In elderly men, failure to empty is due either to bladder-outlet obstruction or to a poorly contractile bladder. Failure to empty is easily diagnosed by an elevated post-void residual volume (PVR). Bladder outlet obstruction may be due to prostatic enlargement – benign or malignant, urethral stricture or bladder-neck contracture, as seen after prostatectomy. Patients with outflow obstruction may present with irritative symptoms i.e. frequency, urgency, urge incontinence, and nocturia and/or obstructive symptoms i.e. hesitancy, intermittency, decreased force of stream, and terminal dribbling. Long-standing outlet obstruction may produce bladder decompensation and overflow incontinence, a process that usually is chronic. These patients report small amounts of urine lost throughout the day.

Poor bladder contractility may be primary (idiopathic) or secondary – a neurologic lesion or chronic outlet obstruction from the prostate or prolapsing cystocele. In an acontractile bladder (also called detrusor areflexia), one cannot demonstrate any muscle contraction during attempted voiding on urodynamic study – also seen in long-standing diabetes or after radical pelvic surgery [18].

Failure to store is secondary to bladder overactivity, sphincter insufficiency, or both. The bladder may contract at inappropriate times, causing a sudden abrupt urge to void (urgency). If the urethral sphincter cannot maintain closure at the time of the contraction, incontinence results (urge incontinence). The two types of urge incontinence are motor urgency and sensory urgency. Though important conceptually, one can make the differentiation only with urodynamic testing. Motor urgency is present when the patient has an urge to urinate that is accompanied by a urodynamically documented uninhibited (involuntary) bladder contraction. Sensory urgency is present when the patient feels a strong urge to urinate but there is no demonstrable detrusor contraction on cystometrogram (CMG). In our experience, sensory urgency, which rarely causes incontinence (but may cause severe frequency), should alert the investigator to another cause such as stone, cystitis, bladder tumor, etc. Bladder overactivity, which may be spontaneous or provoked, is said to be the most common source of urinary incontinence in elderly men [12]. Stress incontinence in men is seen in less than 1% of men after transurethral resection of prostate (TURP) and in 5–10% of patients after radical prostatectomy [19–22]. Even less common causes of stress incontinence include trauma, radiation therapy for prostate cancer, and recurrent stricture disease.

In elderly women, failure to empty is again secondary to outlet obstruction or a poorly contractile bladder. In women outlet obstruction is most common after previous bladder surgery i.e. incontinence surgery or urethral dilation or in those with a large cystocele.

In elderly women failure to store urine is secondary to bladder overactivity, sphincter insufficiency, or both. Such overactivity is the most common cause of urinary incontinence in elderly women, stress urinary incontinence (SUI) is second.

Female stress incontinence which embraces a spectrum of urethral sphincteric dysfunction, conceptually can be subdivided into anatomic stress incontinence (also called simple stress incontinence) and intrinsic sphincteric deficiency (ISD). Anatomic stress incontinence is associated with hypermobility of the bladder and bladder neck. Simple incontinence consists of urine loss during provocative maneuvers such as running, lifting, coughing, etc. By definition, ISD implies some functional damage to the urethral sphincteric mechanism, and these patients almost always have *severe incontinence* with a history of some risk factor associated with urethral sphincteric damage. Risk factors for ISD include prior bladder or pelvic surgery, neurologic disease, pelvic radiation and trauma. It is critical to identify the patients with ISD because they require different treatment than those with 'simple' anatomic stress incontinence. Although additional urodynamic testing is required to make this differentiation a careful history can help to determine whether additional testing is required.

Elderly men and women may have both a failure to store and a failure to empty. This difficult condition, called detrusor hyperactivity with impaired contractility (DHIC), represents the coexistence of detrusor overactivity causing urgency and frequency, and concurrently a bladder that is poorly contractile. Typically DHIC causes urgency, frequency, weak flow rates, and high PVR volume [23]. Some authorities believe that DHIC is the most common form of bladder overactivity in the elderly [24].

History

The history and physical examination remain the cornerstone upon which a urologic diagnosis rests. With geriatric patients, it may be helpful to have a family member present during the interview. A detailed history is a search for an overt or a less obvious cause of incontinence, and it helps one to decide whether additional tests are necessary.

A voiding diary provides useful information on urinary frequency, nocturia, and the number of episodes of urine loss in the incontinent patient. No attempt should be made to alter voiding patterns or fluid intake. In the absence of diuretics, the volume of urine output is a good indication of the patient's fluid intake.

Voiding Symptoms

To evaluate the incontinent patient it is necessary to establish the baseline voiding symptoms. Urgency may be secondary to abrupt sensation of bladder discomfort, or as a conditioned response from the fear of urine leakage. Symptoms of urgency must be probed carefully because they are not sensitive indicators, nor are they specific for bladder overactivity. Again one must consider functional factors such as the patient's mentation, mobility, motivation and access to a toilet. The symptom of urgency that immediately precedes an abrupt gush of urine must be differentiated from the sense of urgency that arises from the patient's fear of incontinence.

Frequency of urination (> 7 diurnal voids), which is common, may simply reflect excessive fluid intake, diuretic medication, or dietary stimulants such as caffeine. Many patients choose to void frequently to avoid incontinence of any kind. Urinary frequency may indicate pain with low-volume bladder filling (inflammation), bladder overactivity, reduced bladder capacity, poor compliance (a 'stiff' bladder), incomplete bladder emptying or even complete urinary retention with overflow incontinence. Again, one must consider bladder irritation secondary to infection, stone, malignancy or external mass.

Nocturia may be secondary to detrusor overactivity, reduced detrusor capacity, excessive urine output or a primary sleep-related disorder. A voiding diary may assist in differentiating these processes. Daytime frequency without nocturia may suggest a psychogenic component, increased fluid intake, timing of diuretic medications or intake of dietary stimulants such as caffeine.

In the patient with urinary incontinence, one must not ignore bladder-outlet obstructive symptoms i.e. decreased force of urinary stream, hesitancy, sensation of incomplete bladder emptying, and post-void dribbling. These symptoms may be present in patients with a poorly contractile bladder from diabetes mellitus or from various neurologic disorders. Although women with a large cystocele may complain of bladder- outlet obstructive symptoms (secondary to urethral hyperangulation), men are far more likely to have obstructive symptoms associated with urinary incontinence. Usually incontinence associated with benign prostatic hyperplasia (BPH) reflects bladder over- activity secondary to bladder outlet obstruction.

Urinary Incontinence

In both men and women, urinary incontinence may be approached conceptually as a failure to store or failure to empty, or a combination of the two. After listening to the chief complaint, directed questions identify whether the incontinence is related to urgency symptoms suggesting bladder overactivity, or provocative maneuvers suggesting stress incontinence and some degree of urethral dysfunction. Basic questions for all patients include the duration and characterization of incontinence, precipitating events and previous incontinence treatments and their effect. What is the frequency and severity of incontinent episodes (daily, weekly, or rarely)? What types of physical activity typically result in urine loss (aerobic exercises vs. quiet walking)? Are protective pads used (panty liners, maxi pads or diapers)? If so, how many pads are used daily, and when changed are the pads wet, damp or dry (changed by habit)?

Past Medical History

Such history provides information on past and present medical disease, past surgical history, obstetric and gynecological history, current medication use, alcohol and drug use i.e., tobacco and caffeine, and drug allergies – including Latex. Knowledge of the medication(s) used is particularly relevant in the geriatric patient; important medications include diuretics, alpha adrenergic agents – agonists or antagonists that may affect bladder-neck tone, and estrogen in the postmenopausal women. Additional focused questions probe for factors other than lower-urinary-tract dysfunction, which may contribute to the development of incontinence, for example, the diurnal variation in urine production seen with congestive heart failure (mobilization of peripheral edema when supine), diuretic use, and the polyuria seen with poorly controlled diabetes. Simple recommendations like use of a bedside commode, timing of diuretic use or encouraging better management of peripheral edema or diabetes mellitus may bring significant improvement.

In the review it is critical to ask about past history of radical pelvic surgery – radical hysterectomy or abdominoperineal resection, prostatectomy – for benign or malignant disease, bladder-neck suspension procedures, or spinal surgery. As noted earlier, women with severe incontinence must be probed for risk factors of ISD.

Often, from the history alone one can classify the type of urinary incontinence. Then the physical examination may uncover specific findings, which support or contradict the diagnosis suggested by the history. One should exercise caution when definitively classifying a type of incontinence based on clinical evaluation alone because in nearly 50% of cases it will be wrong [25, 26]. Often one needs further radiologic or urodynamic evaluation.

Physical Examination

The urologic examination of the incontinent patient must be done in a stepwise fashion, namely a methodical abdominal examination, a directed pelvic examination, either female – vaginal, associated vaginal pathology, bimanual, or male – genitalia, rectal, prostatic, bimanual and a gross neurologic examination.

Initial Evaluation

In the initial evaluation, one inspects the abdomen for obesity, previous surgical scars, or an abdominal or inguinal hernia. The abdomen is palpated to assess for pain or for a suprapubic mass – such as a distended bladder or a pelvic tumor. Usually suprapubic percussion is better than palpation in detecting a distended bladder. One inspects the back and spine for skeletal deformities, scars from trauma or from previous surgery.

Female Pelvic Examination

Proper lighting is mandatory for a speculum examination. Two posterior halves of a vaginal speculum are used sequentially for exposure (Fig. 1). The vaginal introitus is inspected for atrophic vaginitis or stenosis – both common in the elderly. A methodical vaginal examination addresses three distinct areas in a systematic fashion: the anterior vaginal wall, the vaginal apex, and the posterior vaginal wall.

The anterior vaginal wall is assessed by pressing a single posterior one-half of a vaginal speculum along the posterior vaginal wall (vaginal floor). Urethral induration may be a sign of chronic inflammation, urethral divertic-

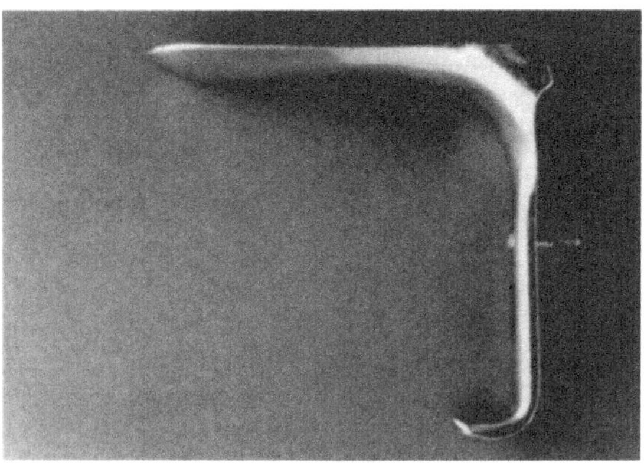

Figure 1. The posterior half of a vagina speculum. Using two of the posterior half speculums allow excellent sequential exposure of the anterior vaginal wall, vaginal apex and posterior vaginal wall.

ulum or tumor. Pale, thin, shining vaginal mucosa or loss of rugation may indicate atrophic vaginitis; in elderly women, such vaginitis is a potentially reversible cause of urinary incontinence. A fixed and scarred anterior vaginal wall in the presence of severe incontinence suggests surgical urethral damage and ISD. Bulging of the anterior vaginal wall at rest when the posterior wall is stabilized usually indicates a cystocele.

One evaluates the vaginal apex by placing a second posterior one-half of the speculum along the anterior wall, noting the position of the cervix or, in post-hysterectomy patients, the apical vaginal cuff. One refers any suspicious vaginal mucosal findings or cervical abnormalities for gynecological evaluation.

The posterior vaginal wall is assessed by placing one-half of a Graves speculum along the anterior vaginal surface. A posterior vaginal wall bulge, seen after stabilizing the anterior vaginal wall, suggests rectocele or an enterocele.

The female pelvic examination is concluded with a bimanual examination to detect any mass or tenderness of the vaginal wall, bladder, uterus, adnexa or other pelvic structure. Any abnormal pelvic findings may require radiologic evaluation. During the rectal examination, look for gluteal asymmetry, sphincter tone, fecal impaction and rectal masses. Pay special attention to the patient's ability to voluntarily contract and relax the levator muscles.

As part of a complete speculum examination, ask the patient to perform the Valsalva maneuver or cough with a full bladder to detect urine leakage, the 'stress test' (Fig. 2). If there is leakage coincident with the cough, it probably is secondary to incompetent bladder outlet. Incontinence a few seconds after the cough may be secondary to an uninhibited detrusor contraction (triggered by the cough) rather than to bladder-outlet incompetence and may indicate further urodynamic testing.

Male Pelvic Examination

A male pelvic examination includes assessment of the external genitalia and perineum, a digital rectal examination (DRE) and neurologic examination. The DRE should assess the size of the prostate and search for any abnormality that suggests prostate cancer. Remember there is little correlation between the estimated prostate size and voiding symptoms. Finally, during the examination, test the anal sphincter tone and integrity of sacral innervation.

Post Void Residual Volume

The post-void residual urine volume (PVR) is essential for all incontinent patients. One can obtain a PVR volume be urethral catheterization or by office ultrasound (our preferred method). The post-void residual volume provides additional information on voiding efficiency and bladder capacity. In an alert patient, a true PVR volume is determined immediately after voiding;

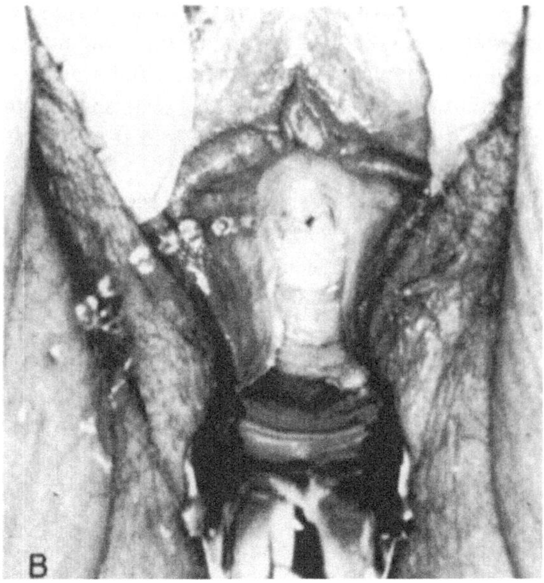

Figure 2. Urine loss concurrent with a provocative maneouver such as a cough suggests some component of urethral dysfunction. Leakage a few seconds after the cough may indicate an over active bladder.

in the demented patient a PVR volume may be determined after an incontinent episode.

Neurologic Examination

The neurologic examination is divided into four parts: (1) mental status, (2) sensory function, (3) motor function, and (4) reflex integrity. Begin with simple observation of the patient for signs of neurologic disease such as dementia, paresis, plegia, and tremor, and the degree of immobility – cane, walker, wheelchair. Mental status is assessed by observing the patient's level of consciousness, orientation, speech pattern, memory and comprehension. Sensory examination includes testing for position, vibration, pinprick, light touch and temperature of specific dermatomes i.e. T4–5 (nipples), T10 (umbilicus), L1 (base of penis, upper scrotum, labia majora), L1–2 (midscrotum, labia minora), L3 (front of knee), S1 (sole and lateral foot), and S3–5 (perineum and perianal skin).

Sensory evaluation also assesses the cutaneous sacral reflexes. The sacral nerve roots (S2–S4) innervate both the external urethral and the anal sphincters. Clinically the external anal sphincter represents all the perineal striated muscles and may be taken to predict urethral sphincteric function. Stimulation of the anal reflex (S2–S5) by lightly stroking the mucocutaneous junction of

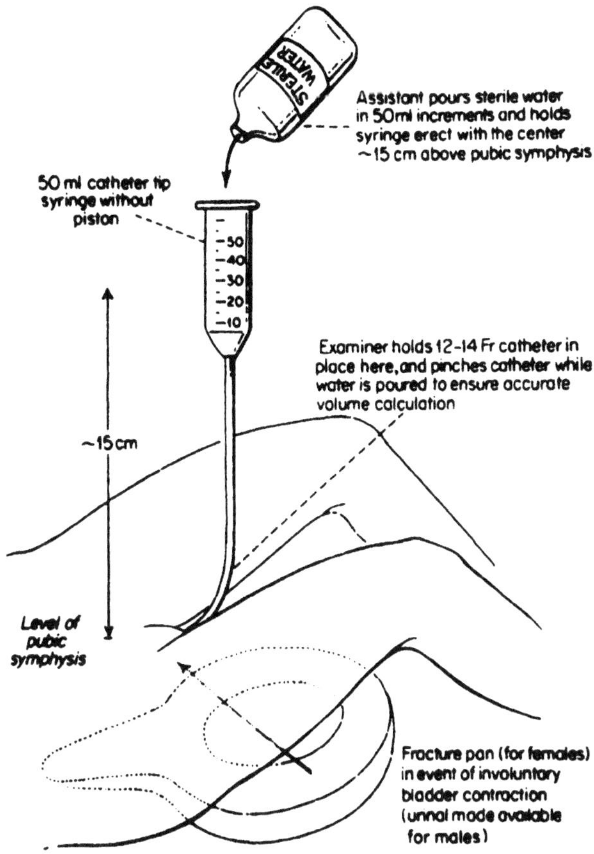

Figure 3. Technique for simple bedside cystometry. (From Ouslander JG, et al., J Am Geriatr Soc 1989; 37: 706.)

the perianal skin causes a visible contraction of external anal sphincter ('anal wink'). Absence of the anal wink reflex usually suggests sacral nerve disease, except in the elderly patient in whom absence of the anal wink is not always abnormal. Then a finger is placed in the rectum to assess sphincter tone and volitional contraction. Usually voluntary contraction of the external anal sphincter indicates normal integrity of pelvic-floor innervation and the conus medullaris. Absence of, or a decrease in sphincter tone, or of voluntary anal contraction may reflect a sacral or peripheral nerve lesion and usually indicates absent conal activity. The presence of anal sphincter tone in the absence of a voluntary anal contraction indicates a suprasacral lesion.

The bulbocavernosus reflex (BCR) refers specifically to the contraction of the bulbocavernosus muscle, however this reflex often is used to test the innervation of all perineal striated muscles. The BCR, a local sacral spinal cord reflex arc, reflects activity in S2–S4. In men, the BCR is elicited by squeezing the glans penis, which causes a reflex contraction of the external anal sphincter. In women, the glans clitoris is used. Absence of the BCR after any of these maneuvers may indicate sacral nerve damage (the BCR should be absent in all patients with a complete lower motor neuron lesion). However, the BCR may be absent in up to 20% of neurologically normal females.

Additional Testing

Every patient should have a urinalysis and a serum creatinine for renal panel. If the patient is confused or the voiding record suggests polyuria, serum electrolytes, calcium, and glucose should be checked. Urologic evaluation is necessary in patients with sterile hematuria or elevated post-void residual volumes – those residual volumes greater than 200 ml. Patients who have had surgical therapy and yet remain incontinent, or who have a new post-operative symptom, such as new urgency or obstructive voiding symptoms, should be evaluated. So also should those with severe incontinence – more than two wet episodes per day, or in patients who have tried simple interventions – behavioral modification and or medical therapy, and have not responded. Urodynamic testing remains the cornerstone of evaluation. Although its precise role in the elderly is not yet clear, its results are reproducible, it is feasible and it is safe in the elderly [11].

Cystoscopy is useful to assess urethral stricture, to evaluate the bladder mucosa and rule out such lesions as tumor, calculi, and foreign bodies. In men, one assesses prostatic size and other indicators of bladder-outlet obstruction. Clinical correlation always is required to interpret cystoscopic findings.

Uroflowmetry, a simple, non invasive test, assesses the rate and volume of a patient's void. This test may help when the parameters are normal, a high flow rate and normal volume, but is more difficult to interpret when the flow rate is low or the volume is low. However, the low flow rate may be secondary to either a bladder-outlet obstruction – from the prostate, urethral stricture, etc. or from a weak, decompensated bladder muscle, from diabetes, neurologic lesion, chronic obstruction, etc. Finally, information about uroflow is valid only when a post-void residual is done to assess the completeness of bladder emptying.

Cystometry is a functional test of bladder storage and emptying. Simple bedside cystometry may be performed in 15–20 minutes (Fig. 1). Bedside cystometry should include: (1) volume at first urge to void ('I am beginning to feel a little full'), (2) presence of any involuntary bladder contraction – e.g. a continuous upward movement of the water column that often is associated with leakage around the urethral catheter, (3) amount of fluid loss with the involuntary contraction, and (4) functional bladder capacity – the volume instilled before an involuntary contraction or when the patient reports a strong urge to void. Simple bedside cystometry can identify bladder overactivity but cannot differentiate the various subtypes of bladder overactivity.

This is particularly important in the elderly man where bladder-outlet obstruction is a common cause of bladder over-activity. More sophisticated urodynamic testing is required to (1) differentiate the causes of urge incontinence, (2) document stress incontinence and the degree of urethral dysfunction, (3) assess the role of bladder-outlet obstruction, and (4) correlate anatomic abnormalities with functional status.

Therapy

Treatment of urinary incontinence in the elderly must be individualized because factors outside the urinary tract limit its feasibility and efficacy. Usually first-line therapy is non-invasive management of urinary incontinence except for the female with severe incontinence secondary to ISD, those with associated pathology that will require surgical correction – such as a large cystocele, vaginal-vault prolapse, or uterine descensus, and the man with severe post-prostatectomy stress incontinence, without associated bladder dysfunction. However, non-operative therapies, even when not first-line therapy, are useful adjuncts for successful postoperative management if surgery ultimately is required. Most treatments discussed in the next few sections may be applied to both men and women.

Behavioral Therapy and Biofeedback

Behavioral therapy for urinary incontinence, which is effective and carries minimal risk, usually is employed as first-line therapy alone or in combination with another therapy. In general, all patients will receive some type of behavioral modification, regardless of whether additional therapies are planned or have been instituted. Behavioral modification includes changes in the daily urination routine including timed voiding, avoidance of known stimulants like caffeine, and restriction of total fluid intake. The authors recommend limiting fluid intake to 1000 to 1200 ml/day unless contraindicated for reasons such as a history of urinary stones, infection, or diabetes with polyuria. Fluid restriction may be effective for many patients, particularly those with minimal to moderate symptoms. Many 'bladder training' programs include habit training, timed voiding, and scheduled 're-training'. Combining fluid restriction (to reduce total urine output) with a timed voiding program (to frequently empty the bladder) can minimize bladder filling to the volume that 'triggers' an uninhibited contraction in urge incontinence, or being so full as to promote urine loss with stress maneuvers. In a prospective, controlled trial of bladder training in elderly women (timed voiding, volitional inhibition and charting) for urge and stress incontinence Fantl demonstrated a 75% improvement and a 12% cure [27]. These behavioral modifications play an important part in the management of less severe stress and urge incontinence.

The etiology and severity of incontinence may help determine whether behavioral therapy alone will be effective. For example, behavioral therapies alone are likely to fail if a patient has had previous surgery that damaged the urethral sphincteric mechanism (men after prostate surgery, women after bladder-neck suspension) and has severe incontinence requiring multiple pads per day. However, an elderly patient with urgency symptoms who drinks a lot of fluids and caffeine daily, may gain relief from simple advice including fluid restriction and avoidance of caffeine. Urgency symptoms will require a dedicated component of behavioral modification, often in addition to medical or some alternative therapy. In contrast, usually only mild forms of stress incontinence will respond to behavioral modification alone, severe forms often require surgery or an alternative but still invasive therapy.

As a treatment for urge incontinence biofeedback depends on the patient's ability to recognize, and then suppress, the uninhibited bladder contraction while voluntarily contracting the sphincter – to prevent the incontinent episode until the bladder contraction is suppressed. An effective biofeedback program, which is labor intensive, requires a motivated patient. Cardozo reported a 40% cure and an additional 20% improved using CMG feedback for idiopathic bladder overactivity [28].

Pelvic Floor Exercises

A useful adjunct in both men and women with stress incontinence is to augment urethral closure by voluntary contraction of pelvic floor muscles. Basic exercises may be done routinely without the aid of complex feedback or expensive devices. Patient motivation is critical to any pelvic-floor exercise program. Pelvic muscle exercises can decrease incontinence substantially in motivated and cognitively intact older women [29]. However, its efficacy is limited in severe incontinence, relapse rates are high, and long- term follow-up data are sparse.

Catheterization and External Devices

Bladder catheterization is used in different patient populations with urinary incontinence, often inappropriately. Patients who require some form of urine collection include many in nursing homes, the mentally impaired, the immobile and patients with total incontinence, usually from overflow. Catheterization options include internal – clean intermittent, indwelling urethral, or suprapubic or external devices such as condom catheters. The object of any therapeutic program is to make the patient catheter free; however, in some situations, catheters are the most realistic alternative.

Indwelling urethral catheters have little place in the outpatient management of urinary incontinence. Most patients can perform clean intermittent catheterization (CIC) or have family or other supports to perform CIC for them. Though 40–80% will have evidence of bacteriuria, symptomatic infections are seen in less than 2% [30, 31]. The complications of indwelling urethral catheters, which increase with duration of catheterization, include infection (urethritis, cystitis, pyelonephritis, and sepsis), stones, and urethral erosion. When the patient needs a chronic indwelling catheter, use the suprapubic approach, because the incidence of significant bacteruria is less than with indwelling urethral catheters, and it avoids local complications such as urethritis and erosion.

External devices include condom catheters, penile clamps, female collection devices and female occluding devices. Condom catheters may cause skin irritation and erosion and external female devices are difficult to use. Penile clamps should be avoided because they can cause skin erosion, urethral injury, or contribute to deterioration of the upper tracts. One female occlusive device consists of a small triangular foam pad, with a layer of hydrophilic adhesive that is placed in the vestibule creating a seal over the urethral meatus. Though 80% of patients who use this device reported reduced incontinence, further clinical evaluation is needed [32].

Absorbent pads and undergarments may provide comfort and convenience when used temporarily. Unfortunately, for many, these garments constitute the principal method of management and, involve great associated expense.

Pharmacologic Therapy

The anticholinergic and antispasmodic agents are helpful to patients with incontinence from uninhibited detrusor contractions but have no role to play in genuine stress incontinence alone. However, drugs that augment outlet resistance such as the tricyclic antidepressant imipramine, the estrogens and alpha agonists may be useful in genuine stress incontinence. Clinically, these agents are most useful in less severe incontinence and generally are used in combination with behavioral modification programs, such as fluid restriction and timed voiding.

Integral to successful management of urge incontinence is pharmacologic depression of the uninhibited detrusor contraction. The goal of therapy is to prevent or delay the uninhibited detrusor contraction in the storage phase of filling, yet maintain complete emptying with micturition. This may be difficult, particularly in men with some component of bladder-outlet obstruction or in women with elevated postvoid residual volumes. Such patients risk urinary retention with anticholinergic or antispasmodic agents and must be approached cautiously, or else start pharmacologic therapy in conjunction with intermittent catheterization to monitor postvoid residual urine volume.

Anticholinergics

Atropine and atropine-like agents inhibit the acetocholine neurohumoral effector mechanism for detrusor contraction thus depressing true involuntary bladder contractions of any etiology. They increase the volume at which the first unstable detrusor contraction is triggered, decrease the strength of the contraction, and increase total bladder capacity. Accordingly, a useful adjunct to anticholinergics is a behavioral modification program such as timed voiding or a toileting regimen to encourage bladder emptying before the patient reaches the volume stimulating urge and UI. Propantheline bromide (Pro-banthine) is the most commonly used antimuscarinic anticholinergic.

Anticholinergic side effects often limit patient compliance. Thorough discussion of the expected side effects are useful with management advice such as oral lozenges for dry mouth and artificial saliva in severe cases.

Musculotropic Relaxants

The musculotropic relaxing agents are direct-acting, smooth muscle relaxants but also have anticholinergic activity and local anesthetic properties. Oxybutynin chloride (Ditropan) is used most commonly in the management of urgency and UI. Tolteradine, a new agent, has an efficacy similar to oxybutynin but is reported to have fewer side effects, particularly dry mouth. Other musculotropic agents with less potent anticholinergic activity include dicyclomine hydrochloride (Bentyl) and flavoxate hydrochloride (Urispas). Clinically these agents are less effective but may benefit elderly persons, who cannot tolerate the stronger agents. The side effects of the musculotropics are primarily anticholinergic.

Tricyclic Antidepressants

The tricyclic antidepressants, particularly Amipramine (Tofranil), facilitate urine storage. Imipramine decreases bladder contractility and increase(s) outlet resistance at the bladder neck and proximal urethra. Because they have different mechanisms of action, tricyclic antidepressants may be synergistic to anticholinergics and musculotropic agents, however, the anticholinergic side effects are often additive. One needs to exercise clinical judgment in the use of tricyclic antidepressants, they are contraindicated in those on MAO inhibitors and should be used cautiously in the elderly person with cardiac disease because of the risk of myocardial depression and conduction disturbances.

Estrogens and Alpha Agonists

Estrogens have well recognized effects on the urethra and bladder neck, particularly in postmenopausal women, although their mechanisms of action are poorly understood. Urethral-outlet resistance is said to be increased by proliferation of the submucosal vascular plexus, enhanced 'mucosal seal' and augmented response to endogenous adrenergic stimulation, either by increase in the alpha-receptors or enhanced receptor function. Alpha agonists, such as phenylpropranolamine, used alone may be effective in genuine stress incontinence by enhancing proximal urethral-outlet resistance. However, patients should be warned to expect clinical relapse when the medicine is discontinued. Estrogens are useful in managing detrusor instability particularly in elderly women with atrophic vaginitis, but the mechanism is unclear.

Surgical Treatment of Stress Incontinence

Stress Urinary Incontinence: Surgical Therapy in Men

Male urinary incontinence often follows sphincteric damage during prostatectomy; it occurs in less than 1% after transurethral resection and in 5–10% after radical prostatectomy. Genuine SUI, which is associated with sphincteric incompetence, is treated by augmenting sphincter function or artificially increasing outlet resistance. Proper diagnostic evaluation of the male with incontinence must include urodynamics to establish the presence of sphincteric insufficiency and to exclude bladder dysfunction.

Periurethral Injection

Gax-collagen (Contigen), a gluteraldehyde cross linked natural substance derived from bovine skin, being studied as a treatment for both male and female SUI. The Gax-collagen is thought to be replaced by natural collagen via a 'remodeling process' after 4–6 months. Cystoscopically controlled injections are placed at multiple positions just proximal to the membranous urethra until the operator can see that the lumen is coapted. One must weigh the advantages of this outpatient procedure under local anesthesia against the cost of the collagen and the need for re-injection if the response is limited. The efficacy collagen injection in men has been disappointing.

Artificial Urinary Sphincter (AUS)

Sphincteric incompetence has been managed using implanted artificial prosthetic devices for 40 years. Patients must be screened to ensure they are mentally and physical capable of using an AUS. The artificial sphincter is effective in managing incontinence secondary to urethral sphincter deficiency after prostatectomy. Total continence can be achieved in 81%, and 95% of the patients achieve socially acceptable continence [33]. Complications include sphincter malfunction, infection, and erosion.

Stress Urinary Incontinence: Surgical Therapy in Women

Anatomic ('simple') incontinence may be treated with a variety of therapies depending on the severity of the incontinence, presence of associated cystocele or other pelvic pathology and most important, the patient's motivation and compliance. Patients should understand that behavioral modification and pharmacotherapy, while it may be effective, must be continued indefinitely or relapse is likely.

Anatomic incontinence can be managed surgically by means of retropubic bladder suspension or a vaginal-approach pubovaginal sling. Both these procedures are effective, the vaginal approach sling has the advantages of reduced post-operative morbidity and shorter hospital stay. We will discuss the sling procedure further under the management of intrinsic sphincteric dysfunction.

Intrinsic Sphincteric Deficiency

For restoration of continence, intrinsic sphincteric deficiency resulting from denervation, previous periurethral surgery, trauma or radiation requires external compression to increase outflow resistance. Treatment options include periurethral injection for 'bulk enhancement' (Teflon®, collagen, fat), artificial sphincter or pubovaginal sling.

Periurethral Injection

Periurethral injection of bulk-enhancing materials, which increases outflow resistance, is not indicated for routine or 'anatomic' SUI because the urethral closure mechanism is not compromised. However, periurethral injections may be used in elderly women with intrinsic sphincter deficiency; it may be performed in the office with relative ease and has a very low morbidity. In contrast to our experience in men, periurethral injection is a viable alternative in the elderly female.

Pubovaginal Sling

In patients with severe incontinence secondary to ISD, the urethra may be 'fixed' in the retropubic space from scarring or urethral hypermobility. Restoration of a hypermobile or poorly supported and damaged urethra to the retropubic position will not achieve continence because the primary deficit is not one of anatomic support but of intrinsic urethral damage. The sling procedure creates a 'hammock' under the urethral sphincteric mechanism, providing a 'back-board' against which the urethra is compressed during provocative maneuvers. In contrast to 'routine' bladder suspension, this floor of support provides excellent continence in patients with ISD. The many varieties of the sling procedure include anterior rectus fascia, fascia lata of the thigh, dermis (skin), vaginal wall, dura mater and synthetic material, and most recently, treated cadaver fascia. We have used treated cadaver fascia almost exclusively in the last 1 $^1/_2$ years, it has the advantage of reliable strength and its use avoids the additional dissection required to harvest native fascia. Pubovaginal slings cure incontinence in 84–96% of patients with SUI [34, 35].

Augmentation Cystoplasty

Augmentation cystoplasty has emerged as the definitive management of severe, refractory hyperreflexia/instability and or poor compliance only since the widespread acceptance of intermittent catheterization [36]. Although a detailed discussion of augmentation cystoplasty is beyond the scope of this chapter, the goal of the augmented bladder is to create a pain-free, adequate capacity reservoir that stores urine at a low pressure. Segments of bowel (ileum, colon and stomach) may be used to augment bladder capacity and Benson and Olsson have reviewed and described the many configurations of intestinal segments [37].

Summary

Urinary incontinence is abnormal at any age. Its prevalence increases with age due to functional impairments and concurrent medical disease. A detailed history and physical examination is essential to evaluate these patients. Urinary incontinence is treatable in all age groups with a logical, multifactorial and persistent approach.

References

1. Figures obtained from the 1990 U.S. Census Bureau.
2. Torrey BB, Kinsella K, Tueuber CM. An aging world international population reports. Series P-95, no. 78. Washington DC: U.S. Bureau of Census, 1987.
3. Verbrugge LM. The dynamics of population dying and health. In: Lewis SJ, editor. Aging and Health: Linking Research and Public Policy. Chelsea, MI: Lewis, 1989.
4. O'Donnel P. The Aging Population. In: Furner ES, Grant MD, Brody JA, editors. Geriatric Urology, 8.
5. Herzog AR, Fultz NH. Prevalence and incidence of urinary incontinence in community dwelling populations. J Am Geriatr Soc 1990; 38: 275.
6. Urinary Incontinence in Adults. NIH consensus conference. JAMA 1989; 261: 2685.
7. Hu TW. Impact of urinary incontinence on health care costs. J Am Geriatr Soc 1990; 38: 292–295.
8. Resnick NM, Geriatric incontinence – geriatric urology. Urol Clin N Amer Feb 1996; 23:61: 55–74.
9. Elbadawi A. Pathology and pathophysiology of detrusor in incontinence. Urol Clin N Amer 1995; 22: 499–512.
10. Resnick NM, Elbadawi A, Yalla SV. Age and the lower urinary tract: What is normal? Neurourol Urodyn, in press.
11. Diokno AC, Brown MB, Brock BM, et al. Clinical and cystometric characteristics of continent and incontinent noninstitutionalized elderly. J Urol 1988; 140: 567–571.
12. Resnick NM, Yalla SV, Laurino E. The pathophysiology of urinary incontinence among institutionalized elderly persons. NEJM 1989; 320: 1.
13. Baldassare JS, Kaye D. Special problems in urinary tract infection in the elderly. Med Clin North Am 1991; 75: 375–390.
14. Ouslander JG, Schapira M, Schnelle JF, et al. Does eradicating bacteriuria affect the severity

of chronic urinary incontinence in nursing home residents? Ann Intern Med 1995; 122: 749–754.
15. Robinson JM. Evaluation of methods for assessment of bladder and urethral function. In: Brocklehurst JC, editor. Urology in the Elderly. New York: Churchill Livingstone, 1984; 19–54.
16. Resnick NM. Geriatric medicine. In: Isselbacher K, Braunwald E, Wilson JD, et al., editors. Harrison's Principles of Internal Medicine. New York: McGraw-Hill, 1994; 30–38.
17. Resnick NM. Voiding dysfunction in the elderly. In: Yalla SV, McGuire EJ, Elbadawi A, Blaivas JG, editors. Neurourology and Urodynamics: Principles and Practice. New York: MacMillan Publishing Company, 1988; 303–330.
18. Ganabathi K, Zimmern PE, Leach GE. Evaluation of Voiding Dysfunction in Geriatric Urology; 203–219.
19. Smith RB. Complications of transurethral surgery. In: Smith RB, Skinner DG, editors. Complications of Urologic Surgery: Prevention and Management. Philadelphia: Saunders, 1976; 277.
20. Chilton CP, et al. A critical evaluation of the results of transurethral resection of the prostate. Br J Urol 1978; 50: 542.
21. Crawford ED, Kiker JD. Radical retropubic prostatectomy. J Urol 1983; 129: 1145.
22. Middleton AW. Pelvic lymphadenectomy with modified radical retropubic prostatectomy as a single operation: technique used and results in 50 consecutive cases. J Urol 1981; 125: 353.
23. Elbadawi A, Yalla SV, Resnick NM. Structural basis of geriatric voiding dysfunction. Ill. Detrusor over activity. J Urol 1993; 150: 1668–1680.
24. Brandeis GB, Yalla SV, Resnick NM. Detrusor hyperactivity with impaired contractility (DHIC): the great mimic. J Urol 1990; 143: 223A.
25. Katz GP, Blaivas JG. A diagnostic dilemma: when urodynamic findings differ from the clinical impression. J Urol 1983; 129: 1170.
26. Wise BG, Cutner A, Cardozo, LD, Kelleher CJ, Burton G, Abbott D. Do detailed symptom questionnaires negate the need for urodynamic investigation? Neuro Urod 1992; 11: 353.
27. Fantl JA, Wyman JF, McClish DK, et al. Efficacy of bladder training in older women with urinary incontinence. JAMA 1991; 65: 609.
28. Cardozo LD, Abrams PD, Stanton SL. Idiopathic bladder instability treated by biofeedback. Br J Urol 1978; 50: 427.
29. Wells TJ, Bink CA, Diokno AC, et al. Pelvic (floor) muscle exercises for SUI in elderly women. J Am Geriatr Soc 1991; 39: 785–791.
30. Rink RC, et al. Intermittent catheterization and the artificial urinary sphincter: compatible techniques in children with neurogenic bladder dysfunction. J Urol. 1985; 133: 352.
31. Bennett CJ, Diokno AC. Clean Intermittent catheterization in the management of the neurogenic bladder in children. J Urol 1984; 132: 526.
32. Newman AK, Smith DA, Harris T, Diokno A. An external female barrier device in the management of urinary incontinence. Neurourol Urodyn 1992; 11: 368(A).
33. Marks JL, Light JK. Management of urinary incontinence after prostatectomy with the artificial urinary sphincter. J Urol 1989; 142: 302.
34. Leach GE, Dmochowski RR, et al. Female stress urinary incontinence clinical guidelines panel summary report on surgical management of female stress urinary incontinence. J Urol 1997; 158: 875.
35. Wright EJ, Iselin CE, et al. Pubovaginal sling using cadaveric allograft fascia for the treatment of intrinsic sphincteric deficiency. J Urol 1998; 160: 759.
36. Linder AL, Leach GE, Raz S. Augmentation cystoplasty in the treatment of neurogenic bladder dysfunction. J Urol 1983; 129: 491.
37. Benson MC, Olsson CA. Urinary diversion. In: Walsh PC, Retik AB, Stamey TA, Vaughn ED, editors. Campbells Urology, 6th edition. Philadelphia, Penn: W.B. Saunders, 1992; 2654.

Access of the Elderly to Dialysis

DIMITRIOS G. OREOPOULOS
The Toronto Western Hospital, Toronto, Ontario, Canada

Many elderly patients, who are suitable for renal replacement treatment, are not referred for a nephrological opinion and so are denied dialysis [1]. This policy may be responsible in a large part for the great difference in the numbers of new patients who present for dialysis in various countries.

Thus in the U.K. [2] of 16 hypothetical patients (most of them elderly), who were described in brief vignettes, on average non-nephrologist consultants and general practitioners considered 6.9 and 7.4 patients respectively as unsuitable for dialysis. This figure was significantly higher than the 4.7 patients considered unsuitable by nephrologists.

In the U.S., Sekkarie et al. [3], who did a prospective study of 76 primary-care physicians and 22 nephrologists found out that the former withheld dialysis from 22% of ESRD patients, compared with the 7% withheld by nephrologists. In deciding not to refer a patient for dialysis, 25% of these primary-care physicians did not consult a nephrologist and 60% cited age as a reason not to refer. (It should be noted that the Institute of Medicine Committee for the study of the Medicare ESRD program explicitly rejected age as a criterion for patient acceptance).

Non-referral for dialysis also occurs in Ontario, Canada. Among the physicians who responded to the questionnaire circulated by Mendelssohn et al. [4], 14% of family physicians and 45% of internists indicated that they recalled not refering certain patients for dialysis, who died subsequently with ESRD, in the last three years. These physicains based their decision on the wishes of a competent patient (94%), short life expectancy (88%) poor quality of life (87%) and age (64%).

Both increasing age and comorbidity were associated with a greater stated choice of non-referral. Other factors affecting the referral pattern were distance from the dialysis center and overcrowding of the nearest dialysis center. Age increased the non-referral pattern in all these categories.

Low referral by primary-care physicians may be based on inadequate knowledge of the indications for and prognosis of modern dialysis, which then may be imparted unchallenged to the potential patient [4].

In the U.S.A. the expanding role of the primary-care physician and the

Oreopoulos et al. (eds.), Nephrology and Geriatrics Integrated, 199–202.

diminishing role of specialists, a pattern promoted by managed care, undoubtedly will change the practice of medicine in general and dialysis in particular [3].

In the Canadian study mentioned above, 67% of the physicians believed that rationing of health care is occurring in Ontario. I want to stress that this occurs even though the Government of Ontario has no explicit policy to ration dialysis among its citizens who require this treatment.

This shows that physicians are responding to the government's indirect measures to do the rationing, something that the government organizations or the managed-care organizations in the U.S.A. will avoid doing overtly by issuing guidelines for rationing.

In the U.S., the health care providers who compete to obtain the 'business' of the various managed-care corporations (business here, represented by the illness of patients), will have to make a profit by practicing savings in various aspects of their practice, something that they can achieve mainly by decreasing hospitalization rates and by limiting referrals to specialists. Such an approach will fall most heavily on patients like the elderly, who require frequent hospitalization and often have multisystem disease that requires referrals to specialists. Nevertheless, this approach will not be acknowledged as policy by the managed care organization – hence there is created a kind of conspiracy by the managed care and physicians against the elderly and all those who may require expensive care.

I believe that this conspiracy is supported by the use of appropriate vocabulary. Thus we talk about 'managed care' where in essence is 'managed costs'. The patients are consumers and the money spent on them are loss ratio and those who are ravaged by disease or old age are considered as financial burdens. Furthermore, I believe that, with the legalization of assisted suicide and subsequent euthanasia, the elderly with ESRD will be coerced covertly into believing that it is 'the right thing to do' and be encouraged to choose 'death with dignity' rather than submit to the 'indignities of this wretched treatment' as it has been described in a recent article in Lancet [6].

Eventually primary-care physicians will get the message concerning this 'conspiracy' and will do their part: they will stop referring these patients to us, as they have already started doing [3].

The policy of incentives is another more sinister way of encouraging/enticing primary-care physicians to save costs for the managed care corporation. The more the physician saves the greater his/her bonus at the end of the year. I consider this policy a sinister one because it takes advantage of the greed latent in all of us, and it will strike a deadly blow against the patient/doctor relationship.

What Should We Do?

I will repeat here some of the recommendations that Hall et al made to those physicians who want to preserve their patients' trust and be their advocates in a managed-care environment [5]:

(a) Maintain high scientific standards by practicing evidence-based medicine.
(b) Be impartial i.e. use the same clinical criteria for all patients even if they have different insurance plans.
(c) Do not enter into any incentive arrangements that are not in common use elsewhere and that you are embarrassed to describe accurately to your patients.

At the same time insurance plans should be encouraged and, if necessary, required by legislation, to describe to prospective clients their incentive policies; also government should ban and make illegal 'gag' clauses that prevent physicians from protesting or revealing what they believe is wrong with these managed care plans.

Finally when, because of forces beyond our control, we cannot offer a treatment to a new patient, we should not conceal the truth but tell the unpleasant truth that economic policies lie behind our decision.

In conclusion I believe that non-referral of elderly for dialysis occurs in North America and I expect that in the future the elderly will have an even greater difficulty in accessing life-supporting chronic treatment.

I believe that the nephrologists should include in their goals, education of primary care physicians and geriatricians about what dialysis (HD and PD) does and what they can offer in terms of life prolongation and quality of life on dialysis.

With a few exceptions, such as the demented patients or the patient who has less than 2–3 months life expectancy and the patient who requires restrains to be dialysed, the rest should be allowed to decide for themselves whether they want to be dialysed after they have been fully informed.

Finally, I believe that physicians (all of us, nephrologists, geriatricians and primary care physicians alike) should focus and refocus continuously on our primary goal, that is, being our patient's advocate and whenever there is a clash between our patients' interests and ours or those of the organization for which we are working, the interests of the patients always take a precedent, otherwise we are in the wrong profession.

References

1. Feest TG, Mistry CD, Grimes DS, Mallick NP. Incidence of advanced chronic renal failure and the need for end stage renal replacement treatment. Br M J Oct 20, 1990; 301: 897–900.
2. Challah S, Wing AJ, Bauer R, Morris RW, Schroeder SA. Negative selection for dialysis and transplantation in the United Kingdom. Br M J 1984; 288: 1119–1122.
3. Sekkarie A, Moss AH. Withholding and withdrawing dialysis: the role of physician

specialty and education and patient functional status. Am J Kidney Dis March 1998; 31(3): 464–472.
4. Mendelssohn DC, Kua BT, Singer PA. Referal for dialysis in Ontario. Arch Intern Med Dec 11-25, 1995; 155: 2473–2478.
5. Hall MA, Berenson RA. Ethical practice in managed care: a dose of realism. Ann Int Med Mar 1, 1998; 128(5): 395–402.
6. Radcliffe-Richards J, Daar AS, Guttman RD, et al. For the International Forum for Transplant Ethics. The case for allowing kidney sales. Lancet 1998; 351: 1950–1952.

Dialysis Withdrawal

DIMITRIOS G. OREOPOULOS
The Toronto Western Hospital, Toronto, Ontario, Canada

In the U.S. there has been a recent increase in deaths due to withdrawal from dialysis. Thus the percentage of such deaths increased from 9.7% in 1988 to 17.6% in 1996 [1].

Almost all reports of deaths due to dialysis withdrawal confirm that such deaths are much more frequent among the elderly than among younger patients [2, 3].

With the anticipated increase in the number of elderly patients on dialysis (approximately 60% of dialysis patients by the year 2000), in the near future nephrologists will face the issue of withdrawal with increasing frequency [4].

Many authors have described the various types of patients who die as a result of dialysis withdrawal. I will divide these patients into two main categories:

(a) those with decision-making capacity and
(b) those without decision-making capacity.

In Sekkarie's prospective study [5], 37% of those who died after withdrawal from dialysis lacked decision-making capacity.

In those who are capable of making decisions, the patient decides that the quality of life on dialysis is not acceptable and eventually the nephrologist has to comply with the patient's wishes because autonomy overrides all other ethical principles.

On the other hand, I believe that patients, who have lost their decision-making capacities, pose the most difficult ethical and legal problems. An important factor in the management of this group is the presence (or not) of an advance directive and/or the designation of a surrogate decision maker.

Despite all efforts to encourage patients to sign advance directives, only 20% of patients in the U.S. actually give an advance directive [6]. A survey in Pittsburgh showed that many patients were unwilling to sign an advance directive and 50% of these said they feared that, by signing a living will, they might influence the subsequent conduct of their physicians [7]. This lack of trust is particularly prominent among black patients in respect to a predominantly white medical profession [1].

Oreopoulos et al. (eds.), Nephrology and Geriatrics Integrated, 203–205.

Why this lack of trust? I suspect that our actions do not inspire our patients to believe that we will do our best for them when they are no longer able to decide for themselves.

What should we do for the 20% of patients who, in their advance directives indicate that they want dialysis to be continued if they lose their decision-making capacity, or for the patients without an advance directive whose families request the continuation of dialysis?

I believe that, when we encourage a patient to give an advance directive, we enter into a contract that commits us to respect and follow their wishes, whatever they decide. However, it seems that whereas we are prepared to follow their wishes if they ask for discontinuation of treatment, we do not know what to do and we feel very uncomfortable if they ask for continuation of treatment.

If patient autonomy is the primary ethical principle in making such decisions, one should continue dialyzing these patients even if the health-care team believes such treatment is futile. However an increasing number of nephrologist declare that they find it difficult when advance directives clash with their own beliefs [8]; they believe that continuing medical care to a patient in persistent vegetative state (PVS), is futile and offends their moral integrity [9].

I believe that resolving such an ethical dilemma requires patience, understanding and compassion. Indeed I feel a strong sense of impatience on behalf of the physician when I see changes in societal attitudes and principles from one that gives primacy to the principle of patient autonomy, which has governed our ethical decision-making until recently, to a community-based model that values societal objectives and the common good above the wishes of the individual [9–11]. This process was eloquently described by Dr. Callahan in his book *Setting Limits*. As described by Arnold Eiser, under the new circumstances the community shall (should) have the capacity to set, develop and administer guidelines concerning such problem areas of decision making [9]. Such a communitarian perspective holds that the community has an interest in assisting the profession of medicine to maintain its integrity and will not compel it to provide non-beneficial futile medical care [9]. Of course an additional benefit of such a policy is that it saves money because the cost of care for those with an advance directive to discontinue treatment is less than one-third of that of those without such a directive [12].

Under these circumstances, I believe that advance directives would be of no use, in ensuring compliance with the patient's wishes.

The main risk in adopting such an approach is that: (1) some individuals, who believe that they should continue being dialyzed for religious reasons (such as orthodox Jews and some Catholics) may feel that they are being discriminated against, but worse [13, 14], this approach may be used predominantly for economic reasons.

In conclusion, I believe that the expected dramatic increase in the numbers of elderly who suffer from ERDS in the next decade will bring into play economic pressures to make death from withdrawal an increasingly common experience for the nephrologist [15, 16].

References

1. United State Renal Data System. 1966 Annual Date Report. Am J Kidney Dis 1966; 10: 1128–1130.
2. Office Technology Assessment. Dialysis for chronic renal failure. In life-sustaining Technologies and the Elderly. OTA-BA-306. Washington, DC: U.S. Government Printing Office, 1987; 2–7.
3. Port FK, Wolfe RA, Hawthorne VM, et al. Discontinuation of dialysis therapy as a cause of death. Am J Nephrol 1989; 9: 145.
4. Bhatnagar V, Maruenda J, Lowenthal DT. Ethical issues involved in dialysis for the elderly. Geriatric Nephrology and Urology 1998; 8(2): 1–5.
5. Sekkarie MA, Moss AH. Withholding and withdrawing dialysis: the role of physician specialty and education and patient functional status. Am J Kidney Dis March 1998; 31(1): 464–472.
6. Holley JL, Nespor S, Rault R. Chronic in-center hemodialysis patients attitudes, knowledge and behavior towards advance directiveness. J Am Soc Nephrol 1993; 3: 1405–1408.
7. Maiorca R. Ethical issues in dialysis: prospects for the year 2000. Nephrol Dial Transplant 1998; 13(1): 1–9.
8. Rutecki GW, Cugino A, Jarjoura D, Kilner JF, Whittier FC. Nephrologist's subjective attitudes towards end of life issues and the conduct of terminal care. Clinical Nephrol 1997; 48: 173–180.
9. Eiser AR. Withdrawal from dialysis: the role of autonomy and community-based values. Am J Kidney Dis March 1996; 27(3): 451–457.
10. Beauchamp TL. Reversing the protections. Hastings Cent Rep 1994; 24: 18–19.
11. Murray TH. Communities need more than autonomy. Hastings Cent Rep 1994; 24: 32–33.
12. Chambers CV, Diamond JJ, Perkel RL, et al. Relationship of advance directives to hospital changes in a Medicare population. Arch Intern Med 1997; 154: 541–547.
13. Anonymous: Bishops warn against withdrawing life supports. Hosp Ethics 1992; 8: 9–10.
14. Jacobovits I. Ethical problems regarding termination of life. In: Meier L, editor. Jewish Values in Bioethics. New York, NY: Human Sciences, 1986; 84–95.
15. Moss AH, Stocking CB, Sachs GA, Siegler M. Variation in attitudes of dialysis unit medical directors towards decisions to withhold. J Am Soc Nephrol 1993; 4(2): 229–234.
16. Bleyer AJ, Tell GS, Evans GW, et al. Survival of patients undergoing renal replacement therapy in one center with special emphasis on racial differences. Am J Kidney Dis 1996; 28: 72.

Managed Care, Geriatrics, and Nephrology

MARTIN G. WHITE
3525 Turtle Creek Blvd., #20DE, Dallas, TX 75219-5514, U.S.A.

Managed care, geriatrics and nephrology have not yet been integrated although limited, fragmentary efforts in this regard include nephrology consultation, ESRD services, and early efforts in disease prevention.

At present the managed-care industry looks upon nephrology as a consultative resource. However, other than consultation, with the exception of the care of end stage renal disease (ESRD), patients' health plans do not see a distinct role for nephrology either in the commercial (employer sponsored plans) or Medicare (federal senior products) risk book of business. Therefore, if it wants to participate more actively, nephrology must understand managed care's shared risk opportunities and to determine in what way the specialty fits into such activities. Then nephrology must seek actively the right to play an essential role. Figure 1 illustrates the low position of nephrology in the distribution of the health care dollar for a given population of Medicare HMO beneficiaries [1]. As a consequence health plans pay little attention to nephrologists and to nephrology issues.

An essential task for the nephrologist is to understand the vision by which healthcare care is being re-engineered, e.g. the concept that everyone should receive all necessary health care [2]. Society must determine what health care is necessary and how we are to satisfy society's seemingly endless appetite for health-care services. Society does not have sharp focus on this issue and has not allocated funding for universal coverage. Secondly the health care team needs to improve the quality of services it delivers and, at the same time, reduce unexplained variations in services and quality. This translates into a system that will monitor, report, and be accountable for the delivery of health care services both from the professional and consumer perspectives. Improving quality implies that we know what quality is and how to measure it; in many respects, nephrology has identified quality parameters in its management of ESRD. Finally we should provide care efficiently, that is, at the right time, in the right place, in the right amount, and at the right price, so that the customer is satisfied with and confident of the quality of the treatment they receive.

In addition, nephrology must 'right-size' its resources. In this regard, it

Oreopoulos et al. (eds.), Nephrology and Geriatrics Integrated, 207–211.

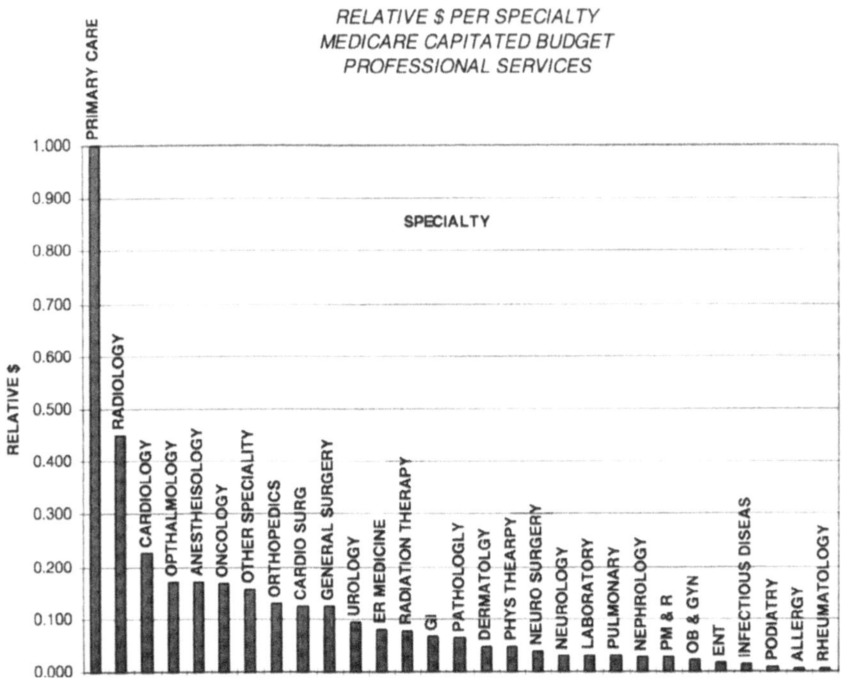

Figure 1. Comparison of medicare risk budget expenditures for all professional services (mental health excluded).

has a distinct advantage over many other specialty areas of medicine, in that its manpower resources are relatively small and predicted to become insufficient in the future [3]. While this issue deserves attention and correction, it also represents a considerable opportunity, namely, to move ahead and incorporate other levels of caregivers into the nephrology healthcare model. This would include redefining the role of the nephrologist, incorporating primary-care physicians into the model, employing and teaming up with advanced nurse practitioners, physician assistants, and others who can participate in the care of nephrology patients [4].

Also nephrology must seek ways to work co-operatively with health plans to better the lives of patients within the managed-care paradigm. We must begin by convincing the administrative and medical leadership of health plans that the nephrologist can make a contribution to the success of these health plans beyond that of providing consultative and ESRD services. For example, it can assist the health plan to carry out a forward-looking analysis of its membership population and thus to anticipate and modify looming co-morbidities. Also we can help them develop rational and practical protocols to identify, monitor, and treat hypertension.

Finally we must understand the focus of the customer and cater to his/her needs if we are to create value for the present and the future. Nephrology has been in the business of treating renal diseases. Its customer orientation has been to care for and comfort those with renal disease, but not to meet traditional customer expectations. It is a 'sickness' specialty. Consumers want to avoid sickness. The challenge to nephrology is to reorganize itself so as to provide the service of prevention.

An informal survey of the corporate medical directors of nationwide health plans, who provide services to the senior population revealed little interest or attention directed toward the specialty of nephrology or to renal disease [5]. When rank ordered from their perspective, nephrology is near the bottom both in the provision of clinical services and in professional remuneration. ESRD services are the only nephrology activity they consider by even a few of the plans. The interest of health plans should increase as governments remove restrictions on HMO Medicare coverage in the coming years, and by the marketing of commercial products by national dialysis chains and vendors [6], who provide these services and share this risk. Renal transplantation, which has been removed from the local nephrologist's sphere of influence, is largely provided by centers specializing in this procedure. In some instances health plans choose 'Centers of Excellence', which offer 'package deals', and provide outstanding results. While they provide quality service and accountability, these arrangements further remove the patient from the local nephrologist. HMO medical directors view pre-ESRD programs promoted by these national dialysis chains and commercial vendors as a marketing gimmick rather than a valued service, therefore it remains for those providers to establish the value of such programs.

Pacificare©, through its Medicare product, Secure Horizons©, have brought strong focus on the fields of nephrology and geriatrics. In some of its markets, this organization focuses on ESRD case management, the application of guidelines, and monitors and reports on accountability of the various providers. This health plan has a Diabetes Quality Initiative which looks at microalbuminuria [7]. Other health plans, in my informal survey, also had diabetes projects, but none provided any measure of nephropathy. This void further indicates the opportunity for larger participation by nephrology.

To further define the role of the nephrologist, I recommend an approach (Table 1) that illustrates the contribution of nephrologists to hypothetical populations of HMO-insured members. The nephrologist gets involved most directly with a small number of individuals from this population and, in that instance, would be the most appropriate principal physician. However the nephrologist must be engaged with the population as a whole but be focused on the identification of sub-populations, who are at higher risk for developing renal disease. If the nephrologist does not establish his/her role and expertise in dealing with health issues of the larger population, he can expect to be relegated to ESRD care and have little input into the larger issues of population health care management.

To date, nephrology has done little to define its larger role in managed

Table 1. Nephrology Involvement in the provision of medical care to members in a health plan

Nephrology Involvement	100 000 Members	1000 Members	100 Members
Population analysis	Participate in Multidisciplinary teams to evaluate a population.	Participate in Multidisciplinary teams to evaluate a population for high risk patients who demonstrate renal manifestations.	Lead Multidisciplinary team to evaluate population for high risk patients who demonstrate renal failure or other active/progressive renal disease.
Cohort identification	Identify high risk cohort. Identify environmental or cultural risk factors.	Identify high risk cohort. Identify environmental or cultural risk factors.	Identify high risk cohort. Identify environmental or cultural risk factors.
Implement evidence based guidelines	Influence and encourage implementation of evidence based clinical guidelines.	Influence and encourage implementation of evidence based clinical guidelines. Participate in guideline development and implementation.	Lead in the implementation of evidence based clinical guidelines. Participate in guidelines, be held accountable.
Educate the health care team	Educate primary care physicians, advanced practice nurses, physician assistants, public, and patients.	Educate primary care physicians, advanced practice nurses, physician assistants, public, and patients.	Educate primary care physicians, advanced practice nurses, physician assistants, public, and patients.
Monitor quality accountability of health care team and its individual members	Influence monitoring and accountability process.	Influence monitoring and accountability process. Participate in monitoring process.	Lead monitoring and accountability process. Be held accountable for process and outcomes.
Provide necessary medical services	Provide nephrology consultation.	Provide nephrology consultation. Follow patients as a consultant or as per guideline.	Provide principal care physician services. Provide and or direct all necessary services.

care, and has done nothing to define its role in services to the geriatric population provided by managed care organizations. As a result, we have great opportunities to improve the health care of this population, face many challenges, abundant risks and great rewards.

References

1. Data from Southwest Physician Associates Health Organization, Dallas, Texas, 1997 Medicare Data covering 5000 members.
2. Brook RH. Managed care is not the problem, quality is. JAMA 1997; 278: 1612–1614.
3. Neilson EG, Hull AR, Wish JR, Neylan JF, Sherman D, Suki WN. Ad hoc committee on nephrology manpower needs: the ad hoc committee report on estimating the future workforce and training requirements for nephrology. J Am Soc Nephrol 1997 (suppl 9); 8: S1–S4.
4. RPA/ASN. Position Paper. The role of non-physician Medical Personnel in Delivering Nephrologic Care. April, 1996.
5. Personal communication. Interviews with HMO Medicare Regional and National Medical Directors.
6. Hull AR. Testimony of Dr. Alan Hull; National Bipartisan Commission on the Future of Medicare, September 8, 1998.
7. Personal Communication, Sam Ho MD, Corporate Medical Director, Pacificare©.

The Challenges of Geriatric Nephrology Managed Care/Disease Managcment

THEODORE I. STEINMAN
Harvard Medical School, Dialysis Unit, Beth Israel Deaconess Medical Center, Renal Division, 330 Brookline Avenue (FD220) , Boston, Massachusetts 02215, U.S.A.

While the rate of growth of the end-stage renal disease (ESRD) in the United States has slowed from the 8–9% to 5–6% as the 1990s have progressed, the care of the geriatric population becomes an ever-growing challenge. For this population, renal replacement therapy (RRT) invariably means dialysis, either hemodialysis or peritoneal dialysis. Only under unusual circumstances is transplantation an option for the elderly patient with ESRD. Other industrialized nations around the world face similar problems. While this paper deals with ESRD in the United States, the situation here is a template for everywhere else.

The United States Renal Data System (USRDS), a thorough database resource, provides us with the demographic information that challenge the nephrology community. In 1995 approximately 220 000 patients were on dialysis in the United States, 17% were performing peritoneal dialysis and the remainder were on hemodialysis [1]. The incidence rate for ESRD/million population is 253 and the prevalence rate is 967. By the year 2000, it is estimated that approximately 300 000 patients will be on dialysis. Approximately 70 000 patients have had kidney transplant in the past three years and they are covered by Medicare for the first three years after transplantation. Three years after successful transplantation, the patients' insurance reverts from Medicare to their primary insurance.

Table 1 shows that the elderly make up the most rapidly growing portion of the ESRD population. While the incidence rate over the 10 years from 1987–1997 has remained stable under age 65, the group between 65 and 74 years and beyond is growing at an exponential rate. In 1997 the ESRD incidence rate for those 65–74 years of age was 1100/million population; this is almost double the rate in 1987 and over 10 times the incidence rate for those 20–44 years of age. Table 2 provides information about age-adjusted, first-year, death rates for hemodialysis patients from 1985–1995. Especially with regard to the elderly, we need to address the following issues.

1. Optimal strategies to improve care in the geriatric population, especially in a managed-care setting.
2. Who should be initiated and who withdrawn from dialysis. This topic will not be discussed in this paper because it is the subject of the nephrology

Oreopoulos et al. (eds.), Nephrology and Geriatrics Integrated, 213–223.

Table 1. ESRD incidence rates/million population 1987–1996

Age	1987		1997
65–74	600		1100
75+	450		1000
45–64	300		400
20–44	90		100
0–19		Unchaged (< 10)	

Source: USRDS 1997.

Table 2. Adjusted 1st year death rates for hemodialysis patients, 1985–1995

	1985	1995
Age 50	17%	14%
Age 70	31%	27%
Males	22%	19%
Females	21%	17%
Black	16%	16%
White	22%	18%
Diabetes	34%	21%
No diabetes	18%	13%

Source: USRDS 1997.

community's next practice guideline. Criteria are being established to suggest who would benefit from renal replacement therapy. General guidelines should provide a uniform approach where none currently exists. Equally important is providing a support structure for physicians as they establish 'contracts' with patients and their families that allows discontinuation of dialysis when it becomes obvious the patient is not benefiting from dialysis treatments.

3. Pre-ESRD care must receive much more attention if we hope to prevent or slow the rate of progression of ESRD for all individuals. In addition, a more comprehensive system of patient care before the individual reaches the need for RRT will be less costly to the system.
4. Does a disease management model work well for the elderly person with chronic renal failure (CRF)? If so, what specific issues need to be addressed?
5. The cost of care is a major concern for society with limited financial resources available for healthcare, hence the medical community must make the commitment that high quality care be provided at the lowest cost.

Outcome Measures in ESRD That Reflect the Delivery of Quality Care

ESRD affects multiorgan systems and to improve outcomes we must focus on approaches to:

1. Adequacy of hemodialysis;
2. Anemia;
3. Calcium/phosphorous metabolism;
4. Metabolic acidosis;
5. Nutrition;
6. Lipid abnormalities;
7. Vascular access.

While each of these issues is important for care givers, this paper focuses on pre-ESRD strategies in a managed care, capitated environment. The emphasis is on chronic disease management. The Dialysis Outcome Quality Initiatives (DOQI) has addressed many of these issues for the dialysis population, hence I refer the reader to the thorough reviews published under the auspices of the National Kidney Foundation [2, 3].

The Growth of Managed Care

In 1996 Health Maintenance Organizations (HMOs) and Managed Care Organizations (MCOs) provided health care to more than 120 million Americans, including 75% of all U.S. workers with health insurance [4]. The managed care revolution dominates healthcare delivery in the United States, with approximately 28% of all Americans being enrolled in some managed care plan. It is therefore incumbent upon physicians to address the many issues that will impact on patient care, especially in the elderly. Managed care agreements dictate: (1) defined eligibility and required requirements; (2) reporting standards (in many cases); (3) reimbursement for all services (medications, dialysis home health services, etc.). While expenses associated with all aspects of patient care have risen, both inflation-adjusted Medicare and HMOs/MCOs reimbursement has declined. The decreased revenue stream has forced the dialysis industry to focus on economic issues associated with staffing, equipment, laboratory services, ancillary services and marketing tools. While Medicare in the United States covers most of the elderly on dialysis, in the past three years the enrollment of the ESRD elderly into MCO plans has tripled from about 4% to over 12% (1997 through 1999).

The agenda of managed care focuses on three major items: costs, costs, costs. However, a managed care world that is obsessed with costs must verbalize its commitment to quality care for all patients. In particular, the ESRD patient is vulnerable because operators of managed care plans have had little experience with high-cost, chronic illness. The unique level of care necessary to maintain the health of the typical renal patient under the ESRD program when viewed in the context of political realities and budgetary constraints in the public and private sectors, creates a problematic outlook for the future of nephrology [5].

Now government agencies, health care institutions, insurance companies and MCOs set the rules for health care, rendering increasingly irrelevant physicians' authority and patients' rights [6]. In 1996, premium dollars to HMOs/MCOs totaled more that 200 billion and managed care plans are adding new members at a rate of approximately 8 million per year. By the year 2000, 80% of all Americans will be enrolled in managed-care plans. Therefore, it is imperative that the nephrology community understand our current and immediate challenges so we can focus our attention on the delivery of quality care. (See the thorough review by Steinman on 'Managed Care, Capitation and the Future of Nephrology' [7].)

Patients with CRF need access to nephrologists because these physicians can deliver more cost-effective care than internists/generalists [8]. A disease management approach that would work well in ESRD and pre-ESRD is a better alternative than the current piecemeal, reactive healthcare delivery response. Potentially, care from the nephrologist before ESRD develops can slow the progression of disease, or at least better prepare the patient for eventual RRT. Care management will support the nephrologist in his/her role as the principal caregiver for the patient with ESRD [12]. A patient who reaches ESRD in better health due to improved management will cost the program less because he/she will require less hospitalization and will have a lower mortality rate. Therefore in MCOs, patients with chronic renal failure must receive the following:

1. Access to relevant specialists.
2. Early referral to a nephrologist. Adhere to the National Institutes of Health guidelines: a female with a serum creatinine $\geq$ 1.5 mg/dl and a male with a serum creatinine $\geq$ 2.0 mg/dl should see a nephrologist in consultation [13].
3. Each HMO must have a mechanism for providing ESRD patients access to dialysis and transplant providers in their geographic area. All forms of RRT must be available to the patient.
4. HMOs/MCOs must adopt a multidisciplinary approach for care of the ESRD patient. Circular integration (Fig. 1) outlines the coordinated team approach to care; the patient is placed at the center of the hub. All members of the team must relate to and communicate with each other to maximize care for the patient.
5. Vertical integration (Fig. 2) shows all of the services that must be available to the patient to maximize care. Figure 3 illustrates how tasks are assigned around dialysis care issues.
6. Practice guidelines and clinical pathways should be the guiding force for care. Uniformity will reduce unnecessary variances, but still allow an individual approach to each patient.
7. Patient education programs are an integral part of any program. Patients

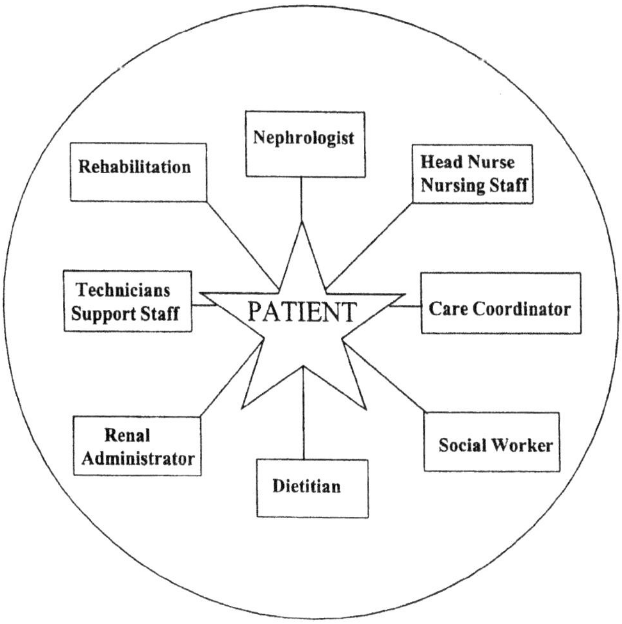

Figure 1. Circular Integration: The health care team relates to the patient in an integrated manner. The patient is the center of the hub and all efforts are directed to improving quality of care and life. All members of the team coordinate care to achieve the desired goals.

need to know what to expect from each member of the renal care team and to understand their own responsibilities for their care.

8. HMOs/MCOs must inform patients of the extent of (and exact limits to) coverage of renal-related requirements.
9. HMOs/MCOs must provide ongoing data to the USRDS system. Only by sharing information can we learn from a comprehensive data base; the end result of sharing will be the best care for the patients.
10. The commitment to quality care must be accompanied by a continuing focus on outcomes research. Continuous quality improvement is the end result of outcomes research. A constant feedback to the nephrologist and other members of the care team will allow for non-threatening improvement in care.

So far managed care has not lived up to its promises and potential and needs to establish its sustainable future. Admittedly, in the United States the healthcare system before managed care was a non-system [14]. However, our system did have committed professionals, caring institutions in various locales, freedom of choice and laws that reflected public confidence. Our baseline system assumed that needed health care services are customary, moral and implied legal rights for U.S. citizen. In contrast, today's version of managed care is characterized by financial and legal manipulation, 'choice' constricted

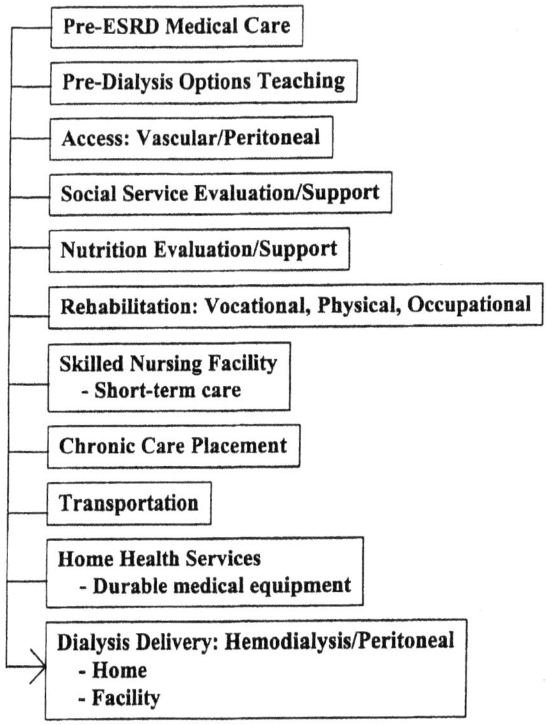

Figure 2. Vertical Integration: The continuum of services which need to be available to the patient with chronic renal failure, beginning in the pre-ESRD period and extending up to dialysis initiation and chronic treatment. Not every service will be used by all the patients.

by provider selection of physicians' panels, and laws reflecting lack of public trust [15]. Managed care can survive its initial foolish years if public policy, legislation and business practices acknowledge: (1) accountability for today's actions and (2) preservation of healthcare resources. The system needs to strike a balance between seeking immediate profit and preserving available resources. A positive development in managed care is the acknowledgement that integrated delivery systems represent an improvement in care. MCOs can survive if they demonstrate that they care as much about patients as profits, that they do not skimp on care, and that they support their share of teaching and research. Also, care of the poor and elderly must be a commitment and physicians need to continuously advocate for this segment of our population. Managing care must offer something special, and this includes controlling costs because good care ultimately costs less.

Dialysis Issues

Task	How Achieved	Primary Responsibility
Dialysis Prescription	Establish goals	Nephrologist
Dialysis Delivery	Each treatment	Nursing/Technician Staff
Adequacy of Dialysis	Monthly lab review	Nephrologist
Social Service	Monthly review	Social Worker
Nutrition	Monthly lab review	Dietitian
Rehabilitation		
-Physical	Establish goals	Physical Therapist
-Occupational	Evaluation of home needs	Occupational Therapist
-Vocational	Employment status	Rehabilitation Commission
Scheduling	Written/Verbal communication	Head Nurse and Secretary
Water Treatment	Maintenance schedule	Technician
Supplies	Order schedule	Renal Administrator

Figure 3. Dialysis care team. Some of the issues which must be addressed on a regular basis. The entire team should meet monthly to review patient programs and dialysis unit issues. A core group of nephrologist, nurse, social worker, dietitian must then sit down together with the patient on a regular basis at least 3 times/year to review goals, progress and achievements. Other members of the care team are added on an as-needed basis.

Disease Management

ESRD is an ideal condition in which to implement a disease-management model. It is easy to identify the ESRD population, the boundaries are defined by the need for dialysis. The entire nephrology community and patients know the parameters of care; they are relatively easy to track because these patients are seen three times per week (hemodialysis) or once a month (peritoneal dialysis). Quality indicators can measure performance and informatics will allow one physician's performance to be compared with that of colleagues in a selected region or nationwide. Core indicators of quality of ESRD care, are accepted throughout the nephrology community, include: Measuring adequacy of dialysis (Kt/V, urea reduction ratio), management of anemia, management of calcium/phosphorous metabolism, treatment of metabolic acidosis, and nutrition (as measured by serum albumin). The following four factors are needed to employ a disease management model [16]:

1. The disease/population to manage.
2. The database needed to plan and manage a program.
3. Costs of caring for potential populations (with a track record of managing these costs in the past).
4. Types of payment and amount available.

Therefore, ESRD is a ideal situation in which to employ a disease management approach. The basis for success with disease management is a fully integrated provider system and a ESRD population who are lifelong users of healthcare. A disease management model will deliver defined regular benefits to ESRD patients, will retain these patients and will attract prospective new patients. ESRD has the longest track record of any disease that is paid on a capitated basis for outpatient care, and experimental programs are underway to determine if ESRD should move into a full global capitation system. Global capitation is a fixed payment to the nephrologist for all services he/she delivers to the ESRD patient, including both inpatient and outpatient care. There is no additional billing allowed by the nephrologist. Therefore, reimbursement must reflect value of the services. Since the government extended the Medicare Secondary Payer (MSP) system for reimbursement from 18–30 months, HMOs/MCOs have faced substantial incremental costs. If ESRD and its current utilization patterns go unmanaged some HMOs may face financial disaster.

Concept of Total Management

Total management uses all cost-effective means for managing disease that maximizes patient care. With respect to the ESRD population, this includes transportation to and from dialysis, physical/vocational rehabilitation, necessary medications (over-the-counter and prescription drugs), food supplements and family/patient counseling. Most important of all for the ESRD population is adherence to the medical regimen, both in and outside of the dialysis program.

These total services can be delivered in an integrated manner only with the services of a care manager (health service coordinator). This is different than a case manager because it is *care* that we are managing. Health service co-ordinators work for the physician as part of the team rather than as an employee of the payer (HMO/MCO). Care management is individualized because the idiosyncrasies of individual patients are recognized in managing illnesses. Each individual and caregiver wants to achieve a maximal sense of wellbeing. However, what the patient is willing to do, based on their fears and expectations, is unique for that patient. An individual approach enhances communication. If the patients perceive that they count as persons, they will participate more fully in group discussions, training, education and similar techniques designed to improve the efficiency of providers.

The manager/health service coordinator helps to 'close the loop' at home. Once the patient leaves the dialysis unit we know little about what is happening in their home environment; circumstances at home may negate the team's goals. A care manager who makes home visits can help the team to understand and neutralize the impediments to care, such as: (1) inability to afford medication; (2) inability to afford prescribed foods; (3) social situations that threaten the wellbeing of the dialysis patient; (4) physical impediments in the home setting; and (5) the degree of the patients' compliance with their own medical care (e.g. are diabetic patients testing their fingerstick blood glucose values as directed). Poor compliance may be due to lack of understanding or lack of motivation and knowing the basis of the compliance issue(s) may allow for focused approaches. In addition, trust develops between the patient and care manager, which improves dialogue and communication. Knowing what motivates the patient helps to improve the patient's care. Caregivers will maximize appropriate services which need to be delivered if they understand the impact of lifestyles, self-monitoring and self-management by the patient. As noted earlier, the ultimate desire is to improve care and lower total costs to the system. Preventive measures can be applied once you understand the patient's entire milieu. If the above described approach can save one or two hospital days per patient/per year, the cost savings will pay for all the services noted while improving quality of life for the patient.

Integrated care can succeed only if there is adequate communication between every member of the team. This in turn requires a database that allows each member to access information that supports their specific role. If the dialysis nurse understands why the patient is gaining excessive weight in the period between dialyses because of difficulties in the home, she can respond to that patient. The ultimate benefit of total disease management is to empower the patient to be an active participant in his/her own care. In the current system of hospital care dialysis units, the patient tends to be in a passive role. Self-advocacy improves overall care and lowers costs. A home-based intervention program reduces the frequency of hospital admissions and out-of-hospital deaths after discharge from hospital [17]. Such a home program can reduce unplanned hospital readmissions, a major component of hospital care costs, since it has been shown that recently discharged patients tend to be non-compliant. Also, it has been noted that 96% of discharged patients have inadequate knowledge about their treatment [18, 19].

Capitation

1997 URSDS data indicates that the population with ESRD > 65 years old have an average of 1.4 hospitalizations per year; the average number of hospital days per year is 11.4 (Table 3). The ESRD population < 65 years of age have an average of 1.3 hospitalizations per year; their average length of stay is 9.6 days. For comparison, the Medicare patients > 65 years of age have an average 7.1 hospital days per year. From 1991–1995, the average number of all hospital admissions for ESRD patients decreased from 1.37 to 1.32 and

Table 3. ESRD and hospitalization

Age	# Hospitalization/Year	Avg. Hosp. Days/Year
> 65	1.4	11.4
< 65	1.3	9.6

For comparison: 7.1 hospital days/year for all Medicare patients > 65 years.
1991–1995: average # of hospital admissions overall decrease 1.37 to 1.32 # hospital days decrease from 12.5 to 10.4.
Source: USRDS 1997.

the number of hospital days decreased from 12.4 to 10.4 days [1]. A global management program can bring a further improvement.

An effective global capitation payment system can be cost-effective only if a disease management program is in place. Without understanding every component of this system and having a detailed communication program, costs for the chronic renal failure population will be difficult to contain. Cost differential between diabetics and non-diabetics, based on age (Table 4), illustrates where cost savings can be achieved with a global disease management approach under a capitated arrangement. This demonstrates the relative difference in the cost of care per ESRD year for diabetics and non-diabetics in the age ranges

Table 4. Relative differences in costs per year of ESRD care for diabetics and non-diabetics in the age ranges 0–9 years is compared to ≥ 75 years. The cost differential falls from $12 000 to $6000 between the lowest and highest age ranges.

Ages	Diabetic	Non-Diabetic
0–19 years	$34 000	$22 000
≥ 75 years	$54 000	$48 000

Sources: HCFA; USRDS 1997.

Table 5. Medicare ESRD managed care capitation demonstration rate cells (of AAPPC).*

	Age	Part A	Part B
Dx: DM	0–19	–	–
	20–64	1.14	1.14
	65+	1.37	1.26
Dx: Other	0–19	0.85	0.95
	20–64	0.76	1.04
	65+	1.13	1.15
Transplant			
All ages and diagnoses		6.24	1.44

* AAPPC = Average annual payment per capita.
Source: Paul Eggers, HCFA.

0–19 years, as compared to > 75 years. The cost differential declines from $12 000 to $6000 between the lowest and highest age ranges [1].

We hope that the Medicare ESRD Managed Care Capitation Demonstration Project [20] will provide the renal community with information about quality care and costs in a capitated system. Table 5 provides rate cells for average annual payment per capita (AAPPC). Rate cells reflect reimbursement, a value of one being Medicare's payment at 100% of the established AAPPC to insurance companies for care of the Medicare patient.

References

1. U.S. Renal Data System, USRDS 1997 Annual Report. National Institutes of Health, National Institute of Diabetes and Digestive and Kidney Diseases, Bethesda, MD, April 1997.
2. National Kidney Foundation. Dialysis outcomes quality initiative, clinical practice guidelines, hemodialysis adequacy, peritoneal dialysis adequacy. Am J Kid Dis 1997; 30: S1–S134.
3. National Kidney Foundation. Dialysis outcomes quality initiative, clinical practice guidelines, management of anemia, vascular access. Am J Kid Dis 1997; 30: S192–S240.
4. Anders G. Health Against Wealth: HMOs and the Breakdown of Medical Trust. New York, Houghton Mifflin, 1996.
5. Swartz K, Brennan TA. Integrated health care, capitated payment and quality: the role of regulation. Ann Intern Med 1996; 124: 442–448.
6. Renal Physicians Association/American Society of Nephrology. Position paper on managed care and nephrology. Washington, DC, December 9, 1995.
7. Steinman TI. Managed care, capitation and the future of nephrology. J Am Soc Nephrol 1997; 1618–1623.
8. Junger P, Zingraff J, Page B, Albouze G, Hannedouche T, Man N-K. Detrimental effects of late referral in patients with chronic renal failure: a case-control study. Kidney Int 1993; 43 (Suppl 41): S170–S173.
9. Ifudu O, Dawood M, Homel P, Friedman EA. Excess morbidity in patients starting uremia therapy without prior care by a nephrologist. Am J Kid Dis 1996; 28: 841–845.
10. ESRD CQI Proposal. Implementation of Health Care Quality Improvement in Medicare's End State Renal Disease (ESRD) Program, Washington, DC, Health Care Financing Administration, 1996.
11. Steinman TI. The dialysis facility of the future: the financial and social environment. Semin Neprhol 1997; 17: 1–8.
12. Holley JL. Nephrologist as primary care providers: a review of the issues. Am J Kid Dis 1998; 31: 574–583.
13. Consensus Development Conference Panel. Morbidity and mortality of renal dialysis in an NIH consensus conference statement. Ann Intern Med 1994; 121: 62–70.
14. Thompson RE. Sustainability as the lynch pin of public policy and industry initiatives. The Physician Executive 1998; 24: 52–55.
15. Maloney FP. The industrialization of medicine. The Physician Executive 1998; 24: 34–38.
16. MacStravic S. Market memo: should providers pursue disease management. Health Care Strategic Management 1998; 16: 19–23.
17. Stewart S, Pearson S, Luke CG, Horowitz JD. Effects of home-based intervention on unplanned readmissions and out-of hospital deaths. J Am Geriatr Soc 1998; 46: 174–180.
18. Editorial. DM carve-outs soften sticker shock of catastrophic care. Healthcare Demand and Disease Management 1998; 4: 81–85.
19. Parkin DM, Henney CR, Quirk J, Crooks J. Knowledge deficit of hospital-discharged patients. Br Med J 1976; 31: 85–90.
20. Eddington B. ESRD managed care demonstration project. Dial Transplant 1987; 26: 162–164.

DISCUSSION / RECOMMENDATIONS / EPILOGUE

Training and Education

LAURENCE H. BECK
Department of Internal Medicine, Cleveland Clinic Florida, 3000 W. Cypress Creek R.D., Ft. Lauderdale, FL 33309, U.S.A.

Our workshop sought to identify educational targets, concluding that the principal target is the nephrology fellow in training. We believe that we can 'capture' the entire spectrum of learners by focusing on the fellows, because of their influence on residents and students. We agreed that we simultaneously need to focus on faculty and practicing physicians. I will outline a proposed plan to accomplish these goals after this introduction.

An additional educational issue concerns managed care. Many health insurance plans and their medical directors reward physicians who ask for fewer consultations or referrals. The improved outcomes that result from synergistic care between nephrologist and geriatrician need to be disseminated to counter such restrictive policies.

Concerning nephrology fellowship training, the new general geriatric requirements of such training programs were planned to be in place in July 1999. However, the next round of geriatric requirements should be made more explicit and more specific. The Residency Review Committee for Internal Medicine (RRC-IM) should revise and expand its text to describe more specific curricular and experiential content.

What is the geriatrics content that should be included in the nephrology curriculum? The knowledge base needs to include physiology, pathophysiology, and the typical geriatric syndromes that have a great overlap with those of nephrology. In addition, each fellowship program should include activities that meet the RRC-IM requirements for experiential learning. A combined three-year nephrology/geriatrics fellowship was seriously proposed.

Experiential learning events will have to be site specific due to the variation in available resources. For example, a geriatrician could regularly schedule attendance at the renal clinic as a consultant; the fellows could 'save up' for him/her their elderly patients with complex and multiple medical problems. Many, if not most, renal programs have an end-stage renal disease multidisciplinary committee that reviews patients who are entering the program and/or patients already in the program who offer on-going management problems. Discussion of such cases would be an effective way of tapping into the geriatrician's knowledge base. Fellows should be encouraged to attend

Oreopoulos et al. (eds.), Nephrology and Geriatrics Integrated, 227–229.

these multi-disciplinary sessions and the geriatrics clinic on a regular basis. On the other hand, we realize that havoc might ensue if cross-disciplinary attendance became the rule for all subspecialties with respect to geriatric learning.

We feel that through individual initiatives, certain centers should consider starting a combined nephrology/geriatrics fellowship that could be completed in three years. At least one individual has created such a combined fellowship de novo, even though there was no formal program in place. Centers of Excellence that have strong programs in each specialty should be encouraged to offer a three-year combined package. To sustain that effort and make it more than just an extra clinical year (with one clinical year each in nephrology and geriatrics), the centers must support either the combined training package through training grant development or copy the program devised for oncology and geriatrics, perhaps with support from a foundation such as Hartford.

It is important to stress that fellows who have gone through such a three year program, two of which are clinical, are unlikely to be prepared for an academic position that would demand scholarly output and publications immediately. Thus these fellows will need post-fellowship support for two or three years afterwards.

The group also spent time addressing the needs of faculty and practicing physicians. CME at national meetings can be utilized; an example is the session on primary care in nephrology that was conducted at a recent American Society of Nephrology (ASN) annual meeting, wherein nephrologists were addressed as primary care physicians for a defined population. We believe that the ASN could have a pre-meeting course or could offer a specific session on geriatric nephrology. Mirroring such an activity at the ASN, the American Geriatrics Society (AGS) meeting should include a session on renal failure in the elderly. As we have learned here, the outcome of such meetings is not just to 'gerontologize' nephrology but to have a two-way exchange in which geriatricians will learn more about appropriate referral and interaction. In nephrology, and probably in other subspecialties, early referral is vital, particularly for the geriatric patient.

Can we develop a presentation package, either on slides or CD-ROM, of geriatric essentials for the nephrologists? Nephrologists do an enormous amount of teaching in the community, at grand rounds at other community hospitals, and at their own institutions. We believe that a group of experts could develop a comprehensive package such as those prepared by the Diabetes Association. I use slides prepared by the University Healthcare Consortium on quality and outcomes, for example, that make informal talks much easier to deliver.

We agreed that we should write editorials that might be published simultaneously in Journal of the American Geriatrics Society (JAGS) and Journal of the American Society of Nephrology (JASN) or the American Journal of Kidney Disease (AJKD); these would focus on training issues in geriatric nephrology. Also nephrologists must write articles or letters for JAGS outlining guidelines for referral and care of elderly patients with renal disease. We also need articles by geriatricians defining a concrete set of knowledge and skills for elderly patients under the nephrologists' care. As we have learned, once the referring physician has sent a patient with end-stage renal disease (ESRD) to a nephrologist, s/he is not desirous of seeing this patient again, appropriately so in many cases.

Each of the relevant professional societies (AGS and ASN) have education committees. Representatives from these societies must get together to discuss joint issues in training. Rather than meeting on a one-time ad hoc basis, a standing committee was proposed, composed of members of each organization who should not only define specific content but also oversee the implementation of those educational objectives. Robert Narins, M.D., who is in charge of the entire postgraduate educational program for the ASN, supports this view; and the 1999 session saw our ideas materialize. Another level of interaction would get representative training program directors together with the program committee.

The National Institute of Aging (NIA) has had (and may still have) an 'add-on' opportunity to permit individuals to join an existing training grant. Thus, if an institution has a nephrology training grant and a coexistent geriatric grant through NIA, there is provision for a one- or two-year 'add-on' to the existing training grant, so long as the total years do not exceed the approved sum of years allowed by the grants. This would be an effective way of 'bootstrapping' to create a combined nephrology/geriatrics training program in the absence of specific external funding for such a combination.

Special Clinical Problems in Geriatric Patients

JIM WINCHESTER
Division of Nephrology and Hypertension, Department of Medicine, Georgetown University Medical Center, Washington DC 20007, U.S.A.

In the care of geriatric patients with renal disease we encourage co-operative efforts, like those recommended by Dr. L. Beck, between geriatrics/nephrology, internal medicine/nephrology, and family practice/nephrology at national, regional, and local levels.

We recommend six initiatives:

(1) A team approach in managing patients should involve allied health professionals. Entry into the team should be flexible; here the word, flexible, connotes co-operation and we do not want to be seen to be taking a patient away from the family practitioner or internal medicine consultant. There should be strong and clear communication between team members, for example; a letter from the nephrologist should go back to the consultant or to the person managing the patient, within 24 hours.

At different stages of the patient's illness, leadership of the team may alternate. Early on the internal medicine practitioner, the geriatrician or family physician may lead while later on as the patient's renal failure becomes more severe, patient management is handled more by the nephrologist.

(2) We also targeted some specific areas in diagnosis and treatment of geriatric patients. We should identify those patients with proteinuria. We should focus on Type-II diabetes, because, as we learned early in this program, almost 80% of all individuals will have diabetes as they grow older. Patients with hypertension also should be identified.

(3) An important way to come to grips with the disease process is to identify promptly those patients who need early dialysis.

(4) Let us banish such terms as end-stage renal disease (ESRD) and pre-ESRD. We believe that they are pejorative terms that signal death. How would you like to be told you have 'end-stage renal disease'? What a horrible terminology. We could adapt Ed Lewis' classification of diabetic nephropathy and speak of 'latent renal disease' to signify 'dip-stick' proteinuria, or 'overt' renal disease when the patient has reduced GFR, bearing in mind that serum creatinine is not a good measure of renal function in elderly patients. That is why we propose the *Cockroft-Gault* formula to correct for age and weight in

Oreopoulos et al. (eds.), Nephrology and Geriatrics Integrated, 231–232.

calculating GFR. In any event we have to find another language for 'end-stage renal disease'.

(5) We need an ombudsman, when rationing and discontinuation of dialysis become necessary. We need a referee to monitor the effects of capitation and managed care on the intake rate of elderly patients requiring dialysis, and to chart our response. The patients and their families must have a court of last resort. Any member of the team could fill this role and this person would lead open discussions on criteria for selection of dialysis.

With regards to functional status we must adopt common criteria for family practice, internal medicine, geriatrics, and nephrology and cease using chronological age as a selection criterion for beginning dialysis.

(6) The sixth initiative is to learn to deal better with end-of-life conflicts that have become so common among the dialysis patients as they get older and lose control. We must get better at caring for the dying patient; wider use of advanced directives would prevent many difficulties for patients and families and also for the treatment team. New information available about dying and the response to stopping dialysis can be helpful both to doctors and to patients and their relatives.

Karl Kjellstrand

The ombudsman needs to be someone outside the system. Whether we like it or not, patients do not trust us as they once did. We need a system whereby any patient receiving care through a big insurance company or HMO has a mechanism of appealing, and not just for end-stage renal disease. The U.S. government is looking at this possibility at the moment. This subject needs wide discussion. If an individual believes his spouse or other relative is being denied end-stage renal replacement therapy, he should have a mechanism of redress outside of the medical profession and outside of the insurance company.

Research: Basic and Clinical

DAVID HUMES, ANDREW LEVEY and KARL KJELLSTRAND
Department of Internal Medicine, University of Michigan Health System, Ann Arbor, MI 48109-0368, U.S.A.

David Humes, M.D.

We review the broad spectrum of research opportunities in aging, in general, and focus specifically on nephrology. I write here about general implementation strategies, and Dr. Levey will describe some of the methods the committee recommends to stimulate geriatric nephrology as a research area.

General Areas Focused on Aging

Organ degeneration is a critical concern for any subspecialty dealing with the aging process. Such degeneration includes dysregulation, especially metabolic dysregulation. An important element in this degeneration is the fibrotic tendency that occurs in all organs with age. We are challenged to understand a growing epidemic of an aging population with end-stage renal disease and their requirements for either pre-ESRD treatment or dialytic therapy.

Clinicians need to understand why elderly patients have fluid and electrolyte imbalance and volume depletion or overload much more frequently than younger individuals. This may be a reflection of a more general neurodegenerative process. These are major opportunities that have not been thoroughly evaluated.

In the kidney the immunologic dysfunction that occurs with aging is reflected in the higher incidence of vasculitis, RPGN, and similar types of abnormalities. We also do not yet know whether the genetics of the aging phenomenon produces a predisposition to sclerotic renal disease. Most likely these matters will be clarified as we better understand the genetic basis of aging in general.

The committee outlined the following specific areas for research opportunities.

Glomerulosclerosis with increasing age. With aging, there is an incremental increase in glomerulosclerosis and scarring. The types of matrixes formed in various renal diseases may differ, although, on simple histologic

Oreopoulos et al. (eds.), Nephrology and Geriatrics Integrated, 233–238.

examination, they look similar. Tubular interstitial fibrosis remains largely unexplored, especially in light of some recent studies suggesting that progressive renal failure correlates more strongly with the amount of scarring in the interstitium than with that in the glomerulus.

The relationship between disease progression and co-morbid conditions, although it is critically important, has not received major attention in studies at the time of writing.

The contribution of exposure to environmental toxins in the development of tubulointerstitial disease has not received the attention it deserves. The elderly have had greater and more prolonged opportunities for such exposure, thereby having a higher prevalence of exposures. Environmental toxin exposure plays a more prominent role in this form of renal disease.

We also need to explore the roles played by cardiac and vascular dysfunctions in the associated cardiovascular genesis of kidney disease.

Finally, acute renal failure is a serious event in the elderly, carrying a high mortality rate. We have not made a serious attempt to understand how or why the elderly are predisposed to this disease process and why their morbidity and mortality rates are so much higher than those of the younger population.

The committee believes we must do better to convert knowledge at the bench to knowledge at the bedside and then to translate this bedside knowledge to improved clinical outcomes. The gaps between each of these successive steps may be related to the lack of a current cohort of junior and senior faculty, who have training in both clinical studies and outcome analysis. This observation suggests a key area for educational initiatives in junior faculty development. Unlike cardiology and oncology, nephrology has not developed a cohort of physicians in academic centers who take a special pride in doing clinical studies. We have a large pre-ESRD and ESRD population base, but we have not identified cohorts of patients within these populations for multicenter studies. Finally, as noted earlier, we are handicapped by a lack of demographic knowledge. How does the epidemiology of renal disease change as we age? How does the anatomical and biochemical pathology change?

Finally, we need better markers in addition to serum BUN and creatinine to track renal dysfunction; we have historically evaluated excretory markers for renal function but have not developed metabolic/synthetic surrogate markers of renal function that could be helpful in further assessing renal disease.

Andrew Levey, M.D.

There are a variety of methodological approaches to these topics, and in my review I will concentrate primarily on the clinical aspects of such studies. Historically, we might compare our efforts in renal research to those in cardiovascular disease before 1948, when the Framingham study was undertaken to map out the natural history of myocardial infarction. At present we are dealing with end-stage renal disease and have an impressive end-stage renal disease registry. We have a great deal of information on end-stage renal disease. However, viewing kidney disease purely from this perspective, is like limiting the prevention of cardiovascular deaths to those who have had their first myocardial infarction. That is, we don't have the same information on the basic incidence, prevalence, and factors associated with chronic renal disease as we have in cardiovascular disease.

Longitudinal studies are described as cohort or case control studies. We would use them to explore the relationships with the initiation and progression of chronic renal disease; within the same cohorts, we would be able to understand the contribution of cardiovascular disease, which seems to be so much a part of the renal disease in these patients. This exploration of relationships might require many studies.

Such longitudinal studies would allow us to document the incidence and prevalence of renal disease and the markers of such disease. The best of the equations to predict creatinine clearance or GFR from serum creatinine do not go beyond the age of 70. A serum creatinine level in an 80- or 85-year old does not translate into any known level of GFR or creatinine clearance. Greater knowledge of the demographic racial and ethnic variations might help us here. Data gained in these studies could become the starting point for pathological studies, studies of nutritional status, studies of genetics and metabolism. Gradually, through these studies we would see more clearly how to select patients for dialysis, especially among the aged; we could explore end-of-life issues even among those who do not make it to 'end-stage renal disease.'

Some might call our work with registries or data bases, cross-sectional studies. Inherently, these are less well organized than the longitudinal studies but help us track, for example, the incidence of acute renal failure. Coronary revascularization is an important issue in these patients, yet we know practically nothing about the underlying coronary lesions, the risks of revascularization, or the outcomes in these patients. Another fertile area for registry study is the pathology of progression of renal failure. Most of the patients said to have diabetic nephropathy have diabetic nephropathy, but there may be pathological changes within the glomeruli, such as mesangial sclerosis. Further study might identify some of the factors that modulate disease progression and response to ACE inhibitors.

The classic vehicle to determining what measures are efficacious is the clinical trial. We need to make fundamental changes in the infrastructure of the clinical trials so that trials can be started more quickly and are more accessible to physicians in practice for patient enrollment. More work is needed in the area of progression of renal failure. As much as we have done to explore the contribution of diabetes and hypertension, we need to do more to understand these leading causes of renal failure in the elderly.

The role of lipid-lowering agents as a modulator of progression of renal disease seems to be a particularly important area for study. In cardiovascular disease, the risk factor approach used by the National Heart, Lung, and Blood Institute (NHLBI) should become the foundation of our studies. Such studies could easily be done in patients with end-stage renal disease because the infrastructure is already there. We have large dialysis groups.

Clinical trials in acute renal failure are bedeviled because we do not agree on the most important outcome. Is it getting out of the ICU? Is it time until recovery of kidney function? Is it survival? Is it getting out of the hospital? Many pharmaceutical companies have tried to generate research interest in growth factors, and some have made an important contribution to studies of protection from sepsis. However, these studies often get bogged down in the implementation stage.

We discussed the value of kindred studies, of susceptibility to renal disease, progression of renal disease, survival with renal disease. We also talked about the broad area of outcomes research and disease management. As Dr. Sherwood has pointed out, we face a second frontier – the translation from clinical trials to disease management.

Concerning implementation, we believe shared funding is essential because these studies are expensive and no one has enough resources to do them on their own. It might be possible to issue a joint RFA from the National Institute on Aging and the NIDDK. This collaboration would call attention to these broad research areas, both clinical and basic. It would create a special study section to review the basic and the clinical grants and assure peer review by experts in nephrology and aging. This approach might jump-start this process because it would get the attention of all investigators.

The National Institutes of Health (NIH) need to partner more effectively with other government agencies, particularly in the care of end-stage renal disease. The Health Care Financing Administration (HCFA) should be closely involved. The Agency for Health Care Policy and Research (AHCPR) is involved with outcomes research. The Centers for Disease Control (CDC) needs to be consulted in studies of toxin-related renal disease. With regards to transplantation, Health Resources Services Administration (HRSA) should be involved. The Veterans Administration (VA) also has a research program. In addition to these government agencies, the NIH needs to work more closely with industry and various professional societies in the conduct of clinical trials.

With regards to the development of a core of clinical research investigators, training grants should include 'slots' for individuals who want to do clinical research. We need more fairness in the review of clinical grants, especially to ensure unbiased peer review. Also, we need additional grant mechanisms, specifically to encourage the development of infrastructures for these large multicenter trials.

Lastly, under implementation, the government should establish a program with NIDDK for the prevention, detection, evaluation, and treatment of chronic renal disease (analogous to the Joint National Commission for the Prevention, Detection, Evaluation, and Treatment of High Blood Pressure). There is very limited public awareness about the problem of renal disease. Today everyone knows his or her own blood pressure and their cholesterol level but no one knows his or her serum creatinine level or urine protein. An educational effort coordinated by the NIH similar to the National High Blood Pressure Coordinating Council or the National Cholesterol Education Program is long overdue. The two topic areas for this effort would be chronic renal disease before the stage of end-stage renal disease and end-stage renal disease management. We recognize the contribution of the Renal Physicians Association (RPA) and the National Kidney Foundation (NKF) in creating and distributing practice guidelines, including the popular NKF Dialysis Outcome Quality Initiative (DOQI). These are valuable tools, but their use should be coordinated through the NIH.

How do we assemble a representative cohort of patients with chronic renal insufficiency or of aging patients to study the onset of chronic insufficiency and its progression? This question should be the focus of an NIH consensus conference. A large observational study begins with a representative sample, but unfortunately the "representative samples" we have in our practices are not particularly representative. The samples in HMOs may come closest to being representative but are not organized well enough to support longitudinal research.

The Cardiovascular Health Study (CHS) may provide a model. This four-community effort that focused on cardiovascular disease in the elderly, its onset and its manifestations. This study is about to close. It has had three assessments. Our university is one of the sites. About 8000 individuals were enrolled. Their data embraces renal failure, renal disease progression and indices of renal function, but the data have not been exploited at all. The problem with developing the data is that, if one defines chronic renal disease as end-stage renal disease, one will not find many patients. Also, until recently most clinical trials did not record renal data.

Dr. Karl Kjellstrand

In the same vein, perhaps, it is striking how cultural factors influence kidney disease. For example, when I compared death certificates and chronic dialysis, I found that elderly black women had a very high access rate to dialysis, whereas elderly white women did not. From a cultural standpoint, the black community tends to be matriarchal; the white community is patriarchal. Similarly, how one looks at aging is culturally dependent. If one compares age and discontinuation of dialysis, one finds it goes up steeply with age in all white Western countries. On the contrary, in Japan it falls sharply. Young Japanese frequently discontinue dialysis but older Japanese patients never do.

Dr. Andrew Levey

Existing data bases are local. The Baltimore longitudinal study on aging, which has been in operation for 35 years, has data on renal function. That study showed that GFR doesn't decline in everyone. In some persons it doesn't change, in some it declines a little, and in some it declines a great deal. The data can be followed for clues about where we should go in the future. A similar study in the VA, which is confined to Boston, has the same kind of data, mostly in men. The EP study is longitudinal; we started with older individuals but now have gone on long enough to have longitudinal data that are available for analysis. A rural aging study is going forward in Iowa, which might shed light on urban versus rural toxic exposures, etc. Kidney disease is not a primary focus of this study, but there are probably some data that would bear on progression.

All such efforts require a faculty across the country that is interested in geriatrics and nephrology, in outcomes and epidemiology. Such people are unique, and we must train more of them.

Epilogue

ROBERT LUKE[1], WILLIAM R. HAZZARD[2] and
DIMITRIOS G. OREOPOULOS[3]
[1] *University of Cincinnati Medical Center, Department of Internal Medicine, Cincinnati, OH 45267-0557, U.S.A.;* [2] *J. Paul Sticht Center on Aging, Wake Forest University School of Medicine, Winston-Salem, NC, U.S.A.;* [3] *The Toronto Western Hospital, Toronto, Ontario, Canada*

Robert Luke, M.D.

My task is to briefly review outcomes of the conference. Bill Hazzard will then discuss outcomes from the geriatric point of view. All of you have made presentations of high quality and I assure the geriatricians that the nephrologists have learned a great deal about geriatrics and what it can do for us.

We need volunteers to write about what geriatricians and internists who read our editorials should understand in terms of renal disease. We should teach the more frequent measurement and proper interpretation of serum creatinine and also educate patients and physicians about prevention of ESRD, especially in diabetes mellitus. It is important that nephrologists begin to contribute more to geriatric journals.

The ASN, RPA, and NKF all will include instructional elements about geriatrics in their meetings. We must also address family physicians.

Geriatric meetings should include a session about 'What every geriatrician should know about nephrology'. It is quite clear that the population served by these two specialties overlaps and that our science overlaps. We can give geriatricians an opportunity to look at chronic renal failure and uremia, which appear to be, to some extent, an accelerated aging process.

We may also be able to study renal damage susceptibility genes in a specific way. With respect to examinations, the ABIM is ensuring that the age groups dealt with in the questions are appropriate for the populations that doctors care for. As a matter of policy the NBME will include many questions concerning the elderly. Also, the ASN program directors' group will set up a joint task force to facilitate the incorporation of a geriatric curriculum into renal fellowship training.

In terms of research, the idea of registries (for example acute renal failure) sounds very interesting and NIH could facilitate this. The concept of a Joint National Commission (JNC) for the prevention of renal disease should include the support of the Council of the American Kidney Societies. NIH could put together such a JNC to educate physicians and patients on the importance of proteinuria, serum creatinine, blood pressure, and diabetes. We hope that an

Oreopoulos et al. (eds.), Nephrology and Geriatrics Integrated, 239–243.

RFA from NIA and NIDDK – Renal program for the study of aging in the kidney may be issued. Congress should respond to our conservative forecast that 600 000 people will be on dialysis by the year 2010 – a huge burden for Medicare funds. I believe that we can make a strong case by focusing on this burden and by emphasizing that we know nothing about the whole cohort of patients who are developing end stage renal disease. Prospective preventative and risk factor studies are much needed. Renal investigators should direct some grant application towards the NIA.

It would be wise to involve geriatricians in the care of ESRD patients both for evaluation and management of dialysis patients in capitated care systems as well as in managed care in general and for end-of-life issues. Often the nephrologist approaches the elderly patient on dialysis with multiple problems and wonders how much of the illness is uremic in origin and how much is not. We need to learn to focus on function; what can the elderly person do and how can we improve that degree of function?

The idea of the 'senior citizen group' of older people donating cadaveric kidneys to other older recipients with end stage renal disease is intriguing. We will also see more transplants from emotionally related donors as well as from older donors.

With respect to capitation, our discipline should endorse the concept of an independent ombudsman. We are going to need one. When rationing comes in some form or other, the rights of the elderly must be defended. We need to work more with HMOs and the larger insurance companies to emphasize risk factors in disease management programs for the prevention of ESRD.

We are very hopeful that one outcome from this meeting will be a book on Geriatric Nephrology to be edited by Dr. Oreopoulos.

Finally, about terminology, I would suggest that the categories of renal impairment be divided into chronic renal insufficiency, which is potentially reversible, and chronic renal failure, which is not reversible.

Bill Hazzard, M.D.

During this conference we have broached but not yet fully engaged the relationship, the similarities and the analogies between nephrology and geriatrics. I sense this to be a double-edged sword. For the renal specialist it would be easy to say 'We are nephrologists. We care for patients with end-stage renal disease. They have multiple co-morbidities, and a shortened expectation of life. They need team care and we do that. So in effect we already are practicing geriatric nephrology'. The geriatricians for their part might say, 'We care for our stable patients with multiple co-morbidities; that is what we do if they have serious kidney disease, we manage them as one of these problem areas. So in effect we already practice geriatric nephrology.' Indeed, there are enormous numbers of similarities between the two disciplines. Both nephrologists and geriatricians practice team care, delegated care, collaborative care, and care management. However, we can also learn much from each other. Concerning the dialogue and these similarities, we have not yet wrestled with the issue of very old people with end-stage renal disease or even with progressive renal disease. We have, however, initiated an important dialogue toward greater collaboration. The focus on function is the mantra of geriatric evaluation and care, and this, as a common focus, can become a major force to strengthen our collaboration.

The disciplines of nephrology and geriatrics both deal with people at the end of life. By definition, end-stage renal disease signals the end of life unless dialysis is instituted and maintained. Most people with ESRD will die within two weeks if they don't have this intervention. Geriatricians deal with people who are very frail; many of them would and do die within two weeks, even with intervention. This burgeoning frail, dependent, multiply disabled, dying population need so much care, just as do those of any age with ESRD.

To some extent nephrology has both the blessing and the curse of having carved out end-stage renal disease as its territory. It is possible for nephrologists to say, 'We've got so much to do . . . just caring for these tremendously challenging patients. We are overwhelmed just providing this kind of care. We simply don't have enough manpower to take on all the additional burdens of truly all people with renal insufficiencies, and we don't have enough people in training.' You hear that same cry from geriatricians, only several times over. We turn out 100 geriatric fellows a year. You turn out about 300 nephrology fellows a year. Your number of ESRD patients is growing progressively. Our number of geriatric patients is growing dramatically and your population of ESRD patients is growing older with each passing year. How can both disciplines cope with these challenges? We are both struggling, though you would seem to enjoy a relative advantage, for it has seemed to me, while a medicine department chair, that nephrology is becoming a subspecialty favored by internal medicine residents because it offers a clearly defined future and a certain stable and predictable (albeit suboptimal) funding base. Geriatrics doesn't offer that at this point. Medicare reimbursement for the services of geriatricians simply does not pay a living wage, and lacking a procedure like dialysis, relatively favoured in Medicare reimbursement, geriatricians serve at best as a 'loss leader' for health care systems attempting to secure a favoured position in the growing Medicare market in the U.S.

Given these realities, perhaps it would be tempting for nephrology to withdraw within that secure funding base and carry on with business as usual without embracing the additional challenges of geriatric renal care. However, business as usual risks stagnation of the field and lost opportunity for leadership. Our academic research and education agendas in both fields have suffered because of the overwhelming responsibility to provide care, a predicament to which both nephrology and geriatrics are equally vulnerable. Both disciplines must thus resolve to preserve sufficient academic energy and time to advance geriatrics *and* nephrology, optimally and in concert in addressing the needs of aging patients with failing renal function in the context of the multiple co-morbidities that ultimately came to affect almost all elderly persons.

The NIA, the NIDDK, academic institutions around the country, and the Hartford Foundation in their enlightened thinking about the future care of the elderly all face similar challenges. We need to get the best and the brightest into our training programs. We need to sustain them in the best way possible through academic initiatives. We are always in a continuous process of recruiting, training and nurturing young professionals through our programs. Both of our fields share this enormous challenge and we will do well to work closely together in this effort.

In yet another way geriatrics and nephrology share a common dilemma. Both disciplines agree that with respect to end-stage disease, the real damage is done before these folks get to the nephrologist or the geriatrician and hence the greatest opportunity to prolong vitality and life of high quality may be in the hands of those who provide care in a preventive mode. How do we husband our limited energies and focus educational efforts in prevention on the large numbers of physicians, nurse practitioners, nurses and others who care for people who are not yet end-stage? How can we get primary care physicians and other health care professionals to assist us in this effort to prevent or delay altogether end-stage renal disease through cholesterol reduction, hypertension management and all the other steps in prevention of renal failure as well in all other consequences of time – age – related declines in cardiovascular health and function? I don't believe either field has done more than scratch the surface in their efforts to delay and prevent the delayable and preventable in their domain. We need systems to support the continuity of everything we do. We both have an enormous investment in these systems. Clearly both nephrologists and geriatricians must develop collaborative relationships that will extend preventive gerontology and related research to populations not yet at end stage and under physicians delivering primary care. Thus, in planning our next summer's meeting with general internal medicine, we will put the emphasis on reaching primary care physicians and others acting well before our end-stage management.

All in all, I am reassured that such multidisciplinary collaboration across the continuum of health, disease, and aging is something good, something valuable, indeed something magic. In these days together at the Gerontology Education Retreat we are trying to capture the spirit of the exciting opportunities in all aspects of gerontology and geriatrics. It is hard to describe this spirit until you feel it. It was hard to describe this magic to the trustees at the Hartford Foundation, yet to their credit, they bought into it, and it is enormously encouraging that the Hartford senior management and its leaders are here with us in Jasper.

Our goal in this project is to bring together the best and the brightest in each subspecialty to spend five full days discussing gerontology and geriatrics in their discipline in a way that they may not have thought about in the past.

You people have done that with a spirit that has been as strong as at any other subspecialty meeting we have had so far.

The formula we have used for these conferences begins by engaging the leadership of the field. We gratefully recognize Robin Luke and Larry Beck, our co-chairs, for their valuable leadership throughout. Also we thank the group who met in Cincinnati last November to plan this conclave, the members of which include Wendy Brown, Chris Abrass, Dick Glassock, and Bob Narins in addition to our co-chairs. You identified and secured the most important people to be here. You identified the movers and the shakers. Thank you, thank you, thank you. I also want to acknowledge Donna Regenstreif, Cori Rieder and Norman Volk, for their enduring support and enlightened leadership of the Hartford Foundation in this continuing experiment. Finally, we thank Nancy Woolard for everything she has done and continues to do for us and for this project, for which she is heart and soul.

Dr. Dimitrios G. Oreopoulos

I want to thank John O. Godden, M.D. for his help in editing all manuscripts before their submission to the publisher, my secretary Ms. Sandra Medeiros for retyping all edited manuscripts and coordinating their collection, and finally our publisher, Mr. Olaf Blaauw, for his commitment to the production of this volume.

GPSR Compliance

The European Union's (EU) General Product Safety Regulation (GPSR) is a set of rules that requires consumer products to be safe and our obligations to ensure this.

If you have any concerns about our products, you can contact us on ProductSafety@springernature.com

In case Publisher is established outside the EU, the EU authorized representative is:

Springer Nature Customer Service Center GmbH
Europaplatz 3
69115 Heidelberg, Germany

Batch number: 10584469

Printed by Printforce, the Netherlands